THE HISTORY OF AMERICAN NURSING

Edited by
Susan Reverby, Wellesley College

A GARLAND SERIES

THE PRACTICAL NURSE

Dorothy Deming

GARLAND PUBLISHING, INC.
NEW YORK • LONDON
1984

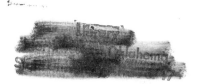

For a complete list of the titles in this series see the final pages of this volume.

This facsimile was made from a copy in the Yale University School of Nursing Library.

Library of Congress Cataloging in Publication Data

Deming, Dorothy.
   The practical nurse.

   (The History of American nursing)
   Reprint. Originally published: New York : Commonwealth Fund, 1947.
      1. Practical nursing—United States.   2. Practical nurses—Training of—United States.   I. Title.   II. Series.
   [DNLM: 1. Nursing, Practical.   WY 195 D381p 1947a]
   RT62.D46   1984   610.73′0693   83-49138
   ISBN 0-8240-6509-3 (alk. paper)

The volumes in this series are printed on acid-free, 250-year-life paper.

Printed in the United States of America

THE PRACTICAL NURSE

LONDON
GEOFFREY CUMBERLEGE
OXFORD UNIVERSITY PRESS

The Practical Nurse

BY DOROTHY DEMING, R.N.

Consultant in Public Health Nursing, Merit System Unit,
American Public Health Association; Formerly
General Director, National Organization
for Public Health Nursing

NEW YORK

THE COMMONWEALTH FUND

1947

PUBLISHER'S NOTE

The Commonwealth Fund is glad to make this book available as a contribution to the better distribution of nursing care, but publication does not necessarily imply nursing care. The author has had entire freedom and is wholly responsible for all statements of fact and opinion.

PUBLISHED BY THE COMMONWEALTH FUND

41 EAST 57TH STREET, NEW YORK 22, N.Y.

————

PRINTED IN THE UNITED STATES OF AMERICA
BY E. L. HILDRETH & COMPANY, INC.

TO MARY M. ROBERTS

*whose courageous writing and speaking
have interpreted nursing to the public
and the public to nurses, for the benefit of the sick and of all who are concerned with their care*

Preface

ALTHOUGH people have welcomed the help of practical nurses in caring for the sick since the dawn of history, it is only within the last ten years that the nursing profession as a whole has formally recruited their services for hospital and home duties and taken official cognizance nationally of their training. In view of this increasing interest, it seems desirable to review and size up the factors in the situation, especially as the acceptance and use of practical nurses are at an all-time peak due to professional nursing shortages. What are the advantages in the use of this group which should be carried over from war experiences into normal times? Are there dangers in this development? What are the safeguards to effective service?

A second consideration in assembling this material is the pressing need for information on how and where practical nurses are actually being used, how and where they are being prepared, what they are being paid, and how their services are controlled—all pertinent information for those concerned with legislation governing practical nurses, with recruiting and guiding them in their choice of jobs, and with setting standards for their services in homes and hospitals.

We need to estimate how many and what kind of practical nurses the public will employ.

There are undoubtedly many untilled fields of usefulness for practical nurses. Suggestions in this book may open the way to others and may offer to administrators who have not as yet employed this type of worker some evidence that the properly prepared practical nurse can be an asset in the care of the sick.

So far as is known, no book on this subject has been written. The data and discussions on the multiple problems involved are scattered through articles in professional journals and occasional paragraphs in textbooks and buried in the reports of past national studies and surveys. An earnest effort has been made to read all these sources and cull those references which seem most significant. Lists of source material are appended to each chapter.

Finally, the most urgent and fundamental reason for this book is the conviction that patients need and deserve the best practical nursing care they can get. It is the responsibility of professional nurses to see that they get it through properly trained and supervised practical nurses. Patients have always wanted and will always want practical nurses for certain types and stages of illness. Hospitals, notably those for chronic and mentally ill patients, have always depended on an attendant or practical nursing type of care. This book attempts to show that a new and desirable kind of practical nurse can be developed who will be a partner of the registered nurse—and a welcome one—in giving care to the sick at home and in all types of hospitals. It faces the reality that the practical nurse is here to stay. Recognition of her place and assistance to her in rendering effective service are long overdue, as the facts assembled here show clearly. It is hoped that this book will offer a basis for the "next steps" in such assistance and recognition.

In a rapidly growing profession such as nursing, no one person would dare to chart the course of future events. The road ahead holds many uncertainties. There is, therefore, no attempt to say that this or that will or should happen to practical nurses, unless past evidence and experience point definitely to a probable outcome or to a desirable safeguard to service. The attempt has been to round up past experience, current practice, and the best thinking on the subject, in the hope that the public, especially doctors, hospital administrators, and registered professional nurses, will recognize the important service which practical nurses can render during illness, when they are properly prepared, licensed, placed, and supervised. Their contribution has been too long disregarded and allowed to grow without safeguards to the patient. It is the author's hope that the material presented in these pages will show that both the needs and the safety of sick people call for the use of practical nurses under controlled conditions. This is a responsibility to be met primarily by the nursing profession who can in turn enlist the active support of the medical profession and an informed public.

D. D.

October 1, 1946

Acknowledgments

THIS book represents the thinking of literally hundreds of people speaking to me directly or through their letters, published articles or books. It would be impossible to thank them all in print, but special appreciation and gratitude are expressed to Katharine Shepard, Superintendent of the Household Nursing Association of Boston, a pioneer educator in the field of practical nursing; to Hortense Hilbert, formerly Associate Director of the National Organization for Public Health Nursing and present Director of the Bureau of Nursing, New York City Department of Health; and Ellen G. Creamer, Director of Nursing, New York Post Graduate Medical School and Hospital, New York, all three of whom have given me encouragement, wise counsel, and constructive ideas. The assistance of the national nursing organizations and of *The American Journal of Nursing* in making the reports of studies and their files available to me is warmly acknowledged, as is the help of the federal agencies which, through correspondence and arrangements for visits, supplied information of typical attendant problems. The directors of the schools for practical nurses, the executive secretaries of state boards of nurse examiners, registry directors, hospital administrators, public health nurses, industrial nurses, and the practical nurses themselves have all shared generously in giving answers to many searching questions, as have several families where practical nurses were on duty. Without their unfailing interest and frank expressions of opinion, the book would not have materialized. It tries to transmit their impressions and reports accurately and fairly.

Contents

CHAPTER ONE

The Practical Nurse and the Care of the Sick

MY FATHER used to say when one of us children was sick, "We'll get Miss Nellie to come in for a few days. She's a great hand with sickness and will relieve your mother." And Miss Nellie would come. I think father paid her two dollars a day and her "keep." She would take the spare room and nurse us back to health—or if the patient had something "catching," nurse and patient shared the spare room. I don't suppose she knew much about "nursing technique." I know she had never had a course in anatomy or physiology, let alone chemistry, physics, or biology, but she knew how to give a child a bed bath, an enema, an inhalation, or a mustard plaster, and how to concoct soft, palatable foods and pleasant tasting drinks which would slide painlessly down sore throats to cool and nourish feverish bodies. My uncle had a long siege with carbuncles, big discharging abscesses on his neck (from which I supposed they got their name) and Miss Nellie stayed, faithfully poulticing, bandaging, boiling clothes, and burning soiled dressings. Once she stayed at a neighbor's three months when old Mrs. Smith had a stroke.

I remember the day our family doctor stepped into the hall, closed the spare room door, and said gravely, "She is very sick. You will have to have a trained nurse. I will send one in tonight."

We did not go to hospitals in those days. There were just two kinds of nurses, the trained or graduate nurse and the household, village, or practical nurse. The former had two years of training in a hospital and wore a white uniform and cap. The latter was any capable woman, seldom with any training, and she wore any kind of comfortable dress or apron that would wash. Either nurse lived in the home for as long as she was needed, and the trained nurse received $25 to $35 a week. A few communities were lucky and had a "district" graduate nurse who came in by the hour to give special treatments or, if you were poor, to nurse you free of charge—the forerunner of our modern visiting or public health nurse. This was the picture of nursing in the early 1900's.

Today, the situation surrounding the employment of nurses is about as complicated, confusing, and unsatisfactory to the public as it could well be. Discoveries in diagnostic procedures, new treatments, advances in obstetrical and surgical care, all calling for expensive and elaborate equipment available only in hospitals, clinics, and a few doctors' offices, have sent patients by the thousands into hospitals and stepped up the "training" of nurses to education on a professional level. The specialization of medicine and surgery also has its counterpart in nursing and we have the surgical nurse, the pediatric nurse, the psychiatric nurse. Graduate, registered, or professional nurses no longer nurse for $30 a week. Their usual charge at this writing in the large cities is a dollar an hour—more for the care of communicable diseases or mental cases—and they prefer eight-hour shifts. Our homes are smaller, our servants fewer, more of us live alone, and full-time "private duty" nursing by a professional nurse in homes, except for short periods of very serious illness or in the homes of the very wealthy, is rapidly becoming a thing of the past.*

In the hospital, in peacetime, if a person is critically ill or in need of constant attention, as during the first few days following surgical operations, he receives "special nursing"—a professional nurse is assigned full time to give care at a charge of $6 to $8 for eight hours of duty. As the patient recovers, he is turned over to the floor or general duty nurses (sometimes the students), staff nurses paid by the hospital whose expense is included in the bill for the hospital room or ward bed.

All this is expensive business. The bill for hospital nursing alone can run as high as $175 a week if full-time service is needed (the hospital usually adds a charge for the nurses' meals). It is no wonder prepaid hospitalization plans that provide a few days of special nursing and pay a part or all of the hospital bill are popular.†

Meantime, what has happened to Miss Nellie's services? Several significant developments: attractive opportunities in the field of business and industry have made it harder to find experienced, competent women who will care for patients not in need of professional nursing; the advancement in professional nursing has left less and less time for bedside nursing of an elementary type and there is a great unfilled need

* In 1927, 54 per cent of the professional nurses were engaged in private duty; in 1943, only 26 per cent (1), and much of the service is now in the form of special or private duty nursing in hospitals.

† At this writing, these plans do not cover the expenses of home nursing. There are one or two exceptions to this statement, notably the Group Health Cooperative of New York City.

for it among patients in both homes and hospitals; Miss Nellie's rather casual, informal, and unstandardized occupation of neighborly nursing has necessarily advanced to a level where it, too, cries out for training courses, practice under supervision, and formal organization. "Where can I get a reliable, well-trained practical nurse to help out when I come home from the hospital with my baby . . . to care for my bedridden father . . . to help me with my two children laid up with grippe . . . to care for me until the cast is off my leg?" cries Mrs. Public, while from the hospitals comes the call, "We need trained and licensed practical nurses to relieve the professional staff of a thousand and one simple nursing duties among convalescents, the mentally ill, the aged, the chronically ill, and in our maternity wards and nurseries."

The home patient is the special victim of this change in nursing supply. The services of professional nurses now available by the hour in nearly all our large cities, from visiting nurse associations or from nurses' registries, do not take the place of the home nurse, who stays and helps out with the household. In an effort to fill this gap, a few cities have developed a visiting housekeeper service which provides women with a slight knowledge of simple nursing procedures to run the home during illness. Their aid to date has been primarily to families unable to afford maid service, and there are probably not more than 300 such workers over the country at the present time. Their charges, when not met by a social service agency, have ranged from $2.75 to $4 a day. It is hoped that under peacetime conditions this service will be greatly augmented.* It is much needed. But even this convenience does not provide a skilled practical nurse to whom the doctor can turn over the complete care of his home patient not in need of professional nursing. The reason for employing a housekeeper is to keep house, not to nurse.

Who then is taking Miss Nellie's place?

Thousands of women nursing for hire who are not professional nurses, not visiting housekeepers, not trained or licensed practical nurses. Their services, once limited to simple bedside care of the sick, have been expanded to take in many of the treatments formerly given only by the doctor or trained nurse—hypodermic injections of insulin for diabetes is a good example. They urgently need training to be safe attendants at the bedside.

* New York City has established a service of this type for the clients of social agencies, under the sponsorship of the Welfare Council.

Their selection should be on the basis of their qualifications to nurse, and their employment should be supervised by professional nurses. Thinking also of Mrs. Public's pocketbook, strained by the high cost of illness, it is obvious that if a reliable, qualified practical nurse were available to take over nursing duties appropriate to her skill in hospitals and homes, the expense of nursing could be lightened. It is neither economical nor logical to employ a highly trained and expensively educated professional nurse to give the care that a person with a few months' training can give safely and well under supervision.

Emergencies also offer testimony to the need of this type of worker. When the national organizations were undertaking the recruitment of practical nurses to relieve the wartime shortages of professional nurses in hospitals, the following points were cited as evidence of how much their services were needed (2).

In many hospitals, 10 per cent of the professional nursing staff had volunteered for military service, leaving patients unnursed, aides unsupervised, and treatments incomplete. Many patients were being prematurely discharged from hospitals without nursing care at home. A third of the doctors were in military service, necessitating the transfer of many highly skilled treatments to professional nurses. The uncertainty of voluntary aide service and its probable withdrawal as the war emergency passed emphasized the need for an employed staff upon which the hospital could count.

Interviewed by the writer, prominent physicians in several cities who are calling practical nurses for their private cases and doctors who are acquainted with their work in hospitals expressed warm approval of their work, a constant demand for more of them, and a desire to see registered nurses welcome this type of service and offer help in developing as high standards of performance as in professional nursing.

Typical of the attitude of many state and city medical associations toward practical nurses is that of the New York Academy of Medicine:

. . . the practical nurse has become an indispensable agent in the community organization for the care of the sick. The war has merely accentuated the need of this addition to our nursing personnel, and in our judgment every effort should be made without delay to develop an effective method for the recruitment of women for practical training and for the development of facilities for the training and placement of this auxiliary nursing corps (3).

The attitude of professional nurses toward practical nurses has been shifting over the years. For the most part, it can honestly be said that reluctance on the part of professional nurses to welcome the practical nurse as a partner in caring for the sick has, in the past, had its roots in concern for the safety of patients and quite secondarily, though very understandably, in fear of job competition from an untrained group. Briefly, a few of the most frequently expressed objections to recognizing practical nurses have been these:

There is danger of confusing the public by offering two types of nursing, one of which is totally unregulated and frequently unskilled

It is not nursing service so much as houskeeping service that is needed in time of subacute illness in homes

There are already more persons calling themselves nurses than can be kept busy—a situation which will become more serious as the Armed Services discharge their thousands of semi-trained corpsmen and corpswomen

If men and women have proficiency in nursing, they should be encouraged to become professional nurses

If practical nurses are recognized, hospitals will employ them to save money, curtailing the amount of professional nursing available to and needed by patients

The public cannot afford practical nurses at their present charges any more than they can afford professional nursing service, so there is no economic advantage in training this group

It will be seen that most of these objections would be met if proper preparation, supervision, and legal control of practice were established, and if the group developed standard-making and accrediting bodies to prevent the exploitation inherent in the last two objections.

Those who favor recognition of and assistance to practical nurses point out that many occupations profit by offering the public several grades of labor; that the practical nurse has already entered our homes and hospitals and therefore must enter our legislative programs, educational plans, and employment agencies; that the responsibility for service to sick people is a joint one shared by trained practical and professional nurses alike; that with the increasingly heavy schedule of tests, treatments, and procedures being assigned to professional nurses by doctors, someone adequately prepared must relieve professional nurses of nonprofessional duties or the patients will suffer. It is both an economy and an assurance of better care to train and license practical nurses.

In 1935, the Board of the National League of Nursing Education voted to approve the principle that all persons who give nursing service for hire be licensed, and to disapprove the setting up of schools for the training of subsidiary workers unless there is control of their practice in the state (3).

In 1938, the Joint Boards of the American Nurses Association, the National League of Nursing Education, and the National Organization for Public Health Nursing concurred in these two principles and stated that:

The [national] nursing organizations favor state licensing of all who nurse for hire. . . . It is the responsibility of the nursing profession to outline principles and policies for the control of nonprofessional workers in the care of the sick

The nursing profession is opposed to the establishments of a formal course for nonprofessional workers in the same institution which conducts a state accredited school of nursing for professional workers (4)

The practical nurses themselves are giving evidence of a desire to improve their own standards and secure legal status, and are seeking professional guidance and advice in these matters. Among recent developments are their efforts to organize local and state practical nurses' associations and the founding, in 1940, of the National Association for Practical Nurse Education, to which both practical and professional nurses belong. The alumnae of many of the older schools have been active for years. Recently, with the opening of eight new schools for practical nurses between 1939 and 1945, alumnae activity has become more marked and interest in state organization has developed. One of the most active state groups, Practical Nurses of New York, Inc., was organized in 1940. Michigan, Massachusetts, and Connecticut now have state associations. During the war, practical nursing groups conducted energetic recruiting campaigns, and several of the state associations have sponsored refresher courses for practical nurses without formal training who are licensed under a waiver. These organizations also have publicity and educational committees and their meetings are well attended. One has its own news bulletin. In at least two cities, Buffalo and New York, the practical nurses have considered the establishment of their own registry, and in October 1945, at their own instigation, the practical nurses were influential in persuading the United

States Employment Service to open a counseling and placement service for practical nurses in New York city, under professional nursing guidance.

In localities where licensed practical nurses are working side by side with registered nurses, being taught by them, placed by the same registry, and serving the same community in homes, hospitals, and industries, it would appear to be efficient as well as mutually helpful to have a close connection between the membership organizations. Although practical nurses are not eligible to membership in registered nurses' associations, there are many opportunities to invite the practical nurses to attend nursing meetings that are of general public interest and other occasions when joint action would save time and result in better service to the public. A beginning in joint planning has been made in a few states on the state level (Massachusetts, Michigan, and New York) and practical nurses are represented on a few national committees such as those concerned with legislation and curriculum planning. "There is such a lot we can do together," a practical nurse told the writer, enthusiastically, when asked how she had enjoyed the joint committee meetings. And to the same question about the same meeting, her usually conservative sister, the professional nurse, replied: "That meeting was a revelation to me!"

Are the practical nurses' associations, local, state, and national, to proceed as units independent of registered nurses and their associations? It is a burning question. If they are, the control of standards for admission to their trade, their education, state legislative control and practice will naturally be their own concern and might conceivably be at odds with the desires and interests of the professional group. This is a pretty crucial issue for practical nurses and for the registered nurses and their membership organizations to decide, and calls for immediate leadership from national nursing headquarters. We have been a long time acting upon the recommendations of authoritative and reliable studies of the situation.

The writer believes that once the practical nurses and their training are wholeheartedly accepted as the responsibility of the professional organizations, once they are welcomed as partners in the care of the sick, many of the problems of function, place, and relationship will straighten out of their own accord, while the conditions which have led to past objections will be eradicated by the improved program of training, licensing, and supervision of the group.

For these reasons, and because all the conditions surrounding modern illness call insistently for the provision of a new type of practical nurse, this book attempts to describe the present situation in homes and hospitals and to suggest ways to safeguard the choice, preparation, supervision, legal control, and distribution of such service. Unfortunately, there has never been a study of a community's need for practical nursing service in homes, hospitals (general and special), institutions for the care of the chronic sick, aged, convalescent, handicapped, and agencies in charge of children. No one has an estimate of the number of practical nurses needed in relation to total population, to registered nurses, or to patients in hospitals, or of the amount of nursing time various types of illness require from practical nurses. In the field of professional nursing we have estimates (5) of the number of nurses needed in relation to patient load in hospitals and the number of public health nurses in relation to population, and there have been time studies of both hospital and home care, but until functions are defined, time requirements figured out, and ratios established in practical nursing service, we will not know what our goals are or how we should arrive at them. This book, therefore, deals necessarily with the status quo.

There is nothing new about this problem of practical nursing service. It is among the most frequently recurring subjects in every formal survey of nursing since 1877 and has, so far as the writer has been able to discover, never failed to draw out at least one recommendation definitely favoring its promotion and use for the benefit of sick people. The most important of these studies, now twenty-three years old, devoted pages to the place and function of the practical nurse (6).

At the present time there is ample evidence of a demand for nonprofessional assistance in the care of sick people wherever they may be. The material in this book provides justification for the following statements:

People sick at home need, want, and are seeking practical nursing care. They cannot afford the charges of professional nurses except for short intervals during acute illness or on a visit basis, and for many conditions they do not need professional nursing care.

Hospitals have found that the service of practical nurses spares professional nursing time, and results in better care to patients, less hectic wards, and more satisfied medical staffs and patients.

Institutions where longterm illnesses and subacute conditions are cared for now depend upon practical nurses for 50 per cent or more of the nursing service. This is especially true of federal and state institutions.

There is an increase in the types of cases for which practical nurses are especially fitted—the chronically ill and the mentally ill.

When there are shortages in professional nursing service (war) or widespread reductions in family income (depressions), the use of this service increases.

Public health agencies and many industrial plants are finding practical nurses under registered nurse supervision an assistance in extending service, in relieving the professional staff of some types of routine duties, and in giving better care to patients.

A variety of agencies and institutions are employing practical nurses for simple nursing care and assistance in health supervision, as, for example, homes for the aged, convalescent, or handicapped, homes for children, and doctors' offices.

The establishment of 49 nonprofit schools for training practical nurses and legislative control of their practice in 18 states, one territory (Hawaii), and one city (Detroit) have strengthened the confidence of employers and raised the standards of service.

"That hardy perennial," as Mary M. Roberts calls the question of permitting the practical nurse to have a place in the care of the sick, has been struggling to exist against rough winds and scorching suns for forty years (7). Opinion as to the place of these workers has been unsettled over the years, but in spite of neglect and unfavorable soil the hardy perennial has survived. Mr. and Mrs. Public have decided the matter. They want practical nurses, and Mr. White, superintendent of the mental hospital, depends on their service for 50 per cent of the care in his 2,500-bed institution, while Dr. Black "could not get along without them" in the county tuberculosis sanatorium. Uncle Sam is looking forward to employing many more in federal health and hospital services. So long as there is widespread public demand for a useful product, its sale cannot be prevented except by controlling the conditions on the grounds of public safety—and such control must usually be backed by law. "When you cannot stop a movement, join it," might well be said to the few who still hope to do away with practical nursing.

To make practical nursing a definite asset in the care of the sick, a first step, it seems to the writer, is the complete recognition and acceptance by professional nurses and professional nursing organizations of the practical nurse and practical nursing, wherever they function. The results of this acceptance would be, obviously, establishment of suitable schools of training, promotion of licensure, development of adequate employment centers for the distribution of service, and professional supervision. The national and state professional nursing bodies already have all the experience, machinery, and knowledge necessary to attain these goals. They could secure the funds. All that is needed is the desire to move forward.

What I would plead for today is vision, vision which sees through all the veils of habit and tradition by which we are walled in to the real needs of the human beings in our communities; and the courage to follow that vision and meet those needs (8).

REFERENCES

1 American Nurses' Association, Nursing Information Bureau, cooperating with the National League of Nursing Education and the National Organization for Public Health Nursing, *Facts about nursing, 1943,* pp. 36–37; May Ayres Burgess, *Nurses, patients and pocketbooks;* report of a study of the economics of nursing by the Committee on the Grading of Nursing Schools, New York, the Committee, 1928, p. 249.

2 Recruitment material, Practical Nurses of New York, Inc., letter from the president, March 1944; National Nursing Council for War Service, *Earn and serve in war, in peace; be a practical nurse* [leaflet]. See also General Federation of Women's Clubs, *Practical nurses, a contribution to victory, a preparation for life* [leaflet].

3 *Earn and serve in war, in peace* (note 2), p. 2.

4 "Recruiting student practical nurses," *American Journal of Nursing* 44:200–201, March 1944.

5 American Nurses' Association, *Facts about nursing, 1945,* pp. 62–63.

6 Josephine Goldmark, *Nursing and nursing education in the United States;* report of the Committee for the Study of Nursing Education, New York, Macmillan, 1923, pp. 14–16, 28–29, 164–165, 171–179, 473–482.

7 "Forward in 1937," *American Journal of Nursing* 37:1–5, January 1937, at p. 4.

8 C.-E. A. Winslow, "Organizing for better community service," *American Journal of Nursing* 38:761–767, July 1938, at p. 766.

CHAPTER TWO

Who Is the Practical Nurse?

THE WELL qualified, well equipped practical nurse, prepared for home and hospital service and licensed by the state to practice, has not just burst upon us. She, like her professional sister, has come a long way over a rough road. All nurses were just nurses until Florence Nightingale insisted that a period of training, including instruction and practice, would produce better nurses and give patients safer care. To be sure, during the Middle Ages it was the custom to include in the education of girls of the upper class "some knowledge of medicine, a smattering of surgery, more especially of that branch concerned with the treatment of wounds," and the early metrical romances are full of accounts of fair ladies "physicking and patching up their knights" (1), but we think of the training of nurses in the modern sense as developing in Miss Nightingale's England of the 1850's. This differentiation between trained and untrained nurses marked the birth of the "practical" nurse.

In America since 1870 when the Nightingale methods were accepted by our first struggling schools, there have been two levels of nursing (2). Both have had to fight for a place in the medical world and the fact that professional nurses have won a degree of recognition from the public and legal status in all states only throws into sharp contrast the unregulated practice of graduates from commercial and correspondence schools.

There was a time, not so long ago, when professional nurses had to fight a reactionary group among the medical profession who felt that eighteen months of training for "good sensible girls" was ample to turn out the kind of nurse needed by them in hospitals. Two years of high school was thought to be sufficient preparation, and completion of grade school quite acceptable. These doctors saw only a form of simple manual work in nursing; scientific "trimmings" were unnecessary (3). There are doctors today who feel the practical nurse needs no training other than what can be taught her at the bedside of the patient. Yet these very doctors are demanding more and more of both groups of nurses in the way of treatments, tests, and procedures which require a period of sound education and clinical experience to be performed at all satisfactorily. Looking back, we can see that the early trained nurses were really practical nurses from our modern viewpoint, while the doctors performed many of the procedures now carried on by professional nurses (4). To understand what has happened to nursing, we must understand what has happened to medical science.

The early pioneers in practical nursing demonstrated a genuine love of nursing and a sincere wish to be of service to the sick. Our grandmothers knew and trusted such women, and most middle-aged men and women of today were delivered at home by the family doctor into the kindly hands of Aunt Judy, Mrs. Martha, or Miss Nellie. Lacking in technical preparation though these early practical nurses were, their hearts were in their work (5). Many of us owe our survival to the devotion and homely remedies offered by the Miss Nellies of years ago. Until about 1910 when professional nurses began to be graduated in quantities, widows and spinsters took to the field of neighborly nursing like ducks to water. Here was a genteel, dignified, protected, not too strenuous means of earning money. "Their care was kindly" epitomizes the best of the service (6).

Some idea of how little practical nurses knew can be gained by looking over the home nursing "aids" and "hints" available to families before the first schools for practical nurses were started. Esther Robertson, a graduate of Bellevue Hospital, wrote in 1903 for those unable to afford a trained nurse, "The family nurse must first of all be firm. Do not let the family see if you are frightened." She also advised, "Do not study your own symptoms." Her book contains instructions on giving medicines, including herbs, making dandelion juice, giving "the water cure," and offers chapters on "Receipts," "Death," and "In Danger of Death" in that order. She is careful to issue warnings from time to time: "Remember to look at the little place in the catheter above the eye where germs are apt to collect" (7).

As late as 1938, a doctor, writing to the New York State Board of Nurse Examiners to vouch for an untrained nurse who wished to be licensed under the waiver on the basis of experience, said: "To my knowledge, for over forty years she has officiated as nurse at the bedside of many and attended in numbers of obstetrical cases. No weather was too severe to deter her going to the aid of the sick. She was efficient. I have overtaken her more than once in the wintertime . . . plodding along in men's overalls, hightop boots, lumberjack coat and cap, a little old lantern, old satchel, . . . on the way to the same place I was bound. . . . She has never received enough for her service to purchase an all-round outfit for herself in clothing. She has a bright eye, keen intellect and active body" (8).

Such services cannot be lightly set aside. Their spirit is the essence of all nursing and burns as brightly today in the wards of our modern hospitals, on the battlefields, and in lonely homes beyond the reach of cities. But the most willing and consecrated spirit cannot follow the doctor into the present-day intricacies of medical care without training and practice. Times have changed; the scene and circumstances surrounding sickness have shifted. Mr. Brown, whose dad fought pneumonia at home with whiskey, mustard pastes, and "cupping," propped on pillows by his bedroom window, is now placed in an oxygen tent in a modern hospital, given intravenous feeding, stimulation, and transfusions of plasma or whole blood—if his pneumonia was not conquered in its early stages by the sulfa drugs or penicillin. Baby Brown is born in a "sterile field" in a spotless operating room in the presence of one or two obstetricians, at least two registered nurses, and an anesthetist. The result? A dramatic saving of lives and shortening of illness. Even those who remain at home during illness—and every year sees more of us entering hospitals for care—have homes too small to accommodate a nurse along with the modern paraphernalia of acute illness.

Advances in medical science have complicated every phase of sickness. There are dozens of things we can do to keep well and secure immunity to disease, but once the symptoms of illness develop, a whole dizzy chain of tests, measurements, treatments, and procedures unrolls. Many of these can be carried out only with hospital equipment, nearly all require skilled and experienced technicians to secure reliable results, and all call for expert interpretation. The discoveries of the laboratory have demanded a more highly educated professional nurse to assist the doctor in diagnosis and treatment and have driven out Miss Nellie, kindly, conscientious and deft though she was, to be replaced by the practical nurse trained, in her turn, to assist the professional in giving bedside care and the simpler treatments (9).

Mrs. Schulz has written, "Mothered by religion, fathered by war, nursing found in science a fairy godmother and in the medical profession a wonderful big brother" (10). Many professional nurses throughout the country are now gratefully seeking and finding in the trained and licensed practical nurse a helpful sister.

SOME DEFINITIONS

There has been no completely satisfactory definition of the modern practical nurse. The National Association for Practical Nurse Education states that a practical nurse is a person "trained to care for semi-acute, convalescent, and chronic patients requiring service under public health nursing agencies, or in institutions, or in homes; she works under the direction of a licensed physician or the supervision of a registered professional nurse, and is prepared to give household assistance when necessary."

"Nurse, Practical; Nurse. (medical ser.) 2-38.20." reads the cryptic heading of the definition in the *Dictionary of Occupational Titles* (11). "One who has a knowledge of nursing secured primarily through practical experience, as opposed to Nurse III* who is required to have fulfilled prescribed educational qualifications; legal restrictions often limit scope of practice to patients in private homes. Attends bedridden, convalescent, infirm or mental patients; cooperates with physician by administering medicine, injections, or massages, and recording scheduled readings of pulse and temperature; gives bed baths or helps patient to bathe; changes bed linen; looks after patient's personal appearance by combing hair, manicuring nails, and dressing patient; prepares special diets and serves meals; may feed patient; may accompany patient on walks or automobile drives; may read to patient; performs any other service during day or night to increase patient's comfort."

This last definition is far from satisfactory and is now practically obsolete. It does not describe the licensed practical nurse who is required to fulfill prescribed training and practice and whose function is not in the least limited to private homes.

Because the trained attendant, nurses' aide, or assistant nurse is mentioned so often in this book and because she is so frequently used in the same capacity as a practical nurse, the following definition is added:

"Nurse, aide; hospital attendant; ward helper (medical ser.) 2-42.20. Assists professional nursing staff in hospitals as by perform-

---

* Nurse III is the graduate, registered, professional nurse, formerly known as the "trained nurse" (but not to be confused with the "trained" nurse in New York state, formerly the term associated with nurses trained in psychiatric institutions). She or he is usually a high school graduate, sometimes a college graduate, and always has at least two to three years of nursing education in a school of nursing approved by the State Board of Examiners and connected, usually, with a registered hospital.

ing routine or less skilled tasks in the care of patients; bathes and dresses patients; answers call bells; makes beds; serves food and nourishment; assists patients in walking; gives alcohol rubs and performs other services,* cleans rooms and equipment. A female worker who does not possess training and experience required for professional status. . . . See orderly for male worker" (12).

Legal titles given to the practical nurse are licensed attendant, licensed attendant nurse, trained attendant, practical nurse, nurses' aide, nursing assistant, and vocational nurse.† Of late, the name practical nurse, although it is not entirely satisfactory and is disliked by many who feel it implies that the professional nurse is not practical, has been generally accepted on the grounds that it is most familiar to the public.

For the purposes of this book the name practical nurse refers to a person with specified training of nine to eighteen months, licensed in the state in which he or she is practicing if a state law exists, and serving in homes, hospitals, public health or industrial agencies under the direction of a licensed physician and—desirably—the supervision of a professional registered nurse. Ward maids, orderlies, volunteer nurses' aides, and professional undergraduate students still in training do not fall into this classification of practical nurse. The thousands of men and women nursing for hire and calling themselves "practical nurses" who have no formal training or legal status are not the practical nurses under favorable consideration here, although their numbers, activities, and practices form one of the principal reasons for writing this book.

THE MODERN PRACTICAL NURSE AS A PERSON

Who is the practical nurse of today? Is she young, is she old, what is her education? What did she do before she became a practical nurse—in short, what kind of person is she? What qualifications and training does she bring to this field?‡

---

* This elastic clause is frequently made to cover all the duties of the fully trained practical nurse.

† The term "vocational nurse" has been employed occasionally to designate a vocational type of training as opposed to that on a professional level. The term is unfortunate as both fields of nursing are actually true vocations, and it has not been acceptable to many groups including some practical nurses. It is used in this book only when notations are made from official statements that employ the term.

‡ The feminine pronoun does not exclude men who are practical nurses but is used because the women's group is far larger. In 1940, 96 per cent of practical nurses were women; 57 per cent of attendants, however, were men.

Personal Qualifications

A composite picture of the best licensed practical nurse, in training, at work, or off duty, shows an energetic, wholesome young woman, past twenty-five but not yet fifty (though she may be nineteen, fifty-five, or even sixty), usually in a clean white, blue, or tan washable uniform (13). She speaks quietly, simply, confidently. She gives an impression of reliability and common sense. She is earnest in her answers to questions and makes no effort to appear other than what she is: a well trained assistant in nursing the sick (14). Her hair is usually dressed simply, she wears no jewelry, her shoes have moderate heels, and her hands are firm, capable, clean, with short nails. She appears very much at home at the bedside or in the kitchen and is almost invariably well liked by patients and families. If you are very critical you may find her vocabulary limited, but she is able to make you comfortable during the bad days of grippe, give your bedridden mother exquisite care, serve a delicious meal of leftovers, and keep the children quiet after school. Her outstanding characteristics are reliability, informal friendliness, and common sense.

W. W. Charters writing of "personality" in nursing refers to leadership "in a quiet sense of taking hold and managing things," sizing up situations, improvising, adapting to changes, and showing initiative in getting things done (15). These qualities we expect and can find in trained practical nurses.

Other attributes of a good attendant nurse were described nearly twenty years ago by Thyra Pedersen of the Veterans' Bureau: "A good memory, punctuality, sympathy, adaptability, regard for hospital regulations and pride in personal appearance. Patience with the unreasonable invalid, ability to act fast in emergencies and desire to increase her knowledge of conditions under her care . . ." (16).

If the practical nurse can add to her nursing ability the art of housekeeping in these days of crowded homes, rising costs, food shortages, and changing family habits, she will go far as a successful member of her chosen occupation.

Practical nurses are always urged by their teachers to interest themselves as far as they can in current events, books, movies, and other outside interests. "I had a fine practical nurse the year the doctor made me stay in bed for a heart condition," said a sweet old lady. "The only trouble was she hated cards, never read, and only listened to Mr. Anthony on the radio." Elderly chronic patients and convalescents like to find their constant companions interested in conversation, current events, and diversional occupations. Good manners are an asset. Schools are concerned with assisting students to better themselves in these ways. Training today, therefore, stresses personal conduct and all it implies in good manners, courtesy, and consideration for others— with particular attention to personal hygiene. Most of the schools take pains to see that the students receive help, advice, and information on personal adjustment problems. Reading is guided. A student is taught to organize her own "way of life" happily, to budget her expenses and time. She is aided in an understanding of human relationships and guided in promoting these among the families she serves. Special attention is paid in all schools to the ethical attitude toward the physician, family, visitors, and professional nurses.

In conversation with directors of schools, supervisors, and employers about the characteristics of practical nurses, the following points were called to the attention of the writer:

Practical nurses are—like their professional sisters—likely to forget that in some cases a home atmosphere conducive to recovery is nearly as important to the patient as medicine. The good practical nurse does not shirk homemaking in its best sense.

Patients and families are apt to expect a great deal of their nurses, and early discouragements sometimes floor young nurses. It is in such cases that a skilled supervisor can be of inestimable help to both nurse and family. It is, therefore, customary throughout the practical nurse's training to stress the value of supervision to her, the importance of referring problems to the professional nurse (in the registry, on duty in the ward, or in the visiting nurse association) and of maintaining contact with the profession which can do much for her (17).

Supervisors report that many practical nurses do not take criticism as easily as the average professional student nurse. This is probably because the group is older, and so more tact is called for on the part of the supervisor.

Nearly all practical nurses find record-keeping difficult. It is one of their greatest failings. This report came not from a few, but from fifteen schools, six hospitals, and four visiting nurse associations. Three practical nurses reported record-keeping as the hardest thing they had to do.

Why Practical Nursing Was Chosen

About seventy practical nurses, in homes, hospitals, visiting nurse associations, and schools of practical nursing in seven states, were asked why they had decided to be practical nurses. All but one gave as the primary reason, "I always wanted to be a nurse." Variations of this reason were: "I liked to take care of sick animals as a child"; "I took care of my mother for five years and loved it"; "I took the Red Cross course and liked it so much that I went on"; "I liked being with people"; "I couldn't be a registered nurse so I did the next best thing"; "I saw so much sickness and misery in the old country, I wanted to do something about it"; "I had to earn a living and had no training, but I knew how to care for a family"; "The hospitals needed me"; "I didn't like industry or office work." One keen-eyed nurse replied, "I wanted to be trained to do my job right—for my own protection as well as my patients'." Several nurses had been working in hospitals in non-nursing jobs and liked what they saw of nursing.

Previous Occupations

Before entering practical nursing, a review of school applications revealed, the women applicants had usually been earning their own living; before the war about 50 per cent, now a higher proportion, had been job holders. Employment included such jobs as domestic work, nurses' helper, ward helper, secretary, clerk, waitress, office work, cooking, sewing, teaching, care of children, and factory work. About 10 per cent of the candidates said they had been "at home." Many come from the Red Cross classes in home nursing and nurses' aide work. A few students come from doctors' offices. Occasionally, candidates who have dropped out of commercial and correspondence schools apply, having seen the futility of study without practice in the care of the sick. A rather large number come from schools of professional nursing, but the misfits from these schools are not as a rule successful as practical nurses.

Most instructors prefer those who have not had formal experience in nursing.

Health

It should go without saying—yet it must be stressed—that every candidate for practical nursing and every practicing graduate should be in good health. She must have considerable energy, strong muscles, and calm nerves. A complete examination by a doctor of the school's choice is a usual prerequisite to admission to the approved schools. This examination includes blood tests and an x-ray of the chest, and upon acceptance the student is immunized and vaccinated if necessary. A reexamination after acute illness and upon completion of the course is advised. Correction of defects should be carried out before starting the course. A report of the student's health is sent to the hospital or agency where practice work is being given.

Employment agencies and registries do not require routine pre-employment examinations as a rule. Institutions and public health agencies usually do.

Age

Authorities agree that eighteen is the minimum age at which girls should begin their training for practical nursing, and applicants over fifty find the work difficult. In 1940, the idea of placing senior high school girls under seventeen in hospitals to get practice for credit as a part of vocational training was deplored by the American Nurses' Association if direct contact with patients was involved. Reasons presented were the youth of the girls, lack of all-round preparation, lack of proper supervision while in the wards, lack of continuity in case experience, and some danger to the girls in an age group susceptible to infection—especially tuberculosis, since the wards of our general hospitals may harbor undiagnosed cases.

When asked what age was preferred in practical nurses, employers, registrars, and physicians usually chose the middle years, twenty-five to forty. A few physicians liked the "younger set." The age range in classes and registries was seventeen to sixty, an exception sixty-five. It was not unusual to find a fifth of the registrants over forty-five (18).

As a rule the younger nurses prefer hospital work to private duty in homes. "It's more exciting," "I learn more," "The hours are more regular," "I don't have so much responsibility," "I don't like children" are some of the reasons. Older women who are familiar with home problems, family emergencies, and planning meals fit better into homes. They say hospital work is too hard, the pressure too great, and they like being in charge of a situation. Directors and supervisors agree with these statements; they prefer women under forty-five for hospital work, although the younger ones are sometimes "flighty" and need more supervision. Hospital administrators also report that the presence of energetic young nurses keeps up the patients' morale, and they feel that young practical nurses receive better health and other supervision than they would when working in private homes.

Vocational guidance secretaries think of practical nursing as an ideal field for the older woman, married or unmarried, who is not trained for other work but is mature in judgment, understands people, and knows homemaking. One of the many inducements offered to practical nurses who grow restive at the thought that no career or assured promotion lies ahead is the reminder that practical nurses will be able to work at their job long after they are fifty—provided they are well. It is a type of work which offers adjustable hours and has a "longer span of acceptability" than many jobs for women (19).

Education

Most of the approved schools insist on a minimum of eighth grade education, making only rare exceptions. Schools prefer candidates with less than four years of high school, partly because, if their grades are good, graduates from high school should be urged to go into professional nursing, partly because a high school graduate may be bored by the elementary character of the subject matter offered or may be able to progress faster than her classmates, making an uncomfortable situation for all, including the teachers. The high school graduates who are accepted are usually those whose grades fell in the lower half of their class. Rarely, a girl or woman with college preparation will be admitted to a school when circumstances warrant it. She is given fair warning that she will be irked by the pace of the class and must not display her superior knowledge or ability to learn fast. Such students usually apply because they wish special training quickly (for instance, a missionary returning to her post within a year), are in great need of employment and untrained for other jobs, or are older women unqualified for professional nursing. Older women of superior education usually make excellent practical nurses.

Of a typical cross section of 97 applicants for the New York state schools for practical nursing tested by The Psychological Corporation, New York, in 1944, one per cent had had some college education, 37 per cent were high school graduates, 40 per cent had had less than four years of high school, and 22 per cent had completed the eighth grade.

The mean age of this group was thirty, the range eighteen to fifty-six (20). Seven per cent were between eighteen and twenty. It is possible that in rural states the percentage of high school graduates is lower than in New York.

Between 1940 and 1945, 633 candidates for the schools of practical nursing have been tested by the Corporation. The battery of tests included scholastic aptitude, vocabulary, mechanical comprehension, and common household knowledge. In the scholastic aptitude tests on 80 candidates, a correlation with the subsequent grade given on theory in the schools was .444. As some of these tests were also given to candidates for schools of professional nursing, the writer asked the Corporation if any conclusions could be drawn as to the difference in performance on the tests related to the difference in preparation and perhaps age of the candidates for the two levels of nursing. The following statement was received:

Candidates for admission to professional nursing are younger than the practical nurse groups. Of 5,744 applicants tested for schools in New York state during 1944, the average age was 18 years 7 months. Of this group 68 per cent were less than 19 years old, 29 per cent were 19 to 25 inclusive, and 3 per cent were 26 years old or above. Only one per cent were as old as 30—the average age for the practical nurse group.

The two groups of students are different in their reactions to tests. There are perhaps several reasons for this. The practical nurse group tends to have been out of school for some time and is therefore less familiar with timed standardized tests than the younger group. Because of this, the tests used have been so selected that the speed factor is not high enough to cause undue tension. Rest periods between tests are also a little more frequent and a little longer than for the younger group. There also seems some possibility that since the practical nurse group is not primarily academically minded, previous examination situations may be remembered somewhat unhappily. On the whole, however, after the initial nervousness has worn off, the group makes a satisfactory adjustment to this experience. They tend to be cooperative and eager to do their best.

Performance on tests also is different for the two groups. On tests of scholastic aptitude the practical nurses rate much lower than candidates for professional nursing. The same is true, though to a lesser degree, on a mechanical comprehension test. In contrast, the practical nurses rate higher than do the younger applicants on household knowledge—showing probably the result of greater experience along this line. Their vocabulary knowledge, while it is actually somewhat less than that of candidates for professional nursing, is rather better in proportion to their scholastic aptitude. This is possibly to some extent the result of their greater average age.

The correlation between test results and school grades is very similar in the two groups, and in both cases much like the correlations found in high schools and colleges. Some critical scores, below which applicants do not often succeed in carrying the course, have been tentatively established and we now feel that the battery should prove to be of definite value as one aid in the selection and guidance of students in schools of practical nursing.

It has been hard to find complete reports of actual community situations in which the practical nurses' qualifications are known. In Shelby County, Indiana, in 1929, the surveyor for the Committee on the Costs of Medical Care interviewed 17 "practical nurses." Their average age was over fifty-five—up to seventy-three. Thirteen had grade school education, two had had correspondence school courses, two had worked in hospitals, 13 had had no training. Two "never did housework," several refused contagious cases, one did only obstetrical work. Most of the group were willing to do twenty-four-hour duty. There was no local registry (21).

IMPROVING THE SERVICE OF PRACTICAL NURSES

There are several points at which control over the quality and quantity of practical nurses should be exercised. The first opportunity is at the school door through entrance requirements—educational, personal, and cultural. While eighth-grade education is considered minimal, two years of high school preferable, ability to handle the scholastic program of the school is the real test. Women with high school diplomas received twenty years ago cannot always absorb the lessons, while grade school youngsters do better at mathematics than many college graduates. Sometimes mediocre classroom performance is offset by unusual skill in nursing procedures, tact, maturity of judgment, personal adaptability, and neatness.

The second point of control, after the setting of entrance requirements, is the selection of students. Under present conditions the need to fill classes has led directors of schools to take all those applying except the obviously unfit. In better times when applicants will be more numerous, the director should do a far more discriminating job. It goes without saying that a personal interview is essential, after credentials have been checked. Some knowledge of the principles of guidance is needed, and the director must decide whether to discourage an applicant from taking up nursing of any type, admit her to the school, or urge her to apply to a school of professional nursing. Sometimes her decision cannot be made until the course is well advanced. She owes it to the public and the graduate practical nurses, however, to be ruthless in weeding out candidates unfitted to nurse or to carry the responsibility of a home where there is illness.

The control of numbers at the source—the schools—is also important in preventing overproduction. We have not had to worry about too many nurses since 1940, but it may well be a major problem now that the war is over. How many practical nurses does America need? How many can find employment? Let us not repeat the experience of professional nursing in which we produced in another postwar period, between 1918 and 1928, too many poorly qualified and too few well qualified nurses. Let us not have to discourage young women from entering this field, but try to produce a high grade supply commensurate with the demand.

Hospital administrators do not believe that the practical nurses now on duty will be supplanted by any large transfer of volunteer nurses' aides to a paid basis. They recognize the facts that the practical nurse has a longer preparation, more continuous work in the hospital under supervision, that she belongs to the hospital staff as an employed worker, sharing in appropriate in-service training programs and staff activities, and that she is capable of developing greater variety of skills than the nurses' aide. No very large proportion of volunteer nurses' aides have changed to pay status in civilian hospitals thus far, and it is thought that with the return of nurses from military service, many aides will discontinue their service to hospitals altogether (22). Their great contribution has been in relieving the registered nurses of simple nursing procedures, building morale, and carrying an interpretation of the hospital problems into the community. One of their indirect contributions to nursing has been a convincing demonstration that a nonprofessional but trained assistant has a place in every hospital. Their presence has done much to change the attitude of thousands of professional nurses toward practical nurses.

Too little attention was given in the years between 1910 and 1930 to the inherent personal fitness of the professional student nurse (23).

Mere completion of certain academic work or years of living are not in themselves recommendations for nursing on any level. "Interest tests" and "achievement tests" should be given and every possible question which might give a clue to the suitability of a candidate should be asked and observations should be made in personal interviews, but even then "only the Almighty can say whether she will be a successful nurse." The records are full of paradoxes. Here is a highly successful nurse who gave as her honest reason for entering training, "I want to marry a doctor." She did. Another, who just "loved" nursing and always wanted to care for sick people, left the school after two months of complete failure to adjust to any of the demands made upon her. Until tests—standardized, reliable, and valid—are available to help select practical nurses, we shall have to depend on the applicant's past record with as complete investigation of references as possible, personal interviews, and performance during the school probationary period. Decisions should be made early in the training, because every day adds to the waste of teaching a pupil who is to be dropped later.

Obviously, raising minimum educational requirement is another means of reducing quantity, though in the case of this occupation, not necessarily quality. Unless the field becomes seriously overcrowded, this would appear to be an unwise step, since it might bar older women without high school education who would make desirable practical nurses. It is thought that now the war is over, the younger women dropping out of industry will continue their education, marry, or seek other fields, while the older women who drop out will be likely candidates for the field of practical nursing.

As the Committee to Study Nursing Education stated in 1923, we want this field to attract women and girls of ability and dignity, with a sense of the fitness of things. We will not find them satisfied if we give them only manual, housecleaning tasks suitable for a maid to perform. They must get from the simple care of sick people the zest of nursing service however humble, a "sense of the worth of the contribution which will tend to vitalize training and to satisfy" (24). Is this too high a hope? Hundreds of happy and successful practical nurses testify otherwise.

REFERENCES

1 Lucy Seymer, *A general history of nursing,* New York, Macmillan, 1933, pp. 47–48.

2 The first "graduate nurse" in the United States completed her course in 1872. State Charities Aid Association, *Report of Committee on Hospitals, 1872,* "Training school for nurses," New York, Putnam, 1877, p. 7. "Our experience proves that the better she is educated and the more refined and intelligent she is, the better nurse she makes"; p. 30.

3 W. Gilman Thompson, "The nursing situation," *New York State Journal of Medicine* 21:178, May 1921. See also Isabel M. Stewart, "Which way are we going in nursing," *Survey* 46:409–410, 1921.

4 Edith M. Stern, "Nurses wanted; a career boom," *Survey Graphic* 31:79–81, February 1942. For a description of the "trained nurse, old style," which sounds very much like one of the present-day untrained nurses, see Alfred Worcester, *A new way of training nurses,* Boston, Cupples and Hurd, 1888, pp. 12–13; those interested will find an outline of his course for trained nurses on p. 71 of his book.

5 See, for example, Louisa M. Alcott, *Hospital sketches, and camp and fireside stories,* Boston, Little, Brown, 1872; also, Marjorie Barstow Greenbie, *Lincoln's daughters of mercy,* New York, Putnam, 1944, especially "Scrubbing the lords of creation," p. 102. Two thousand "nurses" served in the Civil War.

6 Cecelia L. Schulz, *Nursing,* Boston, Bellman Publishing Co., 1941, No. 41, p. 6.

7 Esther Robertson, *The untrained nurse,* Boston, Angel Guardian Press, 1903, pp. 20, 144. For other lessons in home nursing of a later period, see "The household nurse," a series in the *New York Sunday American* in 1911; Isabel M. Stewart, *Lessons in home nursing,* Teacher's College Bulletin, Ninth Series, No. 2, September 22, 1917; E. B. Lowry, *The home nurse,* Chicago, Forbes & Co., 1919; Charlotte A. Aikens, *Home nurse's handbook of practical nursing,* Philadelphia, Saunders, 1913. For textbooks published after 1920 see page 345.

Efforts to supply the public with guides to nursing the sick at home are interesting historically but read like children's primers today. Farmers' almanacs, family Bibles, the back pages of old cook books and diaries abound in family remedies and reminders to harassed mothers as to "what to do when." Some of the published material found incidentally in source reading for this book offers such titles as *The secret of health and guide to home nursing* (1860), *Suggestions for the sickroom,* compiled by An American Woman (1876), *On nurses and nursing with special reference to the management of sick women* (1868), *Plain directions for the care of the sick,* by A. P. Turner (1875), *Sunshine in the sick room* (1885), *Handbook of hygienic practice—practical guide for the sick room* (1865), and *Care of invalids*, prepared by the Mutual Life Insurance Company of New York (1904).

8 Comments by Stella Hawkins, *Law and legislation;* report of conference of members of state boards of nurse examiners, in Philadelphia, 1940, New York, American Nurses' Association (mimeographed).

9 W. S. Leathers, "Some problems in nursing education," *American Journal of Nursing* 32:440, April 1932. See also Hugh Cabot, "The changing relation between nursing and medicine," *Modern Hospital* 36:57–60, January 1931; Hugh Cabot, "Future of nursing education," *Modern Hospital* 60:47–48, February 1943; news item, "College women in nursing," *Public Health Nursing* 36:203, April 1944; Dora Mathis, "Nursing service of the future," *Hospitals* 14:39–40, August 1940.

10 Schulz (note 6), p. 6.

11 United States Department of Labor, Employment Service, *Dictionary of occupational titles,* Part I, Definition of titles, Washington, Government Printing Office, 1939.

12 United States War Manpower Commission, Division of Occupational Analysis and Manning Tables, *Dictionary of occupational titles,* supplement, edition 2, July 1943, Washington, Government Printing Office, 1943.

13 The first description of a uniform suggested by a state appeared in 1921: "One piece dress of tan chambray, attached soft white collar and cuffs of white piqué, caps of tan with white piqué turn back band," short sleeves and white bibbed apron, *Registration of nurses and trained attendants,* University of the State of New York, Bulletin No. 2, February 1, 1921, p. 2.

14 One of the most trenchant statements ever made anent the tendency of practical nurses to "overreach" appeared in the *American Journal of Nursing* in July 1903 (p. 828). The editor wrote: "That trained attendants have a place is unquestioned. The difficulty is that they do not remain in that place."

15 W. W. Charters, "Personality in nursing," *American Journal of Nursing* 30:1246, October 1930.

16 Thyra Pedersen, "The ideal attendant," *United States Veterans' Medical Bureau Bulletin* 4:476–477, May 1928.

17 Katharine Shepard, "The attendant in the home," *Public Health Nursing* 11:259–260, April 1919.

18 Information obtained by the writer in visits to registries and hospitals, and from *Study of the subsidiary worker in nursing service in Pennsylvania,* Pennsylvania State Nurses' Association, 1939–1940, p. 40.

19 Hilda M. Torrop, "A plea for the practical nurse," *Modern Hospital* 62:79–80, March 1944.

20 Figures from The Psychological Corporation, 522 Fifth Avenue, New York, 1944.

21 Allon Peebles, *A survey of the medical facilities of Shelby County, Indiana, 1929,* Publication No. 6 of the Committee on the Costs of Medical Care, Washington, the Committee [1930], pp. 65–66.

22 United States Women's Bureau, *The outlook for women in occupations in the medical services; practical nurses and hospital attendants,* Washington, Government Printing Office, 1945 (Bulletin 203, No. 5), p. 10. Reports to the writer from four general hospitals in November 1945 indicated a 25 per cent drop in volunteer aide service since V-J Day.

23 Harlan H. Horner, "Looking facts in the face," *American Journal of Nursing* 33:13, January 1933.

24 Josephine Goldmark, *Nursing and nursing education in the United States;* report of the Committee for the Study of Nursing Education, New York, Macmillan, 1923, p. 477.

CHAPTER THREE

The Supply of Practical Nurses

N° STATISTICS have been compiled to show the number of non-professional nurses in the United States earning their living by caring for the sick. The indefiniteness and variety of titles applied to these workers over the years make a count virtually impossible. Classifications used by the United States Census Bureau have been untrained nurses, practical nurses, children's nurses, attendants, and student nurses. These terms have been combined, separated, and regrouped in nearly every Census. Up to 1940 the Census terms also showed confusion between untrained and trained nurses, between untrained and licensed practical nurses, between undergraduate professional students and practical nurses. Figures are, therefore, far from clear or comparable.

The number of employed "practical nurses" has been put at 200,000 (1) but this is clearly an underestimate of those who nurse for hire, other than registered nurses. The total reported in the 1940 Census under the titles "practical nurses and midwives" and "attendants in hospitals" is 186,656 (2), but there is no count of the untrained and unlicensed people who set themselves up as nurses—probably about 30,000.

The figures since 1880 are as follows (3):

1880		13,483
1890		42,586
1900		103,747
1910		126,838
1920		151,996
1930		153,443
1940 Practical nurses and midwives	91,107	
Attendants in hospitals and institutions	95,549	186,656

Of the 91,107 persons reported as "practical nurses and midwives" in 1940, 3,909 (4.3 per cent) were men and 87,198 were women; of the attendants in hospitals and institutions, 57 per cent were men. Fourteen per cent of the "practical nurses and midwives" were Negroes (4).

There were more practical nurses and midwives in the South than in any other part of the country, fewest in the West. The following table shows the percentage distribution and ratios of practical nurses and of attendants in various sections of the United States (5).

	Total United States	North- east	North- Central	South	West
Percentage distribution of practical nurses and mid- wives	100	27	28	33	14
Number of people per practical nurse or midwife	1,445	1,451	1,675	1,409	1,086
Percentage distribution of employed attendants	100	41	28	20	11
Number of people per attendant	1,378	915	1,511	2,205	1,291

Another source of information regarding the number of employed nonprofessional nurses in the United States is the census of registered hospitals made annually by the American Medical Association. This survey showed that for the four years 1941–1944 the numbers of practical nurses and attendants (not necessarily licensed) employed in the registered hospital were as follows (6):

	Practical nurses and attendants	Practical nurses	Attendants
1941	112,334	17,332	
1942	116,294	22,161	94,133
1943	109,736	17,309	92,427
1944	88,114		

During these years the number of admissions to the registered hospitals went steadily upward and the bed capacity increased. The number of births also was high.

It is interesting to compare these figures for practical nurses and attendants with the 7,822 assistant nurses and 39,657 auxiliaries in England in 1940. The shortage of nursing assistance was reported as acute (7).

In 1943, the Procurement and Assignment Division of the War Manpower Commission made a study of the hospitals in the United States, and the American Nurses' Association shared in the analysis of the findings. The accompanying tables are based on the report of the study as it appeared in *The American Journal of Nursing* (8). The

PERCENTAGE OF TOTAL NURSING CARE GIVEN BY PAID AUXILIARY
NURSING WORKERS IN 1,162 GENERAL AND RELATED SPECIAL
HOSPITALS IN THE UNITED STATES, JULY 1943

	Government	Nongovernment
Hospitals without schools of nursing	44	41
Hospitals with schools of nursing	29	13

study defined auxiliary workers as, "All persons, other than graduate registered nurses, who are employed in the care of the sick, such as so-called practical nurses, attendants, trained attendants, licensed attendants, licensed undergraduate nurses, licensed practical nurses, ward helpers and orderlies, nurses' aides, nursing aides, etc."

NUMBER OF PATIENTS PER FULL TIME PAID AUXILIARY NURSING
WORKER IN 1,162 GENERAL AND RELATED SPECIAL HOSPITALS IN
THE UNITED STATES, JULY 1943

DAILY AVERAGE PATIENT CENSUS	HOSPITALS WITHOUT SCHOOLS OF NURSING		HOSPITALS WITH SCHOOLS OF NURSING	
	Government	Nongovernment	Government	Nongovernment
Total	6.0	6.2	6.4	13.4
Under 25	4.0	4.0	—	—
25 to 49	5.5	5.6	}14.0	12.9
50 to 99	8.8	7.1		15.2
100 to 199	6.3	7.1	11.2	13.4
200 and over	6.0	7.7	6.1	13.5

RATIO OF PAID AUXILIARY NURSING WORKERS TO GENERAL STAFF
NURSES IN 1,162 GENERAL AND RELATED SPECIAL HOSPITALS IN
THE UNITED STATES, JULY 1943

	Government	Nongovernment
Hospitals without schools of nursing	8:10	7:10
Hospitals with schools of nursing	12:10	6:10

Unfortunately, the breadth of the definition of auxiliary worker makes it impossible to draw any conclusions from these statistics regarding the practical nurse's share in service in these hospitals. The study showed that volunteer nursing service played but a small part in most of these hospitals and "paid auxiliary workers" gave more than a third of the total hours of care in hospitals not having schools of professional nursing. Also,

The practice of employing paid auxiliary nursing workers was about the same for all sizes of nongovernmental hospitals, but among governmental hospitals, the per cent of hospitals which employed paid auxiliaries was higher among the larger hospitals

The practice of employing paid auxiliary nursing workers was considerably more prevalent among hospitals without schools of nursing than among hospitals with schools of nursing—81 per cent and 58 per cent respectively

The per cent of the total nursing care given by the paid auxiliary nursing workers was 42 per cent in hospitals without schools of nursing (with two groups giving nursing care) and 17 per cent in hospitals with schools of nursing, that is with three groups giving nursing care

The ratio of paid auxiliary nursing workers to patients was approximately the same for the governmental and nongovernmental hospitals without schools of nursing and for the governmental hospitals with schools of nursing—.16 paid auxiliaries per patient. In the nongovernmental hospitals with schools of nursing the ratio was .07 paid auxiliaries per patient

The ratio of paid auxiliary nursing workers to general staff nurses was highest in the governmental hospitals with schools of nursing in which there were 12 paid auxiliaries for each 10 general staff nurses (9)

The little information that is available about the number of practical nurses working in homes, in general and special hospitals, in industry, and in institutions for convalescence and chronic diseases is presented in the chapters on those fields of service. Suffice it to say here that there are no complete figures.

We do not know what the ratio of practical nurses to professional nurses or to patients is or should be in hospitals or homes for convalescents or the chronically ill. Probably such ratios cannot be determined until the duties that licensed practical nurses may safely perform are defined and their skills made fairly uniform. Until such guides are supplied, every hospital or infirmary for the aged and every convalescent home will continue to be a law unto itself in assigning responsibilities to practical nurses.

No general study has been made recently of the number of practical nurses available in any one state for all types of service. In November 1944 the Illinois State Nurses Committee on Practical Nursing distributed a questionnaire to which 2,670 practical nurses replied. Of this total, 2,271 were employed in institutions and 399 in private duty. One district has 588 in institutions and 42 in private duty. The majority of nurses were over forty, with grade school education. Also, the majority had had correspondence school courses or experience in special hospitals only, and 464 reported no previous training of any kind.

In 13 states in 1944, there were 29,418 licensed auxiliary workers (practical nurses, trained attendants, etc., whatever the legal title) and 17,021 of these had renewed their licenses in that year. Two states do not require renewal. Six states with legal control of title (Georgia, Florida, Indiana, Mississippi, Oklahoma, and Wisconsin) had not set up courses for practical nurses. One state (Missouri) discontinued its courses in 1940. Nineteen states and the territory of Hawaii reported that a total of 31,510 licenses had been issued to practical nurses or attendants from the date of enactment of the laws to the end of 1945 (10).

No figures are available on the number of licensed practical nurses, as distinguished from attendants, ward helpers, and nurses' aides, employed in hospitals and homes in the United States. Reports from state health and welfare departments are usually in terms of registered nurses and nonregistered or subsidiary workers, not licensed practical nurses.

It was possible, however, thanks to the interest of the American Nurses' Association, to secure some data on the licensure of paid auxiliary nursing workers in a representative sampling of hospitals. The figures are shown in the accompanying table. In this sampling, roughly 10 per cent of the paid auxiliary nursing workers were licensed, a higher figure than might be expected if the federal facilities, with their large staffs of unlicensed attendants, had been included.

LICENSURE OF PAID AUXILIARY NURSING WORKERS IN HOSPITALS

| | | PAID AUXILIARY WORKERS | | |
TYPE OF HOSPITALS	NUMBER OF HOSPITALS	Number employed*	Number licensed	Percentage licensed
Total reporting	1,551	38,439	3,628	9.4
General and related specialt	1,162	15,085	1,751	11.6
Tuberculosis	146	2,610	270	10.3
Mental, diagnostic	33	591	62	10.5
Mental, custodial	116	17,571	1,284	7.3
Chronic	27	1,403	122	8.7
Institutional	9	293	48	16.4
All others	58	886	91	10.3

* Both full-time and part-time workers.

† Includes eye, ear, nose and throat, pediatric, maternity, and industrial hospitals.

Table compiled by Louise M. Tattershall from data obtained in the study of hospitals made in 1943 by the Procurement and Assignment Division of the War Manpower Commission (8). Army, Navy, Marine, Veterans Administration, and Indian Affairs hospitals were not included.

If we accept the estimate of persons hiring out as practical or attendant nurses as 200,000 in the United States, two conclusions can be drawn:

The hired care of people ill at home but not employing registered nurses is largely in the hands of untrained and unregulated persons

The approved schools of practical nursing must be graduating a very small portion of the needed number of practical nurses as indicated by the number now employed and as compared to the number of registered nurses being graduated. Five schools for practical nurses reported only 525 students enrolled in 1943, and one state had three approved schools without students. A rough estimate by the writer of the number of nurses graduating from all the 52 approved schools in 1945 was less than 500

THE FUTURE SUPPLY

Dr. Joseph W. Mountin, of the United States Public Health Service, forecasts the national needs for professional nurses in the coming years for a population of 138,000,000, but he gives no estimate of the need for practical nurses although he fully recognizes their place in the future service to sick people. He writes: "Once the stigma now attached to vocational education in professional circles is removed, future efforts to systematize the training of auxiliary workers may be more productive of results than has been the case so far" (11).

Dr. Mountin suggests that a system of vocational education might be developed which would train all nurses below collegiate grade. Under any set of circumstances, he believes, the professional nurses themselves should be the dominant influence in shaping the curriculum and determining eligibility to practice.

Nor did any of the estimates of nursing needs for the duration of the war include practical nursing service (12).

In Dr. Parran's congressional testimony in behalf of a coordinated hospital service plan, he called for the construction of institutions and nursing homes for chronics as well as base, district, and rural hospitals and health centers. Dr. Parran stated that "There is no ready means of determining the number and scope of new public health facilities that will be required in the postwar period. In view of the almost complete absence of these modern facilities, however, the need will be great" (13).

The mercurial changes and extremes to which nurses, along with other essential workers, are exposed make reliable forecasts impossible. In 1929, a year of great prosperity, we had registered nurses in superabundance and out of work, with a growing use of practical nurses; then the depression enhanced the shortage of jobs for both groups, but by 1937, while we were on the one hand reducing professional schools and raising standards, we were finding more work for professional nurses (eight-hour day and Blue Cross program) and increasing approved facilities for training practical nurses under state laws. The war changed all that, and almost overnight we were graduating more registered nurses than ever before in history, lowering entrance standards, reducing the number in training for practical nursing while increasing their jobs, and creating the largest body of unlicensed, nonprofessional caretakers of the sick that we have ever had—WACs, WAVES, Red Cross Aides, and so on. Professional and nonprofessional workers are distributed approximately as follows (14):

371,066 registered nurses and 126,576 professional student nurses
200,000 practical nurses, paid aides, and midwives
181,677 Red Cross Volunteer Nurses' Aides
100,000 attendants, orderlies, and ward maids
187,897 medical technicians and corpsmen in the Army, Navy, Coast Guard, and Marine services

It is no wonder that 30,000 licensed practical nurses and attendants feel insecure and uncertain of the future in competition with more than a million workers in the same field.

It has been estimated that by its tenth year of operation an adequate public health and medical service program would require 180,000 "vocational nurses."* Public funds will be necessary to train them (15).

It is also anticipated that the professionally educated nurse of the future will devote more of her time and effort to strictly professional phases of nursing service and will supervise a larger number of trained assistants in the performance of the simpler and routine nonprofessional nursing activities (16).

In whatever way the problem is solved, warnings from the experience in overproduction of professional nurses are in order (17).

Candidates for training should not be selected at random
Training should not be promoted solely to meet the hospital's need, to fill or support a school, or to respond to the plea of the candidate in need of employment
The practice period should not be permitted to become a means of supplying cheap labor for institutions
Practical nurses should not be produced without state legislative control of their practice
Nurses should not be trained indiscriminately without a study of the demand

* See note on page 15.

This last warning brings up the problem of establishing schools (and increasing the production of practical nurses) in states where there are few hospitals and where supervision of home service is difficult. Especially is this a problem in states without a law to control the practice of these nurses. For example, in New Hampshire, which has no law, only 56,583 patients entered the 42 registered hospitals in the state in 1944; there were even fewer in Vermont, but Vermont has an "approved" school. Nevada has no accredited professional nursing school, Utah has six, Wyoming two (18). Are these states favorable centers to train practical nurses or would training in their institutions fail to offer sufficient and qualified professional supervision? How would schools provide home nursing experience under supervision? The future preparation of practical nurses must be analyzed, not from the point of view of demand and supply alone, but from the angle of adequate training centers, practice fields, and qualified faculty.

It is evident that the findings in this chapter attempting to estimate the existing supply of practical nurses are scattered, unrelated, incomplete for the country as a whole, not representative of a typical community; they cannot be added together because they represent dissimilar units. The unreliability of our present knowledge of the numbers of workers in this field and the lack of uniformity in definitions indicate the crying need for comprehensive studies and surveys on which to build an estimate of future service from practical nurses needed by the public.

REFERENCES

1 Dorothy Deming, "Practical nurses; a professional responsibility," *American Journal of Nursing* 44:36–43, January 1944.
2 United States Bureau of the Census, *Sixteenth Census of the United States, 1940,* Population, Vol. III, The labor force, Part I, U. S. Summary, Washington, Government Printing Office, 1943, Tables 62, 69, 70, pp. 88, 90, 114, 115.
3 The figures for 1880–1920 are from May Ayres Burgess, *Nurses, patients and pocketbooks;* report of a study of the economics of nursing by the Committee on the Grading of Nursing Schools, New York, the Committee, 1928, p. 40; that for 1930 is from Committee to Study the Grading of Nursing Schools, *Nursing schools today and tomorrow,* New York, the Committee, 1934, pp. 30–31, 45; and those for

1940 are from the *Sixteenth Census*, pp. 15, 75, 82–83, 105–106, and Table 59. By 1930, there were 294,186 trained nurses, which was more than the number of untrained nurses. The ratio of both groups to the population of the United States was 1:273.

4 *Census*, pp. 75, 79, and Table 59.

5 United States Women's Bureau, *Outlook for women in occupations in the medical services; practical nurses and hospital attendants*, Washington, Government Printing Office, 1945 (Bulletin 203, No. 5), p. 2.

6 "Hospital service in the United States," *Journal of the American Medical Association* 127:781, March 31, 1945. See also *ibid.* 121:1019, March 27, 1943; 124:848, March 25, 1944.

7 Muriel M. Edwards, "Nursing in Britain, 1937–1943," *American Journal of Nursing* 44:125–133, February 1944.

8 Louise M. Tattershall and Marion E. Altenderfer, "Paid auxiliary nursing workers employed in general hospitals," *American Journal of Nursing* 44:752–756, August 1944. The other parts of the report were as follows: Louise Tattershall and Margaret D. West, "Wartime nursing care in 604 general hospitals," *American Journal of Nursing* 44:211–214, March 1944; Louise M. Tattershall and Marion E. Altenderfer, "Nursing personnel in general hospitals," *ibid.* 44:853–858, September 1944; Tattershall and Altenderfer, "Hours of nursing service in general hospitals," *ibid.* 44:963–966, October 1944.
  Special appreciation is expressed to Louise M. Tattershall, Statistician of the American Nurses' Association, for assistance in rearranging the data to give emphasis to the auxiliary workers.

9 Tattershall and Altenderfer (note 8), August, p. 756.

10 "Trained attendants and practical nurses; the ANA report on licensed attendants and schools for training attendants," *American Journal of Nursing* 44:7–8, January 1944; *ibid.* 46:391, June 1946.

11 Joseph W. Mountin, "Suggestions to nurses on postwar adjustments," *American Journal of Nursing* 44:321–325, April 1944, at p. 325.

12 "Nursing needs and nursing resources," *American Journal of Nursing* 44:431–432, May 1944; news item, "Nurses balance 1946 supply against needs," *Public Health Nursing* 36:595–597, November 1944, at p. 597.

13 Wartime health and education, Hearings before a subcommittee of the Committee on Education and Labor, U. S. Senate, Part 5, p. 1787.

14 Figures were obtained as follows: professional nurses and students

from American Nurses' Association, Research and Statistical Consultant, *Outline of courses for the training of auxiliary workers in the care of the sick by U. S. Army, U. S. Navy, U. S. Coast Guard, U. S. Maritime Service, American Red Cross*, New York, Joint Committee on Auxiliary Nursing Service, November 1945 (mimeographed); Red Cross Volunteer Nurses' Aides and Service technicians and corpsmen from American Nurses' Association, Nursing Information Bureau, cooperating with the National League of Nursing Education and the National Organization for Public Health Nursing, *Facts about nursing, 1945*, pp. 7, 34; practical nurses, paid aides, midwives, attendants, orderlies, and ward maids estimated by the writer (see note 1).

15 George St. J. Perrott, "Content and administration of a medical care program; training of personnel and research," *American Journal of Public Health* 34:1244–1251, December 1944, p. 1248.

16 A. C. Bachmeyer, "Educational function of the hospital after the war," IN *The Hospital Yearbook*, Chicago, Modern Hospital Publishing Co., 1943, pp. 950–951.

17 Harlan H. Horner, "Looking facts in the face," *American Journal of Nursing* 33:18, January 1933.

18 "Hospital service in the United States, 1945" (note 6), pp. 774, 778.

CHAPTER FOUR

The Birthplace of Practical Nursing—the Home

ATTENDANTS, caretakers, and guardians of the sick are mentioned in the earliest records of Greece, but "nurses" as such do not appear in the history of Egypt, India, China, or Rome before the Christian era. Undoubtedly, the home care of the sick was in the hands of mothers or neighbors, sometimes slaves (1). With the coming of the Christian era, when neighbors failed to be neighborly the Christian Church stepped in, and for generations help and sympathy were offered the sick voluntarily by parish members. The modern prototype is the "parish nurse," employed by the church to visit sick members.

Recognition that knowledge of caring for the sick makes for better neighbors came slowly. Phebe, a deaconess in the first century A.D., organized a group of visitors and taught them how to nurse the sick in their homes. She is usually regarded as the first visiting nurse; indeed, the order of deaconesses laid the foundation for the nurse's calling (2).

> For the care of sickness in the home.
> For the care of the home during sickness.

So reads the slogan under which the graduates of the Household Nursing Association of Boston have served for thirty years, expressing succinctly the dual role of the practical nurse as nurse and homemaker. "Nurse the home," Florence Nightingale said (3), for home is where the heart is, the place the lost return to, the refuge of the hunted, wounded, sick, and weary. Sick children, say pediatricians, often do better at home than in the hospital, and we have all seen the pathetic clinging of the aged to the dear familiar things at home.

Of all the fields of service open to the practical nurse, the home is first in importance, need, and fitness. It is here she finds her greatest usefulness and greatest satisfaction. The home is her proving ground, for even though she is supervised by a professional nurse from an agency, it is not like the hospital where someone is always on hand to take over in an emergency and a professional nurse may reassign cases or withdraw her entirely from a situation. Patients at home make many demands which the practical nurse can fill even better than the professional. In the home she is not an "auxiliary" or "subsidiary" worker, to the family she is "the nurse." She can become indispensable in her own right, and has in hundreds of cases.

Furthermore, the home will always be a sure source of employment. Only a small percentage of the families in the United States can afford private registered nursing care, and that only for short periods. In 1940, only one family in ten had a yearly income of $3,000—six out of ten had $1,500 or less (4). Putting it another way, probably only 40 per cent of the families in the United States can afford private registered nurses at a dollar an hour for brief emergency periods of acute illness (5), less than 20 per cent can afford them for longer periods. Professional nursing care in private homes is steadily declining (6). While the increase in hospitalization accounts for much of this change, it is probably true that practical nursing in private homes has not decreased in like proportion, because this service is ideally suited to long-term subacute and convalescent conditions which are not hospitalized. This state of affairs will probably continue, at least until some form of national health insurance meets the costs of medical and professional nursing care for those sick at home as well as for hospitalization.

It is also true that many professional nurses prefer nursing in hospitals. They like the "controlled" hospital situation. It is less difficult to plan a patient's care, there is adequate, suitable equipment to work with, a doctor is always on hand, there is no interruption from other members of the family, children, maids, or friends who run in and out at all hours. The hours of work are more regular and the nurse can sleep in her own bed. In many hospitals, special-duty nurses are paid through the hospital, thus relieving the nurse of bill-collecting. Hospital positions also offer security, some chance of advancement, paid vacations, and sick leave. Thus the field of home nursing is more open to practical nurses than in years past (7). Indeed, some administrators deplore the trend to train and hire practical nurses in hospitals lest they, too, come to prefer that form of service and desert the patients who must stay at home and who need their care so much.

In 1945, the Women's Bureau of the United States Department of Labor, in a "forecast" of employment for practical nurses, indicated that the trained practical nurse has become a permanent institution. The nurse registries have built a body of experience on the distinction between calls that require professional nursing and those for which practical nursing is more suitable (8).

We do not have any complete or recent data on the percentage of disabling illnesses nursed at home by practical nurses, licensed or unlicensed. The facts we have are scattered, localized, and not recent. The most complete are supplied from the study of the Committee on the Costs of Medical Care.* In 1928–1931, 9,000 families were visited periodically as part of this survey of illness (10). The study included rural, urban, and metropolitan areas, all the geographic sections of eighteen states, all income classes, and both native and foreign born. Illnesses of one day or more were recorded. Visits were made at intervals of two to four months for a twelve-month period (11). This report contains the only sampling we have of the use of practical nurses of any type among a limited group of families with illness.

Sixty per cent of the home illnesses (492 per 1,000 persons in the study) disabled people for one day or more, and 26 per cent resulted in 7.7 days of disability per person. However, only 50 per cent of the illnesses caused the patient to go to bed, and of the total sick days only 13 per cent were spent in bed. This might be interpreted to mean that patients were suffering from mild conditions suited to practical nursing care; indeed, the degenerative diseases of old age accounted for an average of 9.6 days per person in bed (12). Minor digestive upsets kept people in bed the shortest time.

Of the total of 32,752 illnesses reported in the periodic canvasses of this study, 11.2 per cent had some nursing care of one type or another. Of these cases with some nursing, approximately half (5.7 per cent of all cases) were hospital cases without a private nurse but with the usual care of the general duty nurses for the ward or floor or wing in which they were located. . . . Of all cases, 2.07 per cent had a graduate nurse, 0.82 per cent had a practical nurse, and 3.70 per cent had a visiting nurse. Of the total cases, 2.77 per cent had the exclusive services for one or more days or nights of a private nurse (graduate or practical) either in or outside of a hospital, and 0.56 per cent had the exclusive services of two or more such nurses during one or more twenty-four-hour days (13).

Of each 1,000 people in the study, 8.6 had practical nursing service, 189 days of practical nursing per 1,000 population. Rates for males

* The study of nursing care of maternity cases made by the National Health Survey in 1939 (9) did not include a report on the service by nonprofessional nurses. For care of chronic illness by practical nurses, see Chapter VIII.

under fifty-five years of age were low, while women of childbearing age used a great deal of service; the female case rate was 2.7 times that for males. About 16 per cent of the cases under care of practical nurses were maternity cases (14).

While practical nursing was available to all those in lower income brackets, even here its use increased with income. The rate of use of practical nursing per 1,000 population among the highest income families was twice that among the lowest. The same variation occurred in the number of days per case. The need of the middle income group—those with income of $1,200 to $5,000, who were neither rich enough to employ private service nor poor enough to secure free care—was made plain in this study (15).

As would be expected, this study showed that in small towns and rural areas a considerable portion of the population used practical nurses when sick. Obviously, professional nurses are also vitally needed, but this finding lends justification to the contention of those concerned with the education of practical nurses that the need for their service is great in small towns and in the country and that therefore their training should include adaptations to rural homes, experience in small community hospitals, and supervision in rural areas.

It will be noted that the report made no attempt to estimate the need for practical nurses but merely described the status quo (16).

The Committee on the Costs of Medical Care recommended that competent nursing aides and attendants—trained and supervised—be provided (17). An "acute situation" existed. "We have been slow to awaking to the needs." Immediate action was urged to control the unregulated practice of nursing (18).

The Pennsylvania survey of subsidiary workers (1939–1940) indicated that in one area, in 161 families, registered nurses gave 13 per cent of the home care, practical nurses 7 per cent, members of the family 80 per cent; in another area, in 25 families, registered nurses gave 15 per cent of the care, practical nurses 10 per cent, members of the family 75 per cent. Analysis by type of case of the care rendered by practical nurses is interesting. In 351 cases, surgical conditions constituted 11.7 per cent, medical 47.6 per cent, obstetrical 37.0 per cent, and pediatric 3.7 per cent; of 213 cases, 63.8 per cent were listed as "mild" conditions, 36.2 per cent as "serious." Some effort was made to find out why families called practical nurses: 294 replied that they could not afford a registered nurse, 214 wanted a nurse for twenty-four hours, and 206 wanted someone to help with the household (19).

Visiting nurse associations can give very accurate reports of the bedside nursing visits made in homes by their practical nursing staffs. The most impressive figure comes from the Visiting Nurse Service of New York City which reports that, of the home nursing visits made by its staff of 140 registered and 18 practical nurses, 6 per cent were made by the latter (20). As this is a professionally supervised program, we may assume that all these cases were suitable ones for practical nursing service.

In Canada, the study of nursing in Ontario in 1938–1939 indicated a definite need for service from practical nurses for patients ill at home. On a given day, of 117 patients of private doctors who were in need of home nursing care, 63 were not receiving it for lack of money to pay for service. An analysis of 381 patients showed that 199 did not need nursing care, 25 were already employing practical nurses, and 41 others were suitable cases for their service. The remaining 116 cases are not accounted for in the report; presumably they were under the care of professional nurses. One doctor pointed out that 95 per cent of his patients could not pay the charges of professional nurses (21).

THE NEED FOR PRACTICAL NURSES

The absence of complete and recent statistical data on the amount of service given in homes by practical nurses is made up for to some extent by the flood of testimony from doctors, families, social workers, nurses, students, and interested administrators of various community and national agencies who, since the late nineties, have studied, written, and talked in no uncertain terms of the need for practical nurses in homes in time of sickness.

Ever since 1900 *The American Journal of Nursing* has been filled with discussion and arguments regarding the place of the practical nurse, the consensus being that there is a place for her. The question doubtless arose as a result of the passage of the first state law for the registration of nurses in 1903. It was a burning issue for some years. At the end of pages of close-printed airing of views and vituperative effort to prove points, the weary editor of the *Journal* exclaimed, "Neither one of these writers has suggested a practical remedy" (22).

"There is an opening" for attendant nurses, wrote "T. C. F.," in practically every town in New England (23). She cited a town of 2,500 people (more in summer), with a hospital of twelve beds, five doctors, and no visiting nurse. The doctors sent to the cities for graduate nurses. Anyone who would "go out" to care for home sickness was kept busy. This was in 1917, but it could be today.

In 1916, probably as a result of war pressures, the American Hospital Association decided to study the grading and classification of nurses. The committee's conclusions regarding the need in homes was that "the needs in sickness in middle class homes are not always best met by a highly skilled graduate nurse, . . . a less expensive worker who can combine ordinary care of the sick with the care of the home is often more desirable, both from the standpoint of economy and efficiency." The report adds that this second type of worker is often pressed into service for which she is not fitted, and, unsupervised, increases her charges to the families. Experience has shown that both these difficulties can be met by proper organization and management. The report warns: "Women of immoral and dishonest character find a ready entrance into the sickrooms of an unsuspecting public." The recommendation to train workers for a two-fold purpose of caring for home and illness was vigorously supported (24).

The tenor of this early recommendation is repeated sometimes almost word for word, in the "Goldmark Report" (1923) (25), in the report of the Committee to Study the Grading of Nursing Schools (1928) (26), in the recommendations of various studies of practical nursing, notably those in New Jersey (27) and Pennsylvania (1938–1940) (19), and in New York at the time of the drafting of the new Nurse Practice Act (1935–1938) (28); in the findings of the Committee on the Costs of Medical Care (1933) (29), and in the recommendations of the Joint Committee on the Use of Subsidiary Workers of the three national nursing organizations (1935–1939) (30). Factual data were provided and mention was made of the need of home nursing care in the National Health Survey made by United States Public Health Service in 1935, and finally the wartime activities of the following agencies have all been concerned with increasing the home nursing service given by practical nurses: American Nurses' Association, National League of Nursing Education, National Organization for Public Health Nursing, National Nursing Council for War Service, American Red Cross, Department of Nursing Education of the United States Public Health Service, United States Office of Education, National Association for Practical Nurse Education, nearly all the various state and local associations of professional nurses, and a few state associations of licensed practical nurses. The Joint Committee on Auxiliary Nursing Service of the national nursing organizations also is currently concerned with these problems. In November 1944, 19 professional state nurses' associations had committees studying various aspects of the problem.

In all these organizations and among the hundreds of nurses and doctors with whom the writer has talked, or whose words she has read, there is general agreement upon these points:

People sick at home need practical nurses for certain kinds of illness and at certain stages

Few people can afford registered nurses for longterm, subacute, and convalescent conditions cared for at home; a less expensive service must be provided

It is desirable that trained and supervised practical nurses be supplied to homes from a reliable source at a price within the average family's budget

Most authorities—but not all—agree that the practical nurse should be licensed to practice by the state

Beyond this common ground, there is great divergence of opinion. How, where, and for how long this individual should be trained, what cases she may accept, what her fee should be, who is to supervise her, and how she is to be found when needed are points on which there are as many opinions as persons expressing them.

THE SUPPLY

The only source of information on the number of practical nurses, licensed and unlicensed, available for service in homes is the professional and commercial employment agencies, but no study of the total registrants, professional and nonprofessional, has ever been made by city, state, or nation.

The demand through the professional registries for practical nurses for both home and hospital service has invariably exceeded the supply in the last few years (31). All registries—including the commercial ones—say they have more requests than they can fill. Some commercial registries apparently take advantage of the labor shortage. In January 1945, a charge of a dollar an hour for practical nursing service was being made in three Manhattan registries; it was rumored that families in Brooklyn were paying $16 a day and that in Buffalo the rate was as high as $90 a week for a practical nurse. This was at a time when registered nurses from professional registries were receiving a dollar an hour for an eight-hour day, in accordance with the rates set by the local district of the State Nurses' Association.

During the years 1939–1943, the registry reports showed a 43 per cent increase in calls for nonprofessional nurses and only a 13 per cent increase for registered nurses. Calls from homes, however, dropped. In 1939, 10 per cent of all calls came from homes, in 1943 only 4 per cent. With the war, the increase in calls for nonprofessional workers in hospitals showed a 66 per cent increase (31).

In 1943, only 55 per cent of all calls for nonprofessional nurses were filled by the professional registries, as against 73 per cent for professionals. Yet the registry reports showed a 20 per cent increase in nonprofessional and only a 7 per cent increase in professional registrants between 1939 and 1943 (31). It was the general opinion of all the registrars consulted personally as well as of hospitals and institutions now employing practical nurses that more practical nurses could be used and were needed. Yet neither registries nor hospitals had attempted a recruiting campaign to secure graduate practical nurses.

In 1944, 26 professional registries reported that 93.8 per cent of their calls for practical nurses were for home service. They filled 57.6 per cent of these and 70.1 per cent of the calls from hospitals (32).

During the first eleven months of 1944, a registry in a city of less than 500,000 reported 193 calls received, 72 filled. Boston reported 781 calls for practical nurses in 1943 of which 179 were filled; the situation was about the same in 1944. Buffalo answered about 10 per cent of its calls, Washington 23 per cent. These are typical of the reports given to the writer.

ATTEMPTS TO MEET THE NEED

Various experiments have been tried in the past in an effort to provide a satisfactory home nursing service for the sick who do not need professional care. A few of these are described in the following pages.

The Waltham Plan

In Waltham, Massachusetts, in 1888, the experiment was tried of sending out undergraduate students during their course of training to nurse in private homes at a reduced fee (33). While it evoked acid criticism from the nursing profession as being educationally unsound, unsafe for pupil and patient alike, and entirely out of place as a basic curriculum activity, the plan had the great virtue of bringing super- vised nursing care to patients who could not get anything better—and who might get worse—and at a price they could pay. If the experience had been given in the first six months after graduation, the program would probably be regarded as progressive even today.*

Visiting Housekeeper Service

A visiting housekeeper, supplied and supervised by a recognized agency to care for the home when there is illness, is a useful and popu- lar aid. A few communities have had such programs for years (34). The housekeepers are trained by home economists, dietitians, and pro- fessional nurses to run the home and give very elementary nursing care of a custodial type.

Undoubtedly, a trained visiting housekeeper working in cooperation with a registered nurse greatly relieves many home situations if the family can afford to hire two workers or if a visiting housekeeper and a visiting nurse can handle the situation. Some dozen cities have offered the housekeeping services in the past to supplement professional nurs- ing service or to assume some of its simpler duties. During the last few years the services have been greatly diminished because of competing wartime jobs. In the New York plan (a W.P.A. project discontinued in 1940), the professional nurses from the Visiting Nurse Service su- pervised the care of the sick in homes where housekeepers were work- ing. No supervised licensed practical nursing service was then avail- able.

Two cases suitable for a visiting housekeeper who has had the equivalent of a Red Cross home nursing course and is supervised by a visiting nurse are cited from the former New York City visiting house- keeper project (35).

A young mother had lost her left arm in a war plant accident some months previously. Her husband was overseas. The visiting housekeeper

---

* Compare "internships," cadet nurses, and public health nursing affiliations by which the student learns on the actual job under supervision—although the consumer usually pays the same price to the agency as for professional service.

stayed with her during the first four weeks of her new baby's life, helping her with his care and the housework until she learned to manage alone.

Mrs. C., who weighed only 90 pounds, was expecting twins. She already had one child. During the last month of pregnancy and the first weeks of the twins' babyhood, the visiting housekeeper helped with the home and the children. The twins were delivered in a hospital.

In neither of these cases was there anyone actually sick or bedridden. A doctor and a visiting nurse were overseeing both cases.

It is difficult to picture practical nurses and visiting housekeepers working together in one home unless the family is large or the patient's care very demanding, for their homemaking services would overlap. If both services are available, the decision as to whether practical nursing or visiting housekeeper service is most needed should be made on the merits of the individual case. It is important to remember that sickness should be the primary reason for calling the practical nurse (36), and that the housekeeper's services to the sick must be kept at the custodial level. Such services have been compared to those of a children's nurse when one of her young charges is mildly ill. Supervision by a visiting nurse is always desirable. In states where all who nurse for hire must be licensed, this precaution of professional supervision is especially necessary. There is general agreement, however, that a well organized and supervised visiting housekeeper service is greatly needed in every community of any size (37). This type of service is one of the benefits of the Beveridge Plan in England (38).

The Brattleboro Plan

The "Brattleboro Plan" (Vermont) approaches the problem from another standpoint. Besides training practical nurses ("attendants") to care for home illness and the home, with placement after a visit from a registered nurse and under her continued supervision, the plan offers both types of nursing as well as hospital care on a voluntary insurance basis, enabling those who join to get, at reduced rates, home nursing service of the type doctor and registered nurse feel is needed. The plan increases the demand for service. Richards M. Bradley, the great proponent of the scheme and irrepressible protagonist for practical nurses, summarized the advantages of the service in Brattleboro as offering appropriate training, placement, and supervision of a skilled type of worker suited to the average rural Vermont family. He felt professional nurses were blind to the needs of thousands of small-town homes and were selfish in not sharing the demand for nursing care with practical nurses trained for the purpose (39).

For those interested in the functioning of this plan, the writer recommends a careful reading of its evaluation by Katherine Tucker and Violet Hodgson (40).

Home Nursing Courses

Some administrators and physicians have believed that an abundant supply of "practically" trained home nurses available at low cost after a very short course would solve the problem of nursing the sick of moderate means and those living in rural areas. Under this plan, each community would train a group of women through classes in home nursing such as those given by the American Red Cross.

While the Red Cross Home Nursing classes undoubtedly increase the skill and knowledge of homemakers, they are not intended to fill a community need through training practical nurses for hire outside their own homes (41). A more fundamental objection to this plan, however, is the fact that sickness is no respecter of persons. The chance that a person lives in a rural area or has a small income is no guarantee against acute illness. There would be few conditions among acutely ill persons safe in the hands of sketchily trained "nurses." The first effort in acute illness should be to provide registered nursing no matter what the cost. "It is the stage or nature of the illness which should determine the type of nurse employed, not the patient's pocketbook" (42).

There has been no formal appraisal of the results of these home nursing courses.

Service from Professional Nurses

Professional visiting nurses are believed by some to be the answer to the need of home patients of moderate means and those who must be given free service at home. However, visiting nurses solve only part of the problem. They do not remain on a case or make visits after six P.M. (although a few associations take confinement cases at night). Their visits do not provide for getting breakfast for the children or seeing that they have their school lunch, washing the family laundry or the baby's clothing, cleaning the house, and settling the patient for the night.

A dramatic and all-too-true scene is described in *Public Health Nursing* for March 1940 (43). "The patient is given her bath and care. She is left comfortable and rested. Then what? The house is unswept. The stove grows cold. The children come home from school hungry. The patient lies fretting. Her bedclothes are disheveled." The work of the visiting nurse is undone.

The visiting nurse associations in most large cities offer service by professional nurses under two plans: by appointment if the patient needs medication or treatment at specified times, and at any time the nurse can fit the visit into her schedule. The latter is, of course, less expensive.

The report of the hourly appointment service tried in Chicago in 1931 showed that many of the home calls could have been successfully and safely handled by practical nurses under professional supervision (44). The type of service needed was well adapted to the abilities of this group, but no organized trained staff was available in Chicago at that time. A central distributing point was needed for all types of service, an end that would have been served by a community nursing bureau prepared to furnish both registered and practical nurses on full time or part time, pay, part pay, or free.

DUTIES OF THE PRACTICAL NURSE

The attitude of all nurses toward household tasks is one of the stumbling blocks in providing continuous home nursing care and is a disturbing problem to teachers, administrators, registrars, and supervisors.

"It is not that we do not want to do housework," a professional private-duty nurse pointed out to the writer. "Many of us are good housekeepers and like it. But if the patient is sick enough to need a professional nurse, our first attention and most of our time must be free to nurse. We can't be running the house on the side. If the patient needs only occasional professional nursing care, such as a daily dressing or treatment, it is uneconomical to employ a professional nurse full time. A visiting nurse can usually be secured to carry out the treatment at $1.20 to $1.50 a visit, with a practical nurse employed full time to run the home and give the rest of the care the patient needs. I spent three years learning to be a professional nurse and put in an extra year in a maternity hospital. It is not good business from anyone's point of view to ask me to take care of a bedridden arthritic patient who needs no special treatments and a family of three—working husband and two boys in high school. Such a family is happily and economically cared for by a practical nurse."

Many practical nurses feel the same way about homemaking. If they are graduates of approved schools they have had fairly satisfactory grounding in the art of homemaking, but they prefer to nurse. Yet in many of our servantless homes today the practical nurse must help with the house and plan and prepare meals. The practical nurses with whom the author talked were not doing much housework because their patients were taking their full time; the scarcity of professional nurses has increased the use of practical nurses for acutely ill patients. Also, families have more money just now; they can go out for some meals, buy delicatessen food, and hire outside help for cleaning, laundry, and other household tasks.

A survey of the homemaking duties carried by 735 graduate practical nurses made in 1944 by the National Association for Practical Nurse Education indicated that many nurses were almost never asked to do routine cleaning and upkeep such as laundering curtains, mending linen, cleaning silver, nor were very heavy cooking tasks expected, such as baking bread, preserving, canning, or serving guests meals (45). However, a good many other simple, essential tasks had to be done, and the list gives a vivid indication of the need to teach the practical nurse to do "everyday things" well. For example, she may be called upon to order groceries by telephone, arrange flowers, read aloud, tell stories to children, clean the bathroom, fold and sort linen. The nurses themselves asked for more help in entertaining elderly people, guiding children in better health habits, planning family schedules, learning to drive a car, making out bills and receipts, even feeding pets. Several asked for more information in caring for obstetrical cases. One nurse commented to the writer on her own discovery that "In the hospital the patient adjusts to the routines laid down by the nurses. In the home, the nurse adjusts to the family."

One has only to read the list of homemaking duties inherent in giving good care to a home patient (see page 251) to hope that practical nurses will never shun this field or believe it to be foreign to their duties in the home if there is no one else to do them. In the beginning, registered nurses found it possible to help out in many small ways in the household. Failure to help when the care of the patient no longer takes full time is one of the reasons why families do not like and can-not afford to call registered nurses (46). The practical nurses' great—their *very* great—asset to the family is the combination of nursing and homemaking skills. It should be fostered, developed, and made their unique and respected contribution to the care of the sick. This writer would go so far as to say that the candidate for practical nursing who refuses to learn or to like homemaking is not fitted for the field.

If the practical nurse refuses to care for the home in time of illness, her place will be taken by the visiting housekeeper. Indeed, many peo-ple believe that practical nursing should in reality be "subprofessional" nursing, based on a two-year course open only to high school gradu-ates, with the visiting housekeepers trained in home nursing to fill the place of the present practical nurse. To the writer, this division seems merely to complicate the situation unnecessarily, for the practical nurse would then be an inferior professional nurse and the visiting housekeeper a poorly trained practical nurse unable to meet many of the nursing demands in homes, and Mr. and Mrs. Public would have to choose between three levels of nurses instead of two.

The nursing duties usually required of the practical nurse caring for sickness in the home are listed on page 248.

TYPICAL PATIENTS NEEDING CARE

Inasmuch as many people are unfamiliar with the difficulties at-tending sickness in the home, a few cases are cited of the work which practical nurses do in typical homes (47).

An elderly woman and her daughter, both ill with grippe, lived in a small apartment in a hotel. The physician ordered both patients to remain in bed, to drink plenty of fluids, and to have a light, nourishing diet. The practical nurse cooked the three meals and waited on the patients. A hotel maid helped to clean the rooms.

The patient was a young mother of two children, whose fractured right leg was in a plaster cast. The family was in average circumstances, with-out a servant. The nurse took entire care of the six-month-old baby and made up his milk formula every morning. The mother was unable to help with the housework; she could only hold the baby's bottle, and sometimes amuse the three-year-old child. The nurse cooked all the meals for the family, kept the five-room apartment neat, and cared for the mother.

An elderly lady, living by herself, found that her activities and amusements were being gradually curtailed by advancing years and hardening arteries. As neither condition is preventable or curable, there was no need for a nurse trained in special forms of treatment. What was essential was that she should be cared for by someone who understood the principles of nutrition and the value of a judicious mixture of rest, amusement, and exercise, and who would apply these principles to the personal problem of her patient. Not only did the nurse perform such technical services as bathing, supervising diet, and relieving various aches and pains with technical skill and wisdom, but she also entertained and amused her patient, and gave her courage to meet the situation bravely and at least with equanimity. No one could have done it better, few as well.

An elderly man, dying of cancer, was too heavy for his wife to lift. With the help of a stalwart practical nurse, he received as dainty and conscientious care as he would have had in a hospital. The doctor was especially pleased with this case, because the nurse had prevented an incipient bedsore. There were no skilled treatments for a registered nurse to carry out.

An elderly man, helpless and bedridden with arthritis, lived with his frail wife in a three-room apartment. The practical nurse spent eight hours daily giving care to the patient, keeping the apartment neat and clean, and preparing meals. The case lasted eight weeks, during which the nurse carried out the following treatments under the doctor's orders: daily bed bath, massage of back, daily dressing of bedsore, enema p.r.n., steam inhalation twice, catheterization once, hypodermic once.

The patient was a young mother returned from hospital following hysterectomy; she was also a diabetic. Her husband was in the Army. She lived with her two little children in a small house at the edge of town. The practical nurse stayed three weeks until the mother was up and about again. She gave insulin, cared for the children, and managed the home. One child was in bed three days with tonsillitis and was given throat irrigations by the nurse.

The patient, a young business woman returned from hospital following complete mastectomy, lived in a one-room apartment. She was ordered to stay in bed one more week. The practical nurse came in from eight to twelve every morning; she gave bath, prepared meals, left supper in the ice box, kept the place clean, and ran errands. The most notable care given in this case, however, was encouragement. The patient was helped to increasing activity, put in touch with an occupational therapist, and given diversions that would use her arms. The nurse also got in touch with friends and arranged a routine for their visits, so every afternoon was pleasantly occupied. The patient recovered her spirits completely and returned to her job in three weeks.

Not all needs are primarily for nursing care in the bedside sense. The provision of hot, nourishing meals for a distracted, grief-stricken family, the tactful supervision and companionship offered an expectant mother threatened with a miscarriage, the helpful, unobtrusive reorganizing of a disrupted home schedule may not be strictly classified as nursing, but these are assuredly comforting, needed, and curative services which must be given intelligently to be effective. "I did not carry out a single nursing procedure on my last case, but the family said I was the best nurse they had ever had," was the surprised comment of a practical nurse who had tided a family over the crisis of a mental breakdown of the breadwinner.

A grateful patient writing of the care of a practical nurse said: "She seemed to me to have not only the necessary qualities for nursing—capability, a cheerful patience and initiative with good sense behind it—but also that kind of eagerness that enlarges service into something more. . . . She gave so largely of herself . . ." (48).

"Wouldn't you like to have one of our graduates in your own home?" was an unexpected question put to the writer in one city. The answer was yes—emphatically.

RELATIONSHIPS

Practical nurses who are graduates of approved schools have had considerable instruction on matters of ethical relationships to doctors, other nurses, relatives and friends of the families in the homes where they serve. If a doctor requests a treatment about which the practical nurse has not been taught, she is urged to be quite frank with him and explain the situation. The right kind of doctor will respect the nurse who tells him this. She is also urged to secure his special orders in writing and never to take his oral orders indirectly from the family or the patient (49). She is given as much instruction as possible in first steps to take in emergencies, the importance of keeping the doctor informed of any change, and in recording in detail her care and observation of the patient.

Toward the registered nurse—her supervisor, wherever she may be —the attitude of the practical nurse, as observed by the writer, is always friendly. She looks to her for advice and guidance, recognizing her wider experience and knowledge. Both nurses should realize that their services have a common aim—the welfare of the patient—and that a happy, smoothly functioning partnership is vital to the composure of the patient and the contentment of the family.

INCREASING AND SAFEGUARDING HOME SERVICE

The undeveloped opportunities for practical nursing service in homes, the neglected cases, and the misunderstanding among doctors and families make it evident that the future growth of practical nursing will depend on adequacy and suitability of preparation, control under state law, supervision by professional nurses, and a concerted effort to interpret to doctors and the general public what is good practical nursing (as distinguished from unregulated service) and its relation to professional nursing.

For the protection of the public a few schools for practical nurses conduct their own registries and maintain professional contact with the home employer.*

Such supervision from visiting nurse associations or registries is the safeguard to practical home care that convinces private physicians that their cases may safely be transferred to practical nurses. Also, patients may be dismissed early from the hospital with the assurance that professional nursing will be continued in the degree needed. On the subject of supervision, Miss Goldmark commented in 1923: "Here we touch on the crux of subsidiary nursing—the irresponsibility of the sickroom attendant" (50).

We demand to know if a piece of jewelry is sterling silver, or the number of karats of gold in it, but we ask no questions about the quality of bedside care. . . . Required supervision preserves and maintains a standard of excellence (51).

REFERENCES

1 Mary S. Gardner, *Public health nursing,* 3d ed. rev., New York, Macmillan, 1936, pp. 3–5.
2 Adelaide M. Nutting, *History of nursing,* New York, Putnam, 1907,

* Protection of the public is discussed at greater length in Chapters XV, XVI, and XVII.

vol. I, p. 102; Clara B. Rue, *The public health nurse in the community,* Philadelphia, Saunders, 1944, chapter I.

3 Quoted by Mrs. John H. Lowman, "Possible amalgamation of visiting, hourly and household nursing," *American Journal of Nursing* 15:975–984, August 1915, at p. 982.

4 "What do practical nurses do?" *American Journal of Nursing* 40:889, August 1940.

5 Margaret C. Klem, "Who purchase private duty nursing services?" *American Journal of Nursing* 39:1069–1077, October 1939, at pp. 1071, 1077. See also Michael M. Davis, "Nursing service measured by social needs," *American Journal of Nursing* 39:35–40, January 1939, at p. 37.

6 American Nurses' Association, Nursing Information Bureau, cooperating with the National League of Nursing Education and the National Organization for Public Health Nursing, *Facts about nursing, 1943,* p. 7. Compare these figures with May Ayres Burgess, *Nurses, patients and pocketbooks;* report of a study of the economics of nursing by the Committee on the Grading of Nursing Schools, New York, the Committee, 1928, p. 249. See also May Ayres Burgess, "Why not improved training for fewer nurses?" *Modern Hospital* 32:58–61, January 1929.

7 A professional nurse commented on this situation: "Our attitude in the matter [leaving home care to practical nurses] . . . is undoubtedly giving work that should be ours into the hands of the trained attendant and leaving a good many of us idle." Also, the attitude of letting families hire an unqualified nurse, because they can't pay registered nursing fees, is taking work away from registered nurses. Catherine De Nully Fraser, "Where are we drifting?" *Canadian Nurse* 27:422, August 1931.

8 United States Women's Bureau, *The outlook for women in occupations in the medical services; practical nurses and hospital attendants,* Washington, Government Printing Office, 1945 (Bulletin 203, No. 5), p. 13.

9 Jennie C. Goddard, *Medical and nursing services for maternal cases of the National Health Survey,* Washington, Government Printing Office, 1941 (Public Health Bulletin No. 264), pp. 5, 37.

10 Selwyn D. Collins, "Cases and days of illness among males and females, with special reference to confinement to bed; based on 9,000 families visited periodically for 12 months, 1928–31," *Public Health Reports* 55:47–94, January 12, 1940 (Reprint No. 2129).

11 Selwyn D. Collins, "Frequency and volume of nursing service in re-

lation to all illnesses among 9,000 families; based on nation-wide periodic canvasses, 1928–1931," *Milbank Memorial Fund Quarterly* 21:5–36, January 1943, at pp. 5, 15, 19. See also "Nursing needs studied in Detroit," *American Journal of Nursing* 34:773–775, August 1934.

12 Selwyn D. Collins, "Duration of illness from specific diseases among 9,000 families, based on nation-wide periodic canvasses, 1928–31," *Public Health Reports* 55:861–893, May 17, 1940 (Reprint No. 2161), at p. 889. See also editorial comment, *American Journal of Nursing* 19:415, June 1919: "Only 10 per cent of the cases of illness at home need skilled nursing."

13 Collins (note 11), p. 10.

14 Collins (note 11), pp. 11, 15, 19.

15 Selwyn D. Collins, "Variations in nursing service with family income and size of city; based on records for 9,000 families in eighteen states visited periodically for twelve months, 1928–1931," *Milbank Memorial Fund Quarterly* 21:188–213, April 1943, at pp. 188, 196, 198, table 4, p. 203.

16 For comments on this report, see "Recommendations of the Committee on the Costs of Medical Care," *American Journal of Nursing* 32:1290, December 1932; Alden B. Mills, "The need for subsidiary workers in nursing service," *American Journal of Nursing* 34:591, June 1934; Margaret K. Stack, "The non-nursed sick and the idle private duty nurse," *American Journal of Nursing* 34:34, January 1934.

17 Alden B. Mills, "Need for subsidiary workers in nursing service," *40th Annual Report of the National League of Nursing Education,* New York, 1934, p. 158.

18 Elizabeth C. Burgess, "The subsidiary worker," *40th Annual Report of the National League of Nursing Education,* New York, 1934 (reprint, pp. 1–2).

19 Pennsylvania State Nurses' Association, *Study of the subsidiary worker in nursing service in Pennsylvania, 1939–1940,* pp. 50, 46.

20 Mary C. Jarrett, *A brief study of counseling and placement of practical nurses in New York state,* New York, Committee for Recruitment and Education of Practical Nurses of New York, 1945, p. 5.

21 "Survey of nursing care for the non-hospitalized sick; nursing service in Ontario," *Canadian Nurse* 36:416–418, July 1940.

22 Editorial, *American Journal of Nursing* 5:703, June 1905.

23 Letter to the editor signed T.C.F., *American Journal of Nursing* 17:45, February 1917.

24 American Hospital Association, *Report of the Committee to Study the Nursing Problem,* Philadelphia, the Association, 1916, pp. 4, 13–14.

25 Josephine Goldmark, *Nursing and nursing education in the United States;* report of the Committee for the Study of Nursing Education, New York, Macmillan, 1923, especially p. 172.

26 May Ayres Burgess, *Nurses, patients and pocketbooks;* report of a study of the economics of nursing by the Committee on the Grading of Nursing Schools, New York, the Committee, 1928.

27 Ella Hasenjaeger, "The subsidiary worker," *American Journal of Nursing* 38:772–776, July 1938.

28 Harlan H. Horner, "A diagram and some prescriptions; summary of the report," *American Journal of Nursing* 34:666–668, July 1934.

29 See especially Mills (note 16).

30 American Nurses' Association, Joint Committee with the National League of Nursing Education and the National Organization for Public Health Nursing, *Subsidiary workers in the care of the sick,* New York, 1940; revised June 1941.

31 "Calls for nonprofessional workers increase," *American Journal of Nursing* 44:478, May 1944. This was borne out by reports from fourteen registrars visited by the writer during 1944–1945.

   In 1917 an examination of representative registries showed an "untold number" of practical nurses, far exceeding the number of graduate nurses. "The demand is so great we are obliged to register them." Frances Stone, "Is there need for another class of sick attendants besides nurses?" *American Journal of Nursing* 17:991–993, June 1917.

32 American Nurses' Association, Nursing Information Bureau, cooperating with the National League of Nursing Education and the National Organization for Public Health Nursing, *Facts about nursing, 1945,* p. 70.

33 Letter to the editor from "A Waltham graduate," *American Journal of Nursing* 5:527, May 1905. See also Alfred Worcester, *A new way of training nurses,* Boston, Cupples and Hurd, 1888; Isabel M. Stewart, *The education of nurses; historical foundations and modern trends,* New York, Macmillan, 1943, pp. 125–128.

34 Detroit, Toronto, New Haven, and Buffalo, to name a few. There were W.P.A. housekeeping projects in nearly all cities of over 50,000 during 1933–1938. See United States Federal Works Agency, *Report on the progress of the W.P.A. programs,* June 1942, Washington, 1943, p. 18.

35 Marie de Montalvo, "When age and illness meet; New York's home care of dependents," *Trained Nurse and Hospital Review*

102:315–321, April 1939, at p. 319. See also Mary C. Jarrett, "Housekeeping service for home care of chronic patients," W.P.A. Project 165–97–7002, New York, December 1938. Housekeeping aides gave assistance to as many as 3,200 cases in New York city on one day, March 12, 1939. In 677 situations the homemaker was incapacitated. There were 240 calls for help at time of delivery, 124 after confinement, 71 during the antepartum period. Montalvo, p. 321. See also Phyllis Garberson, "Mothers of many," This Week, New York Herald Tribune, January 25, 1945, pp. 26–28. These were homemakers under the Children's Aid Society. In 1945 wages were $20 to $25 a week for an eight-hour day.

36 For discussion, see Hilda M. Torrop, "A plea for the practical nurse," Modern Hospital 62:79–80, March 1944.

37 Ira V. Hiscock, Community health organization, 2d ed. New York, Commonwealth Fund, 1932, pp. 252, 276.

38 "The comprehensive health service should include means of giving household help to housewives, where this appears to be necessary to make possible their most effective medical treatment. This would be organized as part of the welfare service of hospitals and given on the recommendation of the doctor who sends her to the hospital." Sir William Beveridge, Social insurance and allied services, New York, Macmillan, 1942, pp. 132–133.

39 Richards M. Bradley, "Household nursing in relation to similar work," American Journal of Nursing 15:968–975, August 1915. Speaking at the eighteenth annual convention of the American Nurses' Association in 1915, Mr. Bradley said: "Open your minds and hearts to the practical nurse and to her problem which is also your problem"; ibid., p. 975. See also letter to the editor, "The attendant, her place and work," American Journal of Nursing 20:154–156, November 1919.

40 In Nursing services and insurance for medical care in Brattleboro, Vermont; a study of the activities of the Thomas Thompson Trust, by Allon Peebles and Valeria D. McDermott, Chicago, University of Chicago Press, 1932 (Committee on the Costs of Medical Care, No. 17), pp. 46–65. See also Bradley (note 39), p. 973; also Richards M. Bradley, "Attendant nurse solves puzzle of household nursing care," Nation's Health 7:735, November 15, 1925; Richards M. Bradley, "Skilled nursing for all," Survey 70:9, January 1934.

41 "Such training must be much more complete . . . and must be conducted according to the recommendations of the American Nurses' Association as to selection, training, supervision, and licensure of

subsidiary workers for the care of the sick. The certificate which is given . . . must under no circumstances be used as a credential to secure paid employment as a nurse, practical nurse, hospital attendant or other subsidiary worker. If the use of the certificate is violated, the Red Cross reserves the right to reclaim it." *Red Cross Home Nursing, Instructors' Syllabus,* Washington, American Red Cross, 1945, p. 2. Some relaxation of this rule was permitted in hiring help for hospitals during the war emergency.

42 Quotation from Annie W. Goodrich made by Edith M. Ambrose, "How and where should attendants be trained?" *American Journal of Nursing* 17:993–1002, October 1917, at p. 1002.

43 "The subsidiary worker in the home," *Public Health Nursing* 32:142–143, March 1940.

44 Miriam A. Ames, "Hourly nursing; a civic enterprise," *American Journal of Nursing* 32:113, February 1932; 32:220–221, March 1932.

45 "Report of job analyses study of the homemaking responsibilities of the graduate practical nurse," New York, National Association for Practical Nurse Education, 1944, p. 2 of section attesting frequency of duties.

46 Among many comments regarding home tasks and registered nursing service, a letter to the editor from "An old nurse" will be found interesting. *American Journal of Nursing* 6:258, February 1906.

47 Actual cases, either visited with a practical nurse by the writer or quoted from case histories on file in New York, Boston, and Detroit.

48 "A worthy competitor," *American Journal of Nursing* 39:437, April 1939.

49 Florence Dakin and E. M. Thompson, *Simplified nursing,* 4th ed., Philadelphia, Lippincott, 1941, p. 6.

50 Goldmark (note 25), p. 175.

51 Lowman (note 3), pp. 978–979.

CHAPTER FIVE

General Hospitals

THE USE of the practical nurse—trained attendant, nurses' aide, by whatever title she is called—has grown up with the hospital, but there can be no doubt that wartime shortages in all hospital personnel have been a determining factor in the increased employment of the practical nurse and have given her an unprecedented chance to demonstrate her usefulness to the hospital.

The medical profession has been consistent in favoring auxiliary nurses. To quote Dr. Frederick T. Hill, "There are many who feel convinced that the attendant nurse has come to stay. . . . She is going largely to replace the nurse in the actual routine care of the patient. . . . If this is so, it behooves the hospitals as well as the nursing organizations to recognize the fact and take steps to control it." Dr. Hill added that adequate preparation, certification, and licensure should be insisted upon (1).

"Perhaps," wrote Dr. Basil C. MacLean, Director of Strong Memorial Hospital, Rochester, N. Y., in 1936, "we should have a nursing profession and a nursing craft. The latter, however, implies recognition, certification and licensure of both" (2).

Nursing is reaching a professional level, concludes the editor of *Hospitals,* "But the patient is still in bed. His proper care involves many procedures which do not demand the skill of a graduate nurse. . . . in one institution . . . as much as 49 per cent of the nursing service can be delegated to properly trained subsidiary workers" (3).

The war has wrought a decided change in the attitude of professional nurses in hospitals toward the employment of practical nurses. Margaret Tracy, Director of the School of Nursing, University of California, speaking from her experience on the West Coast, states: "We need not fear the subsidiary worker. There is a definite place for her services, both in the hospital and in the home. . . . The intelligent use of a subsidiary group in hospitals may help prevent the exploitation of the professional student group and the glutting of the field with poorly prepared practitioners of nursing" (4).

More than a quarter of the forty general hospitals visited by the writer in 1944–1945 had employed practical nurses only since 1940, although it was usual to find that the hospitals which had been used as practice fields for practical students had been employing the graduates for many years.

It may fairly be said that hospital administrators are heartily in favor of such service, provided they can get qualified workers. In employing a nonprofessional staff, they see the importance, in varying degrees, of protecting the safety and welfare of patients, safeguarding the hospital and its medical staff against complaints—or worse, lawsuits—and safeguarding the education of student nurses. Their most frequently repeated plea was for *qualified* practical nurses. At this time when the hospitals' choice is between totally unfit, unskilled workers and no workers, and they engage ward helpers with the almost certain prospect of a 90 per cent turnover, administrators are skeptical of finding satisfactory service. Indeed, most of those with whom the writer talked prefaced all remarks with, "After the war, when . . ."

These opinions of nurses, doctors, and hospital administrators are indicative of an increasing realization of the differences between a highly trained, well educated, professionally prepared nurse and an assistant taught to do a few rather simple nursing duties—but taught to do them in a manner acceptable to a board of licensure. The idea is far from new (5), but its realization and acceptance have been greatly accelerated by the war emergencies.

THE SITUATION TODAY

In 1944, there were 15,060,403 admissions to the 4,833 general hospitals registered by the American Medical Association, and 61.6 per cent of the beds in these hospitals were occupied. Patients stayed an average of 9.6 days in the nongovernmental general hospitals. Of the total of 2,794,800 births in the United States, 1,856,650 took place in the registered general hospitals (6).

The 4,126 nonfederal general hospitals employed a total of 112,276 registered nurses, including those on private duty, and 27,378 practical nurses and attendants. We do not know how many of the latter were licensed practical nurses, or how many had been previously trained for their jobs (7).

According to reports received in 1944 by the writer from the Minnesota State Department of Health, 409 institutions of all types, with

32,062 beds, employed 2,713 nonregistered nurses of all types (attendants, nurses' aides, and practical nurses), while 35 general hospitals with a total bed capacity of 8,247 depended upon 463 registered nurses, 4,242 professional students, and 447 nonregistered nurses (practical nurses not differentiated).

During the week of January 8, 1945, 13 hospitals in an eastern city were asked whether they employed practical nurses. Two with professional schools of nursing had no practical nurses although one director wanted to interview "some good ones" for employment, and one hospital with a school was definitely not in the market. The remaining ten hospitals reported employing 41 practical nurses. The writer found, however, that this total included paid nurses' aides, licensed practical nurses, and graduate nonregistered nurses (two-year course) who had licenses and were classed as "practicals" although they were doing all but a few highly specialized nursing procedures. Nineteen others of this type had not been counted as practicals although they were licensed. "They are better than practicals," the director said. Two hospitals with professional schools of nursing had had a few practical nurses a long time but "did not really want them." All the eight hospitals without professional schools of nursing were using practical nurses. With the exception of one hospital which was not sure, they could and would use more if they could get them. Roughly, then, some 60 nonregistered nurses were serving in ten hospitals.

When hospital administrators throughout the country were asked if they intended to retain practical nurses after the war, all replied they might but in the same breath added the qualification, "unless there are plenty of registered nurses available who need jobs; then it is only fair to give the work to them."

The writer's visits were all to registered hospitals. It is quite possible that a much larger number of practical nurses would be found in the hospitals not registered by the American Medical Association, most of which are not subject to regulations by either city of state authorities.

In an effort to see practical nurses at work, the writer made visits during 1944 and 1945 to some half hundred general and special hospitals of all types employing licensed and unlicensed practical nurses and trained attendants. The accompanying table shows the number of full time general-duty registered nurses and full time practical nurses (exclusive of students) in ten general hospitals of varying size scattered over seven states. Ratios of practical nurses to patients or to registered nurses should not be computed from this table for a number of reasons, the chief of which are:

The term practical nurse covers a wide range of skill, ability, and duties. A well trained licensed practical nurse may be worth two or three of the untrained kind. As an illustration of the general lack of understanding of the meaning of the term: The director of one hospital asked the visitor if she was counting as practical nurses the Girl Scouts who were helping with ward trays and flowers and running errands

There is a wide difference in the responsibilities permitted the practical nurse staff

It is impossible to get any accurate count of the total full time nursing service given by registered nurses. In most hospitals in 1945, registered nurses constituted a very small part of the paid hospital staff, which included part time, full time, part paid, full paid, and volunteer registered nurses from outside the hospital. Mrs. Black, R.N., aged 67, gave back rubs twice a week and was on half pay; young Mrs. White, R.N., was a full time instrument nurse in the operating room as a volunteer. Ledgers are usually kept on the paid time basis, and administrators will say, "We have the equivalent of ten full time registered nurses from outside the hospital, not including the volunteer time"

The presence of student nurses and Red Cross Volunteer Nurses' Aides also confuses ratios.

REGISTERED AND PRACTICAL NURSES IN TEN GENERAL HOSPITALS

Hospital	Bed capacity	Registered nurses	Practical nurses
A	37	10	6
B	60	26	19
C	105	26	19
D	125	28	14
E	250	41	2
F	400	102	18
G	595	300	4
H*	610	280	2
I*	1500	191	20
J*	2000	500	60

* Hospitals H, I, and J are state and city institutions with attendant service in addition to practical nurses.

There seem to be no standard ratios of practical nurses to other hospital personnel, and authorities are reluctant to quote desirable ratios; "we really do not know," they say (8). In search of this information the writer referred to the *Manual of the Essentials of Good Hospital Nursing Service* (9). Three types of nonprofessional workers are listed—orderlies or ward helpers, ward clerks, and volunteer nurses' aides—but practical nurses are not mentioned. Professional personnel includes only registered nurses; student professional nurses are in a classification by themselves.

DUTIES OF PRACTICAL NURSES

The first letter from an attendant nurse ever published by the *American Journal of Nursing* states:

Here are a few most important and extremely safe rules for an attendant to follow: first, she should always obey orders strictly; second, never assume responsibility not expected of her; third, she should be extremely careful in the use of medicines; fourth, take orders from the charge nurse only; fifth, use her brains in planning her work, be able to answer questions intelligently, yet not become self-important; lastly, she should make good. . . . The attendant fills a small but very necessary place in the busy life of a large hospital. . . . Why not develop good attendants, instead of letting bad ones develop themselves? (10).

Twenty-five years later we are beginning to take this writer's last question seriously, for one of the first steps the war forced upon hospitals was the employment of nonprofessional personnel, and the pressing question arose, how can we develop "good" attendants.

Many hospitals started, even before Pearl Harbor, to differentiate professional and nonprofessional jobs. Remarkable discoveries at once were made (11). It was found that registered nurses were still filling inkwells, washing chart desks, scouring bedpans, taking inventories, and cleaning instruments. An era of reorganization of routines, simplification of techniques, conservation of supplies, delegation of duties, and revision of time schedules for nurses, doctors, and patients alike set in. A return to many of these outworn practices will never be justified if we deal honestly with the public's dollar.

Many "household" tasks should not be assigned to licensed practical nurses any more than to registered nurses. They belong clearly to the field of clerical or maid service. The female ward helpers and orderlies may not be needed if there are adequate maid and janitor services, with licensed men and women practical nurses to give all elementary nursing care to patients (12).

What duties may a graduate practical nurse perform safely in a general hospital? Hospital administrators do not know, they only guess from the most recent experience in their own wards. "We believe that" may, in one institution, be followed by a description of duties in nearly all respects those of the registered nurse; in another, of those typical of the Red Cross Volunteer Nurses' Aide. Most frequently, however, the reply given to the writer's question, "What duties do you consider it safe for a practical nurse to perform?" was, "We don't know. Right now we are letting them do. . . ." There is every evidence that the job analysis now being made under the auspices of the U.S. Office of Education will be a welcome tool to these hospital staffs (13).

No treatments are included in the list of duties approved for subsidiary workers by the American Nurses' Association in 1942 (14); even the taking of temperature is omitted. However, the overcrowded and understaffed conditions of civilian wards have necessitated the addition of about fifty duties to those which a nonprofessional worker is permitted to perform, and the list will probably never again shrink to its original size.

The writer visited ten hospitals that employed graduate practical nurses but had no schools of practical nursing or students in affiliation. In general, the treatments which practical nurses were forbidden to perform were:

Intravenous or intramuscular injections
Deep dressings, with drainage or wide surface
Colostomy, colonic, and bladder irrigations
Catheterization
Care of premature babies
Care of maternity patients up to the fifth day
Care of seriously ill patients, all conditions
Care of patients receiving oxygen
Tests for diagnosis or treatment
All treatments involving siphonage, posterial drainage, or suction
All medications other than those simple doses of "household" remedies
      assigned by the head nurse
All elaborate sterile procedures

Some hospital lists forbid internal medications of all kinds, sterile procedures, care of maternity patients and babies until the fifth day, care of premature babies.

It goes without saying that hospitals permitting only a limited list of duties never assign practical nurses to the operating or delivery rooms. Even though they may draw their staffs from local schools of practical nursing, hospitals do not always allow these graduates to carry out the treatments they have been taught. This usually annoys the practical nurses, but the hospital lists stand.

The procedures usually allowed were those taught in the schools of practical nursing (see lists on pages 248–250).

Sometimes a director of nurses asked the writer for advice in deciding what the practical nurses should be allowed to do. When referred to various sources of help, such as the national agencies, the state board of nurse examiners in states with licensing laws, or the approved practical nursing schools, the director would reply, "But our situation is different. Their recommendations do not apply here."

As a rule, the author found the supervisors of practical nurses more fearful of permitting too much than of not getting enough service from this staff. In several hospitals, however, concern for policies, supervision, duties, and performance was very casual. Decidedly, the situation needs to be controlled.

There was particularly wide variation in the duties allowed practical nurses in a large city with several schools of professional nursing, with the tendency toward placing more and more responsibility on this group as registered nurses went into military service. Reactions to the situation also showed a surprising range—from the administrators who were deeply concerned and wondered what constructive steps could be taken to get the situation in hand, to those who commented resignedly, "What else can we do under the circumstances?"

Large general hospitals with acute services are clearest as to the duties to be assigned to graduate practical nurses. The following list was adopted in 1942 by a general hospital in Boston where practical nurses are licensed and under close supervision. They may take full charge of patients assigned to them by the professional head nurse and assist with the care of those more acutely ill.

Make beds
Admit, discharge, and transfer patients

Distribute and collect trays
Fill ice collars, ice caps, hot water bottles
Distribute bed pans to less acutely ill patients
Give morning and afternoon care: hair, nails, teeth (including artificial
    dentures), routine back care
Give baths
Shave patients
T.P.R.'s as assigned by the head nurse
Feed patients
Help patients to the bathroom
Help patients into chairs
Weigh patients
Give simple enemata

Under the supervision of the head nurse or her assistant, the practical nurse may give flaxseed poultices, foot and hand soaks (not to open areas), and hot wet packs.

In the nursery, the following duties are allowed:

Make cribs and beds
Clean and empty cribs
Wash nursing bottles and nipples
Boil equipment (but the equipment is to be removed from the sterilizer
    by the professional nurse)
Wash baby cups
Change thermometer glasses
Clean closet and scrub baby work tables
Sort formulas and have them ready for each feeding
Keep linen supply in nursery
Change babies
Dress discharged babies
Feed P.C. formulas
Give bottle-fed babies 10 P.M. feeding
Bathe babies at decision of head nurse and nursing office

Licensed attendants may give only the following medicines: aspirin, empirin, sodium bicarbonate, cascara, milk of magnesia, mineral oil.

Some of the duties that practical nurses were performing in the general hospitals visited were quite specialized. One was assisting with the Kenny packs (15). Others were in charge of the preparation of babies' formulas, assisting in the supply room (in charge, in one instance), giving general assistance in delivery rooms, especially before patients were brought in.

It has been pointed out that a practical nurse with a detailed introduction to this latter task may take care of small duties in relation to the patient when a registered nurse assigns them, and may answer telephone calls, keep in touch with fathers, care for all supplies and linen, clean up rooms, help move equipment or the patient, and fetch any needed articles outside "clean" areas (16).

Policies with relation to service in the newborn nurseries also varied greatly. It was usual, however, to find that if a practical nurse was employed in the care of the newborn, she cared for normal babies only, was given special instruction for the job, and was not left in charge of the nursery. The United States Children's Bureau states that in general nonprofessional workers employed in newborn nurseries should be assigned to nonprofessional duties. If they are

. . . assigned to the care of newborn infants they should have had instruction and supervised experience in the nursing care of children, during which time they should have demonstrated ability, interest, and a sense of responsibility. Their duties should be clearly defined; they should be adequately supervised, and the work assigned to them should be commensurate with their training.

In planning for the use of part time workers it should be remembered that the fewer the workers that enter a nursery the less is the danger of introducing infection.

Ratio of nurses to infants and hours of nursing care.—At least three hours of nursing care per twenty-four hours should be provided for full-term infants and six hours for premature infants. This will require that at all times, day and night, nurses (or nurses and auxiliary workers) be provided in the ratio of at least one for each eight full-term infants and at least one for each four premature infants (17).

The Michigan State Department of Health issues recommendations for nursing service in hospital nurseries. Non-nursing functions were described as:

1. General cleaning of the nursery including damp dusting of furniture and equipment, washing diaper pails, scales, baseboards, etc.
2. Washing and making up empty bassinets after the discharge of an infant
3. Removing soiled diapers and linen from the nursery to the laundry
4. Washing soiled feeding equipment and removing it to the milk room

5. Distributing and collecting wash water for mothers' hand-washing before feedings
6. Assisting with the weighing procedure by draping the scale, balancing the weights and recording the infant's weight as directed by the nurse or stripping the bassinet and laying the bottom sheet while the nurse weighs the infant
7. Wrapping and autoclaving freshly laundered linen before it is returned to the unit
8. Recording the temperature of the nursery at designated times
9. Making up nursery supplies as newspaper bags, paper squares, cotton balls, etc.
10. Refilling stock bottles and sterile supply cans to be autoclaved (18)

Nonprofessional service permitted trained practical nurses would include "giving basic care to healthy newborn infants, including weighing, feeding, cord care, diaper changing and carrying to mother's room for breast feeding. They should not give care to premature infants or to infants in isolation for infection or suspected infection" (19).

Medical policies in the conduct of cases have some effect also on the duties of practical nurses. For example, in hospitals where normal maternity patients are allowed out of bed five days after the baby's birth and are giving themselves their own baths in bed on the third day after delivery, practical nurses are given considerable responsibility for all the care after the third day.

Certain jobs fall naturally to men practical nurses, besides the care of male patients. Heavy lifting, moving of heavy equipment, assistance with stretchers and stretcher cases, the care of restless or uncontrollable patients, help with plaster casts, splinting, oxygen tents and cylinders, gas apparatus, food trays and carts when other help is short, and, with special training, assistance in the operating and treatment rooms (cystoscopy, x-ray, etc.).

Usually, convalescent cases without complications are assigned for all care to practical nurses.

Practical nurses can be used safely where they can follow standardized routines established by the hospital and understood by doctors, nurses, volunteers, and students. They can be used where no new judgment will be required of them and they are not expected to adapt their routines to a patient's changing condition, but to report that condition at once for further orders. This policy, typical of nearly all the hospitals that have used practical nurses for more than two years, appears to the writer a safe one for the assignment of duties.

Several supervisors amplified this ruling by saying that they impressed upon the practical staff the necessity for following out all details of the routines, for checking the steps with the printed directions frequently, for not trusting their memories but referring to written orders and asking questions of the supervisor, and never being afraid to say "Show me again" or "I don't know how."

It is extremely difficult to make rigid classification of duties to be assigned to a practical nurse in a hospital because circumstances do alter cases. For example: A patient dying of cancer must have a complicated dressing done frequently, day and night; after she has assisted the professional nurse a number of times, may the practical nurse do the dressing alone even though it involves an irrigation which she would not be permitted to carry out on a patient fresh from the operating room? A practical nurse may certainly bathe a convalescent surgical patient recovering from burned hands, although she would not be allowed to render this service to a patient with pneumonia in an oxygen tent.

The necessity for close supervision in order to assign duties safely was evident in all the hospitals visited. Several institutions had ruled that before the head nurse assigns the practical nurse to a new service involving greater responsibility, she must receive approval from the nursing director's office. Putting this another way:

The subsidiary worker can be checked off for "washed patient's face and hands, but it is *our* [professional nurses'] responsibility if, during that process, she failed to notice and report that the patient showed signs of approaching coma or toxic symptoms. Anyone can carry a tray to or from a patient, but the presentation of breakfast to the patient scheduled for a blood sugar test is a matter the head nurse must explain. If food is rejected, the head nurse is expected to know it, but only the intelligent observer who understands the necessity of making that report tells her about it. It all sounds so simple that the full import of all which has been involved in the performance of these simple-sounding tasks will only be realized when the staff nurse departs and someone less skilled takes her place; only when that happens will administrators and medical staffs realize the dependence they have put on the nurses' trained ability to make and report observations which the doctor made in former years. Before that happens, we should go on record as saying that subsidiary workers of this type are not capable of giving safe nursing care (20).

In visiting some forty special and general hospitals employing practical nurses, the writer found them working in every department and in every service, and carrying out all but a very few duties usually restricted to registered nurses. Rarely, however, were they serving in all departments of a hospital—in the majority only at three or four points. For example, in a hospital in New York State practical nurses were employed in the medical, surgical, maternity, and pediatric services and in the operating, delivery, and supply rooms. In another, in Massachusetts, very limited duties were allowed in the medical and surgical floors only. In all the hospitals visited, they were under the supervision of registered nurses. The decision as to which duties to assign and when rested with the professional group.

It goes almost without saying that the writer did not find graduate practical nurses carrying all treatments or all medications in any hospital conducting a school of nursing of either type.

ADVANTAGES OF USING PRACTICAL NURSES

The advantages of securing the assistance of licensed practical nurses on busy wartime wards were evident during the writer's visits and were continually cited by hospital and nursing administrators, the most important result being the improved nursing care of patients. More procedures are being completed on time, patients are getting prompter service, they feel more free to ask for attention, there are less rush and tension on the wards, head nurses feel less pressed and can do more supervision and teaching, and the doctors admit there is less grumbling among their patients (21). It is noteworthy that, except in one instance, the acceptance of the practical nurse by patients was reported to the writer to be universally favorable. A hospital administrator commented, "We had trouble with one patient, who said she was paying for registered nursing service, so why give her a practical nurse. We explained our shortage and she calmed down. Later, we discovered she was herself a retired registered nurse."

What can happen where a hospital is definitely short of registered nurses and has no subsidiary group on which to depend is described by a recent patient: "Luxury aids" to convalescence are "out," he says, meaning alcohol rubs, hot meals on time, beds promptly made, etc. The nurses have no time to talk or explain things. One "contributes by self-help" (22).

One of the many points at which it was evident that a practical nurse would help to raise the standard of care was in service at night, which has for years been inadequate and hurried. Blanche Pfefferkorn cites a case, and the writer was told of a similar instance. "A critically ill patient, operated on during the day was left entirely alone 7:00–9:30 P.M. . . . . Her gown was soaked with sweat, bed tossed, lips dry, she was moaning . . ." "Either," writes Miss Pfefferkorn of these hectic night wards, "routines are omitted for all, or routines are completed and special treatments and critically ill patients neglected" (23).

It is not unusual for the doctor to find the night nurse so busy that she cannot leave her patients to talk with him or receive his orders. A practical nurse, possibly serving as a "floater," able to carry out such duties as the night nurse directs, would mean unutterable relief to her and greater comfort to patients. Night is a difficult time for patients. They grow homesick, afraid, lonely; vitality is at a low ebb, pain continues, and the hours double in length. The hospital itself is not running on all eight cylinders. Anything that will raise the general morale of night service in the hospitals will be welcome to all. This is not a wartime situation but one of long standing.

A decided factor in decreasing the amount of routine bedside care given by registered nurses nowadays, and indicating the need for the service of practical nurses, is the transfer of certain medical duties to the professional nurse. A survey of 14 hospitals in 1943 indicated that the registered nursing staff was taking on more and more of the duties formerly performed by the doctors (a third of whom in the country as a whole were in military service), such treatments as transfusions, dressings, intravenous injections, and as a consequence having less time for nursing patients. Decreased nursing care was particularly in evidence in the maternity divisions of the hospitals, where a reduction of 24 minutes per patient between 1938 and 1943 was reported. Newborn infants received 18 minutes less care per patient. Private patients suffered more than ward patients in this regard. Also, instead of 62 patients to each supervisor as in 1938, there were, in 1943, 107 patients to each supervisor, obviously making for "unstable" and "unskilled" service. General bedside nursing service in the 14 hospitals studied had decreased 30 per cent (24).

Quantity affects quality, and the addition of qualified practical nurses would frequently have more effect on quality than would more professional nurses, who might still neglect routine care. The amount of professional and nonprofessional nursing service is an index of the quality of nursing given by an institution.

Poor teaching of students accompanies pressure of work. Reasons for procedures are not explained, the best way of carrying out a technique is set aside for the quickest way, and any interpretation of what the patient's symptoms mean or may mean just goes by the board. "If I had some help from a practical nurse on this ward, I could assign my professional student full time to watching this burn case. As it is, she is passing bed pans," said the head nurse of the surgical ward of a 250-bed hospital to the writer.

When visiting general and special hospitals, the writer tried to find out whether any study had been made of the time saved the professional nurses by the introduction of practical nursing assistance. It would be an effective argument to use with those who still believe the practical nurse is for emergency use only if such a study showed, for example, that by the addition of one practical nurse for every six professional nurses the hospital was saved engaging ten additional professional nurses in a year and gave better care to patients. Unfortunately, we do not have any data on the proportionate time needed for the two levels of service, nor do we know how much practical nurses can usually do in an hour or even what they ought to do. No standards of service exist by which to judge—or, indeed, even to plan—such a study, and there is natural reluctance to make such studies so long as ward conditions are abnormal.

The economic aspect of nursing service in hospitals is admittedly a knotty problem, and not only from the point of view of the hospital budget. All nursing service has been cheap for years; hospitals have had "an incredibly good bargain" in nursing care (25). It is a good thing that the public is realizing that nursing service will cost them more, but they expect better service for their money, both in skills and in more suitable adjustments to their needs. Wartime emergencies will soon cease to excuse the shortcomings in nursing in the present-day hospital programs. It has long been clear that hospital administrators should not use the public's money to pay nurses at a dollar an hour to carry water, serve trays, arrange flowers, make beds, clean instruments and equipment, transport patients, and watch over convalescent patients, when reliable workers can be obtained to do these jobs for less (26).

DISADVANTAGES AND DANGERS

In the throes of the war emergency, one director remarked a little hopelessly, "If the truth were known, you would find a lot of hospitals using practicals for registered nurses' duties." Directors of nursing as well as superintendents of hospitals in many cities expressed a real fear that practical nurses would learn to do all that registered nurses do and would be willing to work for less. When the supply of professional nurses gets back to normal, perhaps we may hope that such confusion will be at an end.

The indiscriminate use of practical nurses in registered nursing duties is greatly to be deplored. If one hospital allows practical nurses to give all the treatments and medications professional nurses give, those practical nurses will continue to give them in the next hospital to which they go, or—a more dangerous practice—on the next home private duty case, where there is no supervision.

There would seem to be two possible solutions to this bad situation, pending the enforcement of legal restrictions (and differentiation) of those who nurse for hire. One would be a cooperative agreement among local hospitals to restrict the duties of practical nurses to a list, qualified by limitations, based on the curriculum in practical nursing schools; each administrator would be asked to adhere to this standard list, post it, and inform the medical staff. The second would be the establishment of an approved school of practical nursing in the locality, which would raise the standards of the practical nursing group and do something toward setting up practice fields in the local hospitals.

That practical nurses are being asked to assume hospital responsibilities for which they are not prepared was evident in the replies to a questionnaire regarding their duties sent to practical nurses in active practice (27). They indicated a desire to be taught more advanced hospital procedures, such as how to give (presumably assist with) intramuscular injections, chest aspirations, and catheterization. Replies showed that these duties were being taught them by doctors in clinics, homes, and offices. A few quotations are given.

I have been running blood counts
Would like to learn to take charge of the floor
I have full responsibility of hospital and patients in 8 to 12 hour shifts
I tube feed insulin patients, P.R.N. (in a mental hospital)
I need to know how to give anesthesia
I would like to know how to assist at deliveries as I am asked to do so

Doctors are not always guilty of deliberately exploiting the practical nurse, but they are as confused as professional nurses regarding the duties of this group and probably order treatments without realizing that practical nurses are not prepared to give them. If practical nurses can do only elementary nursing, they ask, then must we have two types of nurses for private patients in the hospital? A doctor with a large practice among elderly patients insists practical nurses must know how to catheterize, give narcotics, and care for patients in casts. He is realistic, not unreasonable.

In large hospitals where the lists of duties of practical nurses are posted and closely watched by the registered staff the doctors seldom ask for advanced types of service from practical nurses, but those in private practice and in small hospitals frequently do. An "educational campaign" to explain to all physicians what they may safely expect the licensed practical nurse to know and do should be undertaken as soon as registered and practical nurses know themselves.

All such statements point directly to the pressing need of the forthcoming job analysis to help decide what is the function of the practical nurse in the hospital (28).

The greatest danger in the employment of this group, however, lies ahead, when, if well qualified practical nurses are abundant, some hospital administrators, with an anxious eye on the budget sheet, will hire more practical nurses than are needed for routine duties, at the same time curtailing the more expensive professional staff to the point where the director of nurses finds she has too few of them for the critical services or for the emergencies that are bound to arise among the acutely ill. This is the moment, as small hospitals will tell you, when the practical nurses are pushed beyond their capacities because the overworked professional nurses either resign or succumb to the temptation of teaching the practical nurses their jobs. Registered nurses who have had such experiences are embittered about the whole practical nursing situation. Unfortunate developments such as these can only be prevented by maintaining at all times and at all points an adequate registered nursing staff. The ratio of registered nurses to patients is doubly important in hospitals accepting student nurses of either type. The interpretation of these situations to the hospital administrator rests with the director of nursing service.

Thousands of hospitals benefited during the war by the presence of volunteer nurses' aides. Some administrators may be reluctant to pay for licensed practical nursing service in peacetime and may seek instead untrained, lower paid "practical nurses." This is a special menace in states without legal control of the subsidiary group.

At the other extreme, there are still a few directors of nursing who feel that the employment and recognition of even the best practical nurses will be a detriment to the standards of professional nursing in hospitals. They believe there will be an unfortunate effect upon the recruitment of college graduates for the professional schools. The only reasonable reply to this argument is that, if professional nursing cannot withstand the impact of subsidiary service, then it is not a profession but a trade whose practitioners need only some high school education and a lot of experience in the practice of their skills.

PRACTICAL NURSES VERSUS WARD MAIDS AND ORDERLIES

The place of a qualified practical nurse trained for service in the wards of our hospitals should not be confused with those of orderlies, ward helpers, or maids, whose duties as a rule cannot be described as "nursing."

Because of the lack of practical men nurses, orderlies carry out many nursing procedures for men patients, sometimes very unskillfully, thereby confusing the picture more. It is vitally important that orderlies and ward helpers be trained for their duties, and such training can be given either on the job or in a central training center. Theirs, however, is not the field of practical nursing in terms of a prepared nursing assistant to the professional nurse (29).

There is confusion, also, in differentiating the duties of practical nurses and ward helpers. The University of Colorado prepared, in 1937, a set of duties for ward helpers which included enemas, preparation of patient for operating room, care of oxygen tents, care of anesthesia patients, as well as the usual aide duties. Aides were paid $140 a month, plus laundry and board. "In this program, there is no danger of turning out practical nurses" (30).

In May 1942, the Colorado State Nursing Council for War Service adopted *A Guide for the Use of the Auxiliary Worker,* meaning nurse aides, attendants, ward helpers, and orderlies; practical nurses are not mentioned, but it will be noted that the duties and salaries are typical of those of practical nurses elsewhere. Workers were to be trained on the job, with brief introductory conferences. The booklet is excellently planned and clearly outlined, but it presents an odd mixture of maid duties, a little nursing and no treatments, not even temperatures to be taken or enemas given, although the auxiliary worker assisting the public health nurse in the home is permitted to do several simple nursing procedures, including taking temperature (31).

Evidently the work of the auxiliary worker in Colorado hospitals is not intended to overlap that of a licensed practical nurse. This may augur well for the future licensed practical nurse or may mean that she will have to find a place for herself between the auxiliary worker and the registered nurse. It would seem that a licensed practical nurse already trained to carry out all the procedures listed in this booklet, and many more, would be of greater service, especially to the public health nurses in homes and clinics, than the very slightly trained auxiliary worker. As of January 1945, Colorado has no state law controlling nonprofessional nursing or any approved school of practical nursing, so this policy of conservatism in the duties permitted aides is undoubtedly wise.

SALARIES AND PERSONNEL POLICIES

Salaries of practical nurses in the general hospitals visited in 1944–1945 ranged from $75 a month with full maintenance to $145 without maintenance. Professional salaries at this time ranged from $110 to $175 a month, the latter without maintenance.

Efficiency reports should be kept for the practical nurses as for any other members of the staff, and they should be included in general staff conferences. Confusion is reduced by making them responsible to one person rather than letting any registered nurse give them orders.

Nearly all the general hospitals surveyed have the same personnel policies for both groups of nurses in regard to hours of duty, sick leave, vacations, and so forth.

THE PROBLEM OF UNIFORMS AND CAPS

Policies about uniforms and caps vary greatly in the general hospitals. A graduate practical nurse may wear "all white," with school pin in evidence, the uniform (colored) of her school, or any washable white or colored dress that suits her fancy and meets with the approval of the director of nurses. Some hospitals stipulate that she cannot wear a cap, some insist on a distinctive emblem, initials, or label to differentiate her from a registered nurse. Most registered nurses would prefer that the practical nurses not wear caps—but "it's a free country, and anyone can wear a white cap."

That the uniform is important was proved by the questions raised about it on every visit, by the report that a battle royal had been fought to get the practical nurses out of caps, out of white, or into the hospital color, and by the general tension noticeable when the question was asked. It would seem a most strategic step for licensed practical nurses to adopt a color, one that is universally becoming and different from other nurses' uniforms (not the public health blue, for instance), a becoming cap of the same color, and an emblem standardized as that of a licensed practical nurse (32). A *uniform* uniform would be the best publicity for the trained licensed practical nurse and would settle once and for all, from Maine to Texas, the question, "Is she a licensed practical nurse?" As things are now, her uniform may look like the maid's, the dietitian's, the nurses' aide's, or the registered nurse's.

There is another point in favor of a recognized uniform: The practical nurse would have some degree of protection. As it is now, she is often forced into embarrassing situations by visiting doctors, and occasionally by professional nurses who are in a hurry to get a job done. The doctor often doesn't stop to look at the small insigne or pin, but he would notice the color of the uniform, and the professional nurse would think twice before imposing upon the practical nurse whose distinctive uniform she had always before her.

All this may seem trivial, but to those concerned it is a red hot issue. The writer, a professional nurse friendly to the practical nurses, would beg for a little more diplomacy and forbearance on both sides and the immediate adoption of an "L.P.N." uniform which will become as familiar to the public as the white of the institutional or private duty "R.N." or the blue of the public health nurse.

THE ATTITUDE OF PRACTICAL NURSES IN GENERAL HOSPITALS

Practical nurses, as can be readily understood, are not always happy in their early adjustment to busy hospital wards, especially if their duties are not clearly defined, time is not taken to introduce them to their work, and an effort is not made to make them feel welcome. In talking with practical nurses on duty in several general hospitals, the writer found some who were supremely happy, literally bubbling over with the satisfaction they got from nursing, others who were quietly content, and a few who felt neglected, repressed, and disliked. "They don't really want us here."

It was not unusual to have a practical nurse ask: "Why don't they let me do more? I have been taught to do thus and so." Young nurses are always ambitious and it seems only natural for them to beg to be allowed to help in the operating or delivery rooms, especially when they see the heavy load of work the professional staff carries there. To take the attitude that they have no business even dreaming of such heights, that they are trying to push the registered nurses out of their jobs, or "don't know their place" seems a little unreasonable and harsh. "I want to know how to do more things," a twenty-year-old Irish girl said to the writer. "I've been here a year doing the same things over and over"—and doing them superlatively well, her supervisor confided later. Perhaps better planning, by which the difficulties in jobs are graded (33), and promotion to more and more responsibility as a reward for good work would help keep these energetic young women content and give them a feeling of security and of being wanted. The real truth of the matter is that practical nursing can be developed into a challenging service in its own right under favoring leadership and professional approval.

Sometimes, too, a practical nurse's comment revealed thoughtlessness on the part of her supervisor. "They used to let me sit down and feed the children, or help with charting on the pediatric ward, but now I am on my feet all day. I never sit down—not here!"

A practical nurse, when asked how she "fitted in" at first when her service was new to the hospital staff, told the writer she kept her eyes open, never overstepped her orders, and made herself useful wherever she saw a chance. This nurse also made the sensible suggestion that a head nurse would be wise in not thrusting the hardest jobs at once onto the practical staff—give them easy ones and let the hard ones come as a promotion. In this way, interest would be held and ambition spurred on.

It was suggested by several staff practical nurses that a "manual" of practical nursing duties acceptable to the hospital would assist new staff members.

THE SMALL HOSPITAL

Because hospitals of less than a hundred beds, especially those in rural areas, are peculiarly vulnerable to scarcity in nursing service, they are given separate consideration here.

It has always been difficult for small hospitals to secure enough well qualified nurses. Nurses, like doctors, tend to congregate in the large cities (34); they prefer the professional companionship, the social contacts, and the wealth of clinical experience provided by large cities and large hospitals. Small hospitals, especially those with less than fifty beds, are usually unable to supply experience in quantity and variety and are therefore frowned upon as centers for medical or professional nursing education. They can seldom rely upon service from students (35). In emergencies, the small hospital does not have extra staff to call on, to shift, or to summon from the local registry. Even volunteer service in rural communities is limited compared to a city's resources. Yet of 4,833 registered general hospitals in the United States, 3,079 have less than a hundred beds—2,115 have less than fifty (36). Their problem is greater in proportion, then, than is the larger hospitals'.

Salaries are not usually as high as in urban areas, at least not on paper, but nurses do not always stop to think that $1,500 in a small city or town will go as far as or farther than $1,700 in the city. Small hospitals paid general duty registered staff nurses a medium salary of $117.50 a month in 1943. Top salaries seldom exceeded $170 (37). The writer found salaries for practical nurses in five hospitals of less than a hundred beds ranging from $90 to $125 a month, the latter for experienced staff members. When a specialty was offered, the salary was as high as $135.

Registered nurses are apt not to like rural hospitals for another reason, though this very element appeals to a few—they are required to perform duties of all kinds, including housekeeping. They may even have to cook in emergencies. Little can be done about this, writes Ruth A. Weston, except to provide professional nurses with a better background for performing these tasks (38).

Granting that emergencies are much harder to meet in small hospitals, put a heavier strain on the staff, and call for versatile adjustments to every position in the hospital in a way that almost never happens in a large hospital, still it hardly seems efficient to rely wholly upon registered nurses to fill all jobs in normal times. "We have too many patients to do our work well," is the chief complaint of these rural nurses. Helen Teal points out that one of the "hardships" rural professional nurses must face is the periodic request of the Board or chief doctor to reduce overhead "by the employment of practical nurses." Throughout a very sympathetic and competent article dealing with rural hospital nursing problems, Miss Teal does not once suggest the employment of qualified practical nurses to help out in the many serious crises in small hospitals (39).

A brief study of small hospital nursing service was made by the *American Journal of Nursing* in 1940 (40). In 402 hospitals of less than 100 beds, 4,049 registered nurses were employed, all positions included. A nurse is superintendent in about 80 per cent of these hospitals. Only two of these 402 hospitals were in places of more than 25,-000 population, 85 per cent were in places of 10,000 or less. None had a school of professional nursing. In 69 per cent of the hospitals, registered nurses carried all the nursing care; only 31 per cent employed subsidiary workers. Practical nurses were within this group, but not designated by the title. Voluntary hospitals made up about half the 31 per cent employing subsidiary workers. In 50 per cent of this group there were less than five registered nurses.

Of the hospitals of less than 25 beds, 106 had 5 or fewer registered nurses, 35 had between 6 and 10, one had between 11 and 15; of those with 25 to 49 beds, 34 had 5 or less, 74 had 6 to 10, 36 had 11 to 15, and 14 had 16 or more registered nurses. As division of these staffs into shifts must be allowed for, it would appear that someone besides a registered nurse was giving nursing care in these prewar hospitals.

Authorities state that there should be enough professional nurses to give each patient an average of two and a half to three hours of nursing care in each twenty-four hours (41). Thus, 25 patients would need seventy-five hours of care or at least 9 nurses to cover the twenty-four hours. Even before the war this condition was not met. Small hospitals should make use of attendant service for relatively unskilled service. The least satisfactory method of assisting our hospitals out of financial holes is to employ semi-skilled and therefore cheap assistants (42). Patients' safety must not be jeopardized at any cost.

It would appear that a staff of trained practical nurses assisting the registered staff would be a safe, reasonably economical, though not cheap, solution of the problem of more and better care for rural hospital patients.

One of the ways to relieve the stringencies in small rural hospitals may be through governmental aid.* Future plans for the expansion of service in these centers should outline the place and function of practical nurses. Better equipment, greater centralization of service (such as use of the community hospital as a health center), and adequate salaries would attract more and better nurses of both levels, as well as doctors, to the rural areas.

REFERENCES

1 Frederick T. Hill, "Present and future status of the volunteer and the attendant," *Hospital Management* 56:60, 62, 64, December 1943.
2 Basil C. MacLean, "Nurses—what next," *Modern Hospital* 47:51–53, August 1936, at p. 53.
3 "Nurses and subsidiary workers," *Hospitals* 12:124, March 1938. See also Lucius R. Wilson, "The subsidiary worker in efficient routine service," *Hospital Management* 43:23, 38, January 1937.
4 Margaret Tracy, "Trends in nursing," *Pacific Coast Journal of Nursing* 37:590, October 1941.
5 See American Hospital Association, *Report of the Committee to Study the Nursing Problem*, Philadelphia, the Association, 1916; Josephine Goldmark, *Nursing and nursing education in the United States;* report of the Committee for the Study of Nursing Education, New York, Macmillan, 1923; May Ayres Burgess, *Nurses, patients and pocketbooks,* report of a study of the economics of nursing by the Committee on the Grading of Nursing Schools, New York, the Committee, 1928; Committee on the Costs of Medical Care, *Medical care for the American people;* final report of the Committee, Chicago, University of Chicago Press, 1932 (Committee on the Costs of Medical Care, No. 28).

* For example, the expansion of rural hospitals proposed in pending federal legislation.

6 "Hospital service in the United States, 1945," *Journal of the American Medical Association* 127:771, 779, March 31, 1945. The figure for total births is from the *World Almanac* for 1945.

7 "Hospital service in the United States, 1945," (note 6), p. 781. The writer is glad to report that the Commission on Hospital Care, a nongovernmental public service committee appointed to study hospital service in the United States, is now endeavoring to obtain information concerning the various types of nursing personnel in hospitals, including practical nurses. Further data should be available from this source soon.

8 For time estimates in professional nursing and ratios of nurses to patients, see American Nurses' Association, Nursing Information Bureau, cooperating with the National League of Nursing Information and the National Organization for Public Health Nursing, *Facts about nursing, 1944,* pp. 58–69. In 1941 the New York City Department of Hospitals used a ratio of six to eight hospital attendants to ten practical nurses. See also Mary Ellen Manley, "The subsidiary worker in the nursing care of the sick," *Hospitals* 14:61–64, February 1940.

9 American Hospital Association and National League of Nursing Education, *Manual of the essentials of good hospital nursing service,* Chicago and New York, the Associations, 1942, pp. 12–13, 18–19, 24, 36, 48. The *Manual* is now in the process of revision and will include references to licensed practical nurses, with definition of their place, function, training, supervision, and the personnel policies affecting them.

10 Letter to the editor, *American Journal of Nursing* 20:155–156, January 1920.

11 Virginia L. Christopher, "Economies of nursing service in wartime," *American Journal of Nursing* 44:136–138, February 1944. See also Margaret E. Benson, "Meeting the shortage of nurses," *American Journal of Nursing* 41:1376–1380, December 1941; "A nursing service adjusts to wartime pressures," *American Journal of Nursing* 44:537–540, June 1944.

12 For discussion of orderly service, see Malcolm T. MacEachern, *Hospital organization and management,* Chicago, Physicians' Record Company, 1940; also Margaret Pinkerton, "Subsidiary workers in the general hospital," *Hospitals* 13:31–32, March 1939.

13 For interest in methods of assigning duties, see Manley (note 8), pp. 61–62. A reclassification of duties showed that 180 performed by registered nurses could be done by practicals. In all, some 350 nursing and non-nursing duties may be performed by this group.

14 See American Nurses' Association, Joint Committee with the Na-

tional League of Nursing Education and the National Organization for Public Health Nursing, *Subsidiary workers in the care of the sick,* New York, 1940; revised June 1941.

15 See Inez L. Armstrong, "How we met the poliomyelitis epidemic," *American Journal of Nursing* 44:529–532, June 1944. The *National Foundation News* of the National Foundation for Infantile Paralysis supplied reports on the subject of training aides during 1944–1945.

16 M. Edward Davis and Mabel C. Carmon, *DeLee's obstetrics for nurses,* 13th ed., Philadelphia, Saunders, 1944, p. 236.

17 "Nursing care of newborn infants; excerpts from Children's Bureau Publication 292, Standards and recommendations for hospital care of newborn infants, full-term and premature," *American Journal of Nursing* 43:560–563, June 1943.

18 Michigan State Department of Health, *Recommendations for nursing service in hospital nurseries,* 1944, p. 20.

19 Registered nursing procedures may, of course, be found in the standard textbooks. The reader's attention is called, however, to a typical list of treatments in progress in the wards of Strong Memorial Hospital, for 473 patients. Clare Dennison, "Maintaining the quality of nursing service in the emergency," *American Journal of Nursing* 42:774–784, July 1942, at pp. 776–777.

20 Dennison (note 19), p. 780.

21 Ellen C. Creamer, "Practical nurses; their preparation and sphere," *Hospitals* 13:64–67, August 1939.

22 Ernest R. Groves, "The hospital patient in wartime," *Hygeia* 22:12, January 1944. That these are not purely wartime situations is shown by hospital experience in 1934; see Elizabeth Brannigan, "Boston's experience in training attendants," *Trained Nurse and Hospital Review* 93:230, September 1934.

23 Blanche Pfefferkorn, "A new deal for the patient at night," *American Journal of Nursing* 32:1179–1182, November 1932. For ways of relieving the tired nurse, see also J. J. Golub, "The tired nurse—what can we do for her?" *Modern Hospital* 31:77–81, October 1928, and Joseph C. Doane, "Why a high level of nursing service is needed at night," *Modern Hospital* 37:84–87, October 1931.

24 Lucille Petry, "Increasing and using auxiliaries," *Hospitals* 17:37–40, February 1943, at pp. 39–40.

25 Margaret H. Jackson, "The future of the nursing profession," *Nursing Times* 40:305, April 29, 1944.

26 See Wilson (note 3), p. 38, for discussion of these points.

27 *Report of job analyses study of the homemaking responsibilities of the graduate practical nurse,* New York, National Association for

Practical Nurse Education, 1944 (mimeographed). These quotations are taken from the section marked "Suggestions," pp. 1–8.

28 United States Office of Education job analysis of practical nursing services scheduled for publication in 1947. It will be available from the Government Printing Office, Washington, D. C.

29 For a description of what was taught in one city as standardized duties of ward aides, many of which are also typical of practical nursing functions, see Winifred McL. Shepler, Estelle C. Koch, and James Alexander Hamilton, "Standardized training course of ward aides," *Modern Hospital* 51:65–72, December 1938.

30 Ernestine Bong, "Those subsidiary workers," *Modern Hospital* 49:63–64, September 1937, at p. 64.

31 *A guide for the use of the auxiliary worker,* adopted by the Colorado State Nursing Council for War Service, Denver, 1942, pp. 9–12.

32 See note 13, page 26. The uniform worn by practical nurses in the New Britain, Connecticut, Visiting Nurse Association is described on page 173.

33 Helen W. Faddis, "Experiments in solving the staffing problem," *American Journal of Nursing* 37:991–993, September 1937.

34 See United States Women's Bureau, *Outlook for women in occupations in the medical services; professional nurses,* Washington, Government Printing Office, 1945 (Bulletin 203, No. 3), p. 2.

35 See, however, "Minnesota plans for rural nursing service," *American Journal of Nursing* 44:147–150, February 1944; also A. G. Stasel, "Minnesota leaders outline plan to train both nurses and aides for rural areas," *Hospitals* 17:63–64, August 1943.

36 "Hospital service in the United States, 1945" (note 6), p. 773.

37 "Salaries for professional employees 'going up,'" *Modern Hospital* 62:73–74, January 1944; see also Raymond P. Sloan, "These small hospitals can 'take it'," *Modern Hospital* 62:46–49, January 1944, at pp. 46–48.

38 Ruth A. Weston, "Advanced courses and rural patients," *American Journal of Nursing* 44:735–736, August 1944, at p. 736.

39 For a vivid description of the exigencies of small hospitals, see Helen Teal, "In a small hospital nursing is not simple," *Modern Hospital* 45:57–59, July 1935.

40 "Nursing in small hospitals in small towns," *American Journal of Nursing* 40:1370–1372, December 1940, at p. 1372.

41 *Facts about nursing, 1945,* pp. 62–63.

42 See Henry J. Southmayd and Geddes Smith, *Small community hospitals,* New York, Commonwealth Fund, 1944, pp. 69, 102.

CHAPTER SIX

Mental Hospitals

FOR MANY centuries the care of the mentally ill was in the hands of untrained and semi-trained persons, and even today many people think of a mental hospital as an asylum for the insane or hopelessly demented, served by a staff of custodians, attendants, or wardens whose job is mainly to keep the inmates from escaping or hurting themselves or others. Physical strength was once as much a prerequisite in an attendant as were iron bars in all the windows. If registered nurses were thought of at all in connection with the care of the mentally ill in institutions, it was only as caring for those who were physically ill.

The modern mental hospital has a staff of trained specialists: doctors, psychiatrists, psychologists, registered nurses, occupational therapists, physical therapists, dietitians, medical psychiatric social workers, and attendants. Their aim is to prevent mental breakdown, to treat early deviations from normal behavior, and to initiate treatment to restore those already suffering from some form of psychosis. Our progress in understanding mental disease has changed the whole conception of the function of a mental institution from an asylum or last place of refuge for the hopelessly insane to a hospital where minds are restored to normal functioning. With the exception of those suffering from the mental deterioration of old age, advanced organic disease, or congenital deficiencies, and a small percentage of patients admitted too late for aid, the outlook for the majority of patients in mental hospitals is bright. But it could be brighter.

Few mental patients are treated in their own homes; the majority are admitted to hospitals or private institutions or report regularly to psychiatrists in private practice or special clinics. However, both registered and practical nurses when caring for ill people at home are in a strategic position to observe the early signs of mental maladjustments in members of the family as well as in their patients. They can be of inestimable help in recognizing these signs and guiding the sufferers to expert care (1).

Sensitivity and tact as well as sound fundamental knowledge of steps to be taken must be developed in both professional and practical nursing students. With these needs in view, schools are promoting affiliations in approved mental hospitals for professional student nurses (2), while the schools for practical nurses are beginning to enrich their curricula with more information and reading in the field of mental hygiene. The directors of nurses in mental hospitals advocate a definite period of orientation for all attendants and nurses, students and graduates, no matter what their general background and hospital experience may have been. The more a nurse knows about psychiatric nursing, the better fitted she is to care for all types of patients. Indeed, many nurse educators urge a required—not elective—affiliation with a mental hospital for all types of nurses.

HOSPITALS, PATIENTS, AND NURSES

In 1944, there were 566 mental hospitals in the United States with beds for 648,745 people—37.5 per cent of all hospital beds. These were 95.4 per cent occupied. Thirty-six hospitals had less than 25 beds, but 232 had more than 1,000 beds. There were, in 512 of these hospitals, 4,705 graduate nurses and 32,707 practical nurses and attendants. No differentiation between licensed, trained, or untrained practical nurses and attendants was made in this latter classification, but orderlies and ward maids were not included (3). These few workers are distributed over eight-hour shifts, and no arithmetic is needed to show that mental patients are largely dependent on care from attendants and are woefully in need of skilled professional nursing.

In the study of hospitals in the United States made by the Procurement and Assignment Division of the War Manpower Commission, the "paid auxiliary nursing workers" in 103 mental-custodial hospitals were distributed as shown in the accompanying table (4). These figures show the heavy burden carried by nonprofessional staff and the astounding dearth of professional nurses. Since auxiliary workers as defined in this study included practical nurses, attendants, ward helpers, and orderlies, the report is not helpful in differentiating the work of practical nurses.

A study made in California in 1940–1941 revealed that in the eight state mental institutions caring for 24,000 patients only 18 registered nurses were employed (5). In Minnesota in 1944 there were in eight institutions providing 11,984 beds for mental and epileptic patients 51 registered nurses, 710 nonprofessional nurses, and 113 professional student nurses (6). In January 1945 at Rochester (New York) State Hospital (capacity 3,400) there were 60 registered nurses and 400 attendants on the day of the writer's visit.

PAID AUXILIARY NURSING WORKERS IN 103 MENTAL-CUSTODIAL
HOSPITALS

		GOVERNMENT HOSPITALS		NON-GOVERNMENTAL HOSPITALS	
	TOTAL	Without students*	With students	Without students	With students
Number of hospitals reporting paid auxiliary workers	103	62	41	9	4
Number of paid auxiliary workers to each general staff nurse	17.6	19.0	16.4	12.1	1.8
Number of patients to each auxiliary worker	14.5	14.7	14.3	9.0	4.6
Percentage of nursing care given by paid auxiliary workers	88.3	95.4	81.9	93.1	45.0

* Professional students.
Table prepared by the American Nurses' Association.

Wartime shortages cut registered and attendant nursing staffs by more than half in some mental hospitals (7), but the ratio of all nurses (registered, practical, students, and paid aides) to patients has never been adequate. In 1943 the ratio in 61 hospitals in the United States and Ontario, Canada, ranged from one nurse to 2.12 patients to one to 21, the average in state hospitals being one to 12.22, while the range for registered nurses only to patients was from one nurse to 3.1 patients to one to 2,684 (8).

Most authorities agree that the staffs of registered psychiatric nurses should be increased to provide a ratio of at least one to each 10 patients. Dr. Samuel W. Hamilton, of the Division of Mental Hygiene, United States Public Health Service, speaking at the 1944 annual meeting of the National Committee for Mental Hygiene, remarked that a ratio of one registered nurse to every 25 patients in mental hospitals would be "wonderful." The ratio of attendants to patients should be one to 5 to 7 (9).

Theoretically, three levels of nursing care are needed in mental hospitals:

That given by the professional registered nurse, who supervises all nursing care, serves in admitting, operating, and treatment rooms, and carries out all highly skilled nursing and psychiatric nursing procedures

That given by the practical nurse, who assists the professional nurse wherever needed, is responsible for all simple routine nursing procedures among convalescent, ambulatory, or mildly (physically) ill patients, and supervises attendant services when needed

That given by the attendant, who provides custodial care to all those not in need of special or psychiatric nursing and assumes considerable responsibility for housekeeping services on the wards

In reality, there is great confusion about the duties of the nursing staff, and the term practical or attendant nurse is not found in mental hospitals unless the hospital is conducting a school for the training of this group. But untrained and trained attendants abound, and the line of responsibility between these two classes is vague just as it is vague between the duties of a trained attendant and a licensed practical nurse. Many an untrained male attendant carries on all the nursing procedures permitted a licensed practical nurse and some of the professional nurse's duties into the bargain. A female attendant of fifteen years' experience on a women's ward will be quite capable of carrying out all the listed duties of a trained attendant or practical nurse, for, as might be expected, experience on the job in a mental hospital produces a worker who is superior in her practical handling of patients to the otherwise well trained nurse of any level entering the psychiatric wards for the first time. Self-assurance, freedom from fear, and knowledge of the "ropes" are essential to all workers dealing with these patients, from the doctors and dentists to the gardeners and clerks, but the professional nursing staff is expected to have deeper understanding and greater skill in interpreting the actions of the patients with relation to their prescribed treatment, the stage of the disease, and the prognosis. A superintendent of a state hospital put it this way to the writer: "The seriousness of the shortage of registered nurses in mental hospitals is not physical neglect of the patients—they are still well fed, warm, clothed and housed—but in psychiatric nursing, a level of service the attendant can never attain."

In this chapter the term "attendant" designates anyone not a registered nurse or professional student, orderly, or ward maid who gives nursing care to mental patients. The term covers trained and untrained attendants, nurses' aides, practical nurses, licensed and unlicensed, and "dropped" or dismissed undergraduate students serving under any title except registered nurse.

Most authorities agree that the nursing of the mentally ill in institutions is a highly specialized field, requiring more than the usual skilled nursing techniques. The nurse must keep a jump ahead of the destructive, mischievous activities of the maniac patient, must foresee and prevent suicidal tendencies and planning on the part of the depressed patient, and must understand what may be going on in the brain of the psychopathic patient with involutional psychoses. She must learn how to bring the patient out from hiding under his cover of unreality and teach him to face life anew. She must assist the physician in his effort to lead the patient to recovery whether it be by suggestion or the more drastic therapy of electric shock. To observe keenly and constantly with understanding is vital on a psychopathic ward. In the absence of highly trained nursing specialists, patients may remain lethargic or even retrogress and the objective of the doctor's treatment is delayed, if not lost.

It is partly the lack of this kind of specialized knowledge among attendants and registered nurses that has sometimes caused the medical staff of a mental institution to seek still another grade of help. The Institute of Living of the Hartford Retreat at Hartford, Connecticut, has for some years sought as "psychiatric aides" college and high school graduates and those trained in the arts with satisfactory educational background. This non-nurse aide works as a member of the medical team in caring for patients, yet she is neither registered, practical, nor attendant nurse. Her duties are performed

. . . under the direction and supervision of the doctors and the nursing officers. One of her major functions is to stimulate the interest of the patients who are guests in the educational, reeducational and social programs.

The psychiatric aide also has an opportunity to learn bed-side nursing and home nursing techniques such as taking pulse, temperature or respiration, making records and serving sick trays. She will not be over her depth as she increasingly becomes an auxiliary teacher in a very practical way (10).

Many of the patients in mental hospitals receive only custodial care —shelter, food, clothing, and protection. This is not to say they do not need something more—home life, affection, and simple duties (11), but the problem of caring for hundreds of harmless, irresponsible, dependent mental defectives and elderly people in all stages and with all types of senile psychoses must, in most institutions, be dealt with *en masse*. Recovery for them is not possible. The best that can be hoped for is adjustment to life that will keep them comfortable and contented. The routine of their days is almost unchanging: dressing and undressing, washing, eating, walking, rocking, sleeping. True nursing care is needed only when they are sick. They should be entirely in the custodial care of attendants (or of practical nurses if they are mildly sick) under professional nurse supervision. Also, the attendant who is going to be absorbed in housekeeping duties does not need to be taught nursing treatments. Her duties are the care of beds, wards, closets, linen, supplies, lavatories, dressing rooms, patients' clothing, help on visiting days, assistance at meals, escorting patients to treatment rooms or to the dentist, etc.

The place and function of the attendant in the disturbed and convalescent wards of our mental hospitals are vitally important, but they are hard to define and evaluate because, inevitably, when assigned so much responsibility for the physical care of a patient, the attendant has great influence on his mental state. Just the way a bath is given may fix the patient's mind-set and disturb his emotional balance for the day. In 1918 Annie W. Goodrich said she could not see "the trained attendant caring for the mental patients who can be restored to a good mental condition" (12). Yet today, if these patients were not served by attendants, many of their wants would not be cared for at all, so scarce are professional nurses in our mental hospitals.

A study of attendants in mental hospitals in 1936 led Harriet Bailey to suggest that these workers should be chosen with a view to permanent employment and that they should be adequately prepared and receive advancement. She urged that the general ratio of all types of nurses be raised to one to each six patients. She pointed out, what is evident today with sad frequency, that the fewer the nursing personnel, the more patients must be on restraint or in seclusion and the higher the incidence of accidents (13).

Some mental hospitals have no registered male nurses and women nurses never enter the male division. The care of the male patients is, therefore, wholly in the hands of attendants—trained or untrained, nearly always trained only on the job. Medications and postoperative care are in their hands. This situation leads the American Psychiatric Association to urge provision of a uniform standard of care for men and women patients, centralization of all nursing personnel under competent professional nursing directors, and formal training of attendants (14).

DUTIES OF ATTENDANTS

In order to perform their duties satisfactorily, it is believed that attendants, in addition to good health, some high school education, and a genuine interest in their field, should have a speaking acquaintance with elementary psychology, abnormal psychology, and mental hygiene, should be neat and have a pleasant, prepossessing, yet authoritative manner, and should be keenly observant and alert. They should be taught simple professional ethics and learn to handle situations helpfully and safely and to report intelligently what they have observed and done (15). A worker thus prepared will be of much greater service in relieving the professional nurse, in giving care to patients, and in interpreting conditions to physicians.

In addition to the nursing procedures that a practical nurse with basic training is expected to know, attendants are given instruction in handling untidy, restless, and disturbed patients and those who are bedfast, in feeding, in assistance with tube feedings and with hydrotherapy treatments, and in the use of restraints of various kinds, and are taught what to observe and report about patients.

All personnel must be taught a few simple rules for their own protection and the safety of all, such as checking patients in and out of wards, locking doors, precautions against fire, keeping track of drugs, utensils, keys, what to do in emergencies, and so forth.

As a rule, practical nurses and attendants in mental hospitals do not do any of the skilled nursing procedures forbidden them in the general hospitals. Such treatments as all types of shock therapy, hydrotherapy, gavage, and major surgical dressings are not within the province of the attendant or practical nurse, though she may assist with them under registered nurse supervision (16). The great and regrettable exception to this is on the "men's side." As has been said, in the men's wards in many hospitals men attendants (rarely professional nurses or licensed practical nurses) carry out all the nursing procedures not done by doctors.

In most institutions, the chief or head professional nurse on duty is responsible for nursing care. If she assigns duties not on the approved posted list she must supervise their performance and be held accountable for any mistakes. Unfortunately, professional nurse directors are not always responsible for the work of the attendants, who may be under a matron or directly responsible to the superintendent of the hospital (17).

THE TRAINING OF ATTENDANTS

Above all, it becomes evident that for the safety of the patient, other inmates, and personnel, as well as for the proper psychiatric care of the patient, all attendants, whether they give practical nursing service or only custodial care, must receive training.

One of the first state hospitals to recognize the need of a training course was the Elgin State Hospital in Illinois.* The attendant is given a handbook or manual outlining attitudes, duties, rules of the hospital, and a general description of mental illness and what it means. He or she must learn thoughtful consideration and kindliness and "a trained understanding of the psychotic patient in his relation to the entire state hospital situation in which he is placed. . . . The major portion of many patients' treatments consists of the attendants' attitudes towards them" (18).

The difference in the training given attendants in mental hospitals —often within the same state—is staggering. One hospital trains on the job, in the ward, as the new worker comes in; no one person is responsible for planned program, the teaching is done by whoever is in charge of the ward. Another hospital is clinging to a six-month course although the turnover of employees is so fast and great that every week workers who have not finished the course leave and new workers enter the advanced classes of a course just finishing. Another

* See also the Veterans Bureau plan described on page 192.

hospital appears to be offering a curriculum that is too involved and advanced for the position and its duties, to say nothing of the intelligence of the attendants now applying for work (19).

In June 1942 the Committee on Mental Hygiene and Psychiatric Nursing of the National League of Nursing Education prepared an outline for a course for attendants in mental hospitals (20). The requirements were unusual in that they made high school graduation a prerequisite. The length of the course was six to eight months, and it was to be given only in hospitals approved by the American Psychiatric Association. Recommended content included the usual classroom and ward practice periods, orientation, personal hygiene, behavior, and ward housekeeping—the latter to be ten to twenty hours. The longest time was to be devoted to classroom instruction (60 to 100 hours with additional time for practice) in patient care including special therapies. A careful analysis of the list of procedures taught in this course leaves one with the feeling that the attendant would turn out to be as proficient in this type of work as a licensed practical nurse yet would be lacking in the desirable preparation and training for practical nursing elsewhere. This course is naturally drawn up within the framework of the mental hospital, so that with eight months of training and an additional period (which might be six months to six years) of experience the individual would still be unable to pass a state examination for practical nursing if such an examination happened to feature maternity, pediatrics, nutrition, or household management.

"Affiliations" might be the answer for the would-be licensed practical nurse, as they are for the professional nurse attending a school of nursing in a mental hospital. Or it may be that the "trained attendant" will have to add a definitive adjective or noun—"psychiatric trained attendant," "trained attendant (psychiatry)"—a step involving much complicated legislation. In any case, if the requirements of this suggested course were adhered to, attendants would be overtrained from the standpoint of average performance expected today, and undertrained in the subjects required for licensed practical nurses.

Those familiar with attendants who have had improper or inadequate preparation in the care of mental patients will recognize these shortcomings:

Failure to distinguish between symptoms of mental origin and those due to bodily disease

Failure to distinguish between various types of mental illness, and ignorance of the treatment of each

Lack of a professional attitude, because of ignorance of professional ethics

Favoritism toward some patients and neglect of others, because of inability
or inexperience in controlling personal feelings and prejudices

Regard of their work as merely a means of livelihood, rather than as a professional responsibility

Lack of interest in obtaining results, because attendant's work is often
taken as a last resort, perhaps because of financial need or inability to succeed in work more to their liking (21).

SALARIES

Salaries of attendants, trained attendants, and practical nurses in
mental hospitals have been bettered by the war, although wages are
sometimes lower than those of elevator operators, laundrymen, and
gardeners—60 to 70 cents an hour compared with 75 to 85 cents. Institutions in which attendants, trained or untrained, are under Civil
Service seem to fare somewhat better. (See page 187)

Because salaries and working conditions are poor and hours are
long, desirable workers have not been attracted to this kind of work.

THE FUTURE OF PRACTICAL NURSING IN MENTAL HOSPITALS

Dr. Joseph W. Mountin predicts the need of 30,800 registered
nurses in our mental hospitals within a few years—almost eight times
as many as we have now (22). Will this cut down the trained or untrained attendant service? Will licensed practical nurses with good
basic preparation find a place in mental hospitals, and will the hospitals pay their slightly higher salaries if untrained attendants are abundant at low wages? Will hospital administrators recognize three levels
of care? Will the foster home care of specially selected patients be extended, thus decreasing the hospital load and increasing the responsibility of those who supervise such care? (23) Will the homes of practical nurses be suitable for the placement of selected mental patients?

There is no group of patients more in need of trained nonprofessional service than the mentally ill, and no field of service open to licensed practical nurses about which there is greater confusion. There
seems to be no way of telling whether mental hospitals will adhere to
their present practice of wasting professional nursing time in nonprofessional duties, and either overtraining or undertraining poor at-

tendants, leaving the licensed practical nurse out of the picture entirely, or will assign housekeeping and custodial duties to attendants and employ trained practical nurses, both men and women, to function on a second level of nursing as assistants to the professional staff.* So far as the writer has been able to discover, the present attendant in the mental hospital may be either totally unfit, even vicious, in the performance of his or her duties, or so well trained and experienced in the particular job that the service may be superior to that of an inexperienced professional nurse. The latter situation, however, is extremely rare, the former distressingly common. No mental hospital visited by the writer could report a satisfactory, adequate, or stable attendant service; all confessed to using professional time unwisely. Attendant service was most nearly filling the need of patients where institutions had training courses resembling that for practical nurses but directed toward the situation peculiar to the mental patient, and where custodial care was given by ward maids.

A clearer distinction and division between patients needing skilled psychiatric nursing and those requiring custodial care only would do much to clarify the nursing situation. Such differentiation and classification rest with the medical staff.

Interest in nursing service for the mentally ill on the part of the American Psychiatric Association and of the Division of Mental Hygiene of the United States Public Health Service has done much to bring the plight of the mental hospitals before the public and the professions. Very practical help to mental hospitals in handling the attendant problem is in sight. This help already takes tangible form in two publications—a manual of instruction for attendants prepared for mental hospitals Mrs. Laura W. Fitzsimmons (24), and *The Attendant's Guide*, a handbook of information for attendants in mental hospitals, by Edith M. Stern (25). Both these "tools" offer information ideally adapted to the needs of our hard-pressed mental hospitals and are excellent teaching material for practical nurses.

REFERENCES

1 Mental deterioration among elderly chronically ill people, for example, is frequent. In New York city in 1938, of 1,935 persons over

---

* It is understood that the New York State Division of Mental Hygiene plans to make a definite classification, under Civil Service, for licensed practical nurses in its state mental institutions.

65 years of age who were being cared for at home, 18 per cent showed signs of mental illness or mental decline. Mary C. Jarrett, "Housekeeping service for home care of chronic patients," W.P.A. Project 165–97–7002, December 31, 1938, p. 13.

2 Editorial, "More psychiatric nursing needed," *American Journal of Nursing* 44:723, August 1944. See also Laura W. Fitzsimmons, "Facts and trends in psychiatric nursing," *American Journal of Nursing* 44:732–735, August 1944. In 1943, 54 per cent of the professional schools provided psychiatric experience for their students.

3 "Hospital service in the United States, 1945," *Journal of the American Medical Association* 127:773, 777, 781, March 31, 1945.

4 Louise Tattershall and Margaret D. West, "Wartime nursing care in 604 general hospitals," *American Journal of Nursing* 44:211–214, March 1944; Louise M. Tattershall and Marion E. Altenderfer, "Paid auxiliary nursing workers employed in general hospitals," *ibid.* 44:752–756, August 1944; Tattershall and Altenderfer, "Nursing personnel in general hospitals," *ibid.* 44:853–858, September 1944; Tattershall and Altenderfer, "Hours of nursing in general hospitals," *ibid.* 44:963–966, October 1944.

5 Information from the American Psychiatric Association.

6 Information from Viktor O. Wilson, M.D., Director, Division of Child Hygiene, Minnesota Department of Health.

7 Laura Fitzsimmons, "Report of a survey of nursing in mental hospitals in the U.S. and Ontario, Canada," *American Journal of Psychiatry* 100:623–627, March 1944, at p. 624. See also Dorothy Deming, "Mental hospitals in wartime," *American Journal of Nursing* 43:1013–1017, November 1943, at pp. 1013–1014. In one state institution whose normal quota of ward attendants was 538 there were 168 on duty on the day of the writer's visit; the census was more than 6,000 patients.

8 Fitzsimmons (note 7), p. 623. See also editorial, "More psychiatric nursing needed," *American Journal of Nursing* 44:723, August 1944; and Fitzsimmons (note 2).

9 Quoted by Virginia Calohan, "Psychiatric nursing today and tomorrow," *R.N.—A Journal for Nurses* 8:49–51, 74, 76, 78, December 1944, at p. 49.

10 *Where shall I serve?* Neuro-Psychiatric Institute of the Hartford Retreat, 1944, pp. 5, 32–33 [illustrated booklet]. The Institute of Living, formerly the Neuro-Psychiatric Institute, accommodates 350 "guests" in residence. There is a staff of 600 to 700, mostly doctors, nurses, aides, and teachers.

11 Hester B. Crutcher, *Foster home care for mental patients,* New York, Commonwealth Fund, 1944, pp. 2–3.
12 Annie W. Goodrich, "Position of attendants," *American Journal of Nursing* 18:1009, October 1918. See also Stephen Rushmore, "Community nursing needs," *New England Journal of Medicine,* 217:861–864, November 25, 1937, at p. 862.
13 Harriet Bailey, "Nursing schools in psychiatric hospitals," *American Journal of Nursing* 36:495–508, May 1936, at pp. 507, 501. See also Dorothy Deming, "Mental hospitals in wartime" (note 7), p. 1014; George W. Weber, Robert E. Plunkett, and Frederick MacCurdy, "Problem of control of tuberculosis in mental hospitals with reduced personnel," *American Journal of Public Health* 34:962–966, September 1944, at p. 963.
14 Fitzsimmons (note 2), p. 735.
15 Fitzsimmons (note 7), pp. 625–626.
16 The reader is referred to the *Manual of attendants' duties and instructions* recommended and prepared by the American Psychiatric Association, 9 Rockefeller Plaza, New York 20, N.Y., for the details of procedure and policy in carrying out all duties.
17 Fitzsimmons (note 7), p. 626.
18 Charles F. Read, *Manual for hospital attendants,* State Department of Public Welfare of Illinois, 1939 (revised), pp. 21, 22.
19 Fitzsimmons (note 7), pp. 625–626.
20 "Course for attendants in mental hospitals," *American Journal of Nursing* 42:683, June 1942.
21 Helen Ode, "Subsidiary workers need training for work in psychiatric hospitals," *Hospital Management* 51:51–53, March 1941, at p. 51.
22 Joseph W. Mountin, "Suggestions to nurses on postwar adjustments," *American Journal of Nursing* 44:321–325, April 1944.
23 Crutcher (note 11), pp. 14, 33.
24 Laura W. Fitzsimmons, *Manual for training attendants in mental hospitals,* New York, American Psychiatric Association, 1945.
25 Edith M. Stern, *The attendant's guide,* New York, Commonwealth Fund, 1945.

CHAPTER SEVEN

Tuberculosis Hospitals

NEXT TO mental hospitals, the tuberculosis hospitals of our country have suffered most from wartime shortages. They have faced almost unbelievable difficulties from curtailment in all types of personnel. "If we had plenty of efficient kitchen, ward, laundry, and housekeeping staff," the superintendent of a hospital said to the writer, "we could get by with a 50 per cent emergency cut in nursing personnel, but when our supply of doctors, nurses, maids, cooks, orderlies, and janitors fails and turnover rises 25 per cent, how can a superintendent sleep nights?"

THE SUPPLY OF NURSES

In 1944, there were 79,848 beds for tuberculosis patients in 453 institutions in the United States. These were occupied by an average of 63,025 patients—78.9 per cent occupancy. A total of 4,161 registered nurses and 4,277 practical nurses and attendants were employed in 424 of these hospitals (1). We do not know how many of these last were licensed practical nurses.

The situation regarding "paid auxiliary nursing workers" (attendants, practical nurses, ward helpers, aides, and orderlies) in tuberculosis hospitals in 1943 as revealed by the study made by the War Manpower Commission is shown in the table on page 101 (2).

A series of visits made by the writer in 1943–1944 to 11 tuberculosis hospitals with bed capacities of from 60 to 2,000 (total patients 5,283) showed cuts in normal registered nursing staffs of from 25 to 68 per cent (3). In all 11 hospitals there were, on the day visited, 677 registered nurses (normal 1,312), 706 "graduates,"* practicals, and paid nurses' aides, and 323 students, including 20 practical nursing students. It had been almost impossible to replace registered nurses with trained personnel of any type, so the hospitals had usually trained their own. "We could not get along without our own nurses," was an un-

---

* For the sake of simplification and because "graduates" are not registered, in this chapter they are considered to be in a class with licensed practical nurses unless otherwise indicated.

varying comment. "They know more about tuberculosis than the raw young registered nurses who have had no experience in tuberculosis throughout their training."* Until they were asked to do so, superintendents frequently made no distinction between registered and graduate nurses in reporting to the writer the number on duty. Sometimes reference to the files was necessary.

PAID AUXILIARY NURSING WORKERS IN 146 TUBERCULOSIS HOSPITALS

	TOTAL	GOVERNMENTAL HOSPITALS		NON-GOVERNMENTAL HOSPITALS	
		Without students	*With students*	*Without students*	*With students*
Number of hospitals reporting paid auxiliary workers	122	115	7	22	2
Number of paid auxiliary workers to each general staff nurse	2.1	1.9	2.0	4.2	0.8
Number of patients to each auxiliary worker	11.3	11.1	13.7	9.3	33.1
Percentage of nursing care given by paid auxiliary workers	65.3	66.0	61.2	60.5	18.8

"Students" does not include practical nursing students, only professionals.

The shortages are not related to the size of the hospital, for one hospital of 50-bed capacity was without a registered nurse while one of 60 beds reported 6 registered nurses and no other type. In the first hospital, the doctor must have been burdened with a heavy load of worry and the duty of constant personal supervision of patients. In the second, either a group of workers not called nurses was helping with routines or else some very expensive skilled nursing time was going into manual labor and elementary nursing procedures.

A more recent figure showing dependence on nonprofessional staff comes from Minnesota. In 1944, 13 sanatoria with a total of 1,292 beds

* See footnote on page 107.

(not including one of 697 beds with a basic school of professional nursing) employed 54 registered and 124 nonprofessional nurses (4).

To indicate variations in registered and nonprofessional staffs (for the sake of clarity, considering the "graduate" on a level with the licensed practical nurse as stated above), a random sampling of large and small hospitals in states with and without state laws licensing practical nurses was taken from the 1942 Directory, and it is presented in the table on page 103. It is probably safe to assume 80 to 85 per cent bed occupancy in these hospitals and some reduction since 1942 in the number of registered nurses. As might be expected, "graduates" exceeded registered nurses in the large hospitals in states without a law to license practical nurses, and it is evident that many of the institutions were depending on attendant service of types not designated as "nurses: registered, graduate, or licensed practical." Obviously a hospital of 100 beds, 80 per cent occupied, could not get along with 10 nurses of all types unless all the patients were ambulatory. It must be remembered that 10 nurses must cover day and night service, possibly in three shifts, and that at least one of the 10 will be largely occupied with administrative and supervisory duties.

A random sampling of private tuberculosis sanatoria of more than 10 beds reveals even greater variation in ratios, as shown in the table on page 104. One must conclude that these private hospitals were not occupied to capacity, that they served ambulatory patients mainly, or else that their patients were receiving very meager care. Even if they were only 50 per cent occupied, the registered nurse ratio was below the standard.

Some of these situations are old stories, others have been aggravated by wartime conditions, but all show a confused and frantic effort to supply adequate nursing care to tuberculous patients whose average stay is between three months and a year in our hospitals. In no other type of hospital do circumstances seem to alter the size and type of nursing staffs so directly.

In 1945 the American Trudeau Society recommended that:

Provision should be made for new members of the general duty nursing staff who have not had instruction and experience in tuberculosis nursing, to receive at least a short technical course with follow-up supervision.

. . . Nursing service shall be properly adjusted with respect to the proportion of infirmary, semi-ambulant and ambulant patients, the ratio of nurses for whom shall be not less than 1:3, 1:8 and 1:30, respectively. This is for twenty-four-hour coverage. If thoracic surgery is done at the institution, the ratio of nurses to patients recently operated upon should be not less than 1:2. In calculating ratios of nurses to patients, suitable credit may be given for services performed by orderlies, nursing attendants or other well-trained auxiliary workers (5).

NUMBER OF REGISTERED AND "GRADUATE" NURSES IN A SAMPLING OF
SANATORIA IN STATES WITH AND WITHOUT A STATE LAW
LICENSING PRACTICAL NURSES, 1942

Name of hospital and state	Bed capacity	Registered nurses	"Graduates"
IN STATES WITH LICENSING LAW			
Robert Koch, Missouri	688	82	54
Hopemount, West Virginia	475	20	60
Rutland, Massachusetts	365	22	30
Undercliff, Connecticut	318	55	4
Mount Morris, New York	250	34	26
Gaylord Farm, Connecticut	145	9	10
Hillcrest, California	130	10	2
Cambridge, Massachusetts	100	5	12
Sunny Rest, Wisconsin	85	9	4*
Mt. Pleasant, Maryland	60	10	2
IN STATES WITHOUT LICENSING LAW			
State Hospital, Arkansas	1,155	16	154
Hamilton County, Ohio	583	36	95
Oakdale State Hospital, Iowa	424	13	48
State Hospital, Florida	400	44	20
State Hospital, North Dakota	368	7	36
Allenwood, New Jersey	100	10	7
Mineral Springs, Minnesota	100	8	6
Pembroke, New Hampshire	100	5	12
Douglas County, Nebraska	80	8	5
Macon County, Illinois	80	9	2

Table made from a random sampling from *Tuberculosis hospital and sanatorium directory,* New York, National Tuberculosis Association, 1942.

* "Nursing aids."

NUMBER OF REGISTERED AND "GRADUATE" NURSES IN A SAMPLING OF
PRIVATE SANATORIA OF MORE THAN TEN BEDS IN STATES WITH AND
WITHOUT A STATE LAW LICENSING PRACTICAL NURSES, 1942

Name of hospital and state	Bed capacity	Registered nurses	"Graduates"
IN STATES WITH LICENSING LAW			
Gabriels, New York	112	4	6
Belmont, California	100	5	5
Morningside, Wisconsin	54	3	5
IN STATES WITHOUT LICENSING LAW			
Edward, Illinois	101	12	10
East Lawn, Michigan	95	5	5
St. Francis, Colorado	75	4	13
St. Luke's Home, Arizona	50	2	7
Sacred Heart, Pennsylvania	40	2	2*
Wilmington, North Carolina	40	4	4
Sycamore Hill, New Jersey	34	1	1†

Table made from a random sampling of *Tuberculosis hospital and sanatorium directory,* New York, National Tuberculosis Association, 1942.
* "Nursing aids."
† Student nurse.

In November 1941, 42 sanatoria had a ratio of one registered nurse to 30 or more patients, 6 hospitals had one to 80 or more patients, 2 had no professional nursing at all; only two hospitals out of 247 had been able to maintain the ratio recommended in 1935 by the Committee on Sanatorium Standards of the American Trudeau Society, namely, one nurse to 5 to 7 patients, one to 30 semi-ambulatory patients (6).

Probably no ratio should be stated as desirable until far more study has been made of the duties that can be safely assigned to supervised nonprofessional staff under the varying conditions found in tuberculosis hospitals. Such a study has been recommended (7) and is long overdue.

A few of the factors described to the writer as conditioning the ratios of nurses to patients and of professional to practical nurses are:

Stage of tuberculosis at which the majority of patients are admitted
Ratio of ambulatory to bed patients

Inclusion of general major surgery in the hospital's program of service
Amount of thoracic surgery performed on patients
Policy of the medical staff with regard to the kind, amount, and pace of activities allowed
Presence of a children's division or unit
Number, quality, and reliability of ward maids, orderlies, and other housekeeping staff and their rate of turnover
Amount and quality of nursing supervision
Presence of a body of students, as a school attached to the hospital, affiliates, or postgraduates
Length of time ambulatory patients are held before discharge

Underlying the conditions that are peculiar to tuberculosis sanatoria is the most influential factor of all, common to all hospitals—the supply of nursing personnel on either professional or nonprofessional level. If a hospital can get more of one, less of the other, duties are redistributed to fit the available supply. The ratios of registered and practical nurses have to date been regulated by necessity and not by design.

Even under normal peacetime conditions, tuberculosis hospitals have had difficulty in securing nursing personnel and this difficulty has not always depended upon salary scales. Sanatoria far from town, with meager social diversions, limited chances for professional advancement, and monotonous service demands, find it hard to attract and hold both registered and practical nurses. Fear of contracting the disease keeps many away (8).

In the group of tuberculosis sanatoria surveyed by the American Trudeau Society in 1942, the following evidence of attempting to meet the shortage was given (9):

"We employ relatives of patients and train them as nurses' aides" (200-bed capacity)
"We have been employing practical nurses in place of registered nurses, but have recently found it practically impossible to secure any" (50-bed capacity)
"For our purposes we have found that a good practical nurse is better than a mine-run graduate" (50-bed capacity) (10)
"We have been forced to take girls with no training but with some aptitude and teach them the rudiments of tuberculosis nursing. Almost half prove satisfactory" (50-bed capacity)

"We take anyone to do practical nursing who has a white dress. We recently hired a woman 65 years old and were tickled to death to get her" (250-bed capacity)

"We are having some trouble with the graduate nurses as they are not so willing to work with the practical nurses we are using now" (150-bed capacity)

"For nurses, we are using anything we can get—two-year graduates, practical nurses, nurses' aides" (50-bed capacity)

"In normal times we have 104 nurses, today we have 51 registered, 23 practical, 3 nurses' aides" (400-bed capacity)

"We are using convalescent patients on a part time basis for nursing" (600-bed capacity)

"The turnover is very rapid in nurses' aides. We are unable to obtain enough of them" (300-bed capacity)

In this study, 80 sanatoria reported the use of nurses' aides of some description other than Red Cross, 65 employed practical nurses and attendants, and 2 were employing unregistered nurses—probably students dropped from professional schools (11).

In summary, we may say that tuberculosis hospitals are attempting to replace professional nursing service in three ways.

1. By training ex-patients. This is a time-honored and "logical and economical" way out. Its safety appeals to administrators, who are usually enthusiastic about the results. They never fail to point out that the ex-patient —be she registered nurse or gardener—makes a "good worker" who understands the necessity for precautions, knows the hospital routines, and serves as a morale builder among the patients. Such employment is to the advantage of the workers, they say, because close check is kept on health, overfatigue is avoided, and another breakdown is prevented.

2. By hiring an attendant group and training them on the job. The degree of training varies with the individual's capacity to learn and the time the hospital can devote to teaching. One woman may be "trained up" to function as a very good practical nurse—in tuberculosis. Another stays at ward-maid level.

The training of attendants on the job may be carried on in the wards with patients, or formal classroom instruction may precede and accompany ward service. Educational requirements range from grammar to high school graduation. At Cedarcrest Hospital, Hartford, Connecticut, the war emergency training course for attendants was a year and a half in length with preliminary and concurrent classroom work. Attendants with two years of high school were preferred. Three classes were admitted early in the war to tide the hospital over the shortage, and about 50 students completed the work before the course was discontinued. On the day of the writer's visit, in November 1944, there were 264 patients nursed by 14 registered nurses, 8 special attendants, and 34 nonprofessional students. This hospital reported having 65 graduate nurses (the registered nurses were in this group) and 7 attendants, a total of 72 "nurses," in 1942.

3. By using student service. In the old days, basic schools for professional nursing in tuberculosis hospitals supplied a high grade of assistance in patient care.* At present, professional student service comes mostly through affiliations with schools connected with general hospitals. Schools for practical nurses exist in some tuberculosis hospitals, and practice is offered pupils from "home schools" in several others. On the other hand, 21 of the 49 schools for practical nurses listed by the United States Office of Education were known not to offer experience in tuberculosis nursing in 1945.

None of the three methods of securing nonprofessional nursing service would be as satisfactory as the use of previously trained licensed practical nurses, could they be obtained and given an intensive introduction to the work of the hospital. The suggestion that an affiliation of one to three months in a tuberculosis hospital be offered the practical nurse as a part of her basic training seems in line with the plan for professional students. Such affiliation could be made elective. Or a "postgraduate" course in the specialty could be offered to licensed practical nurses.

Until a supply of licensed practical nurses can be drawn upon, the best we can hope for is enough registered and practical nurses to provide professional nursing care in all skilled medical and nursing procedures for acutely ill patients and health instruction for those able to benefit from it, with practical nursing service for all simple routine duties performed by attendants trained by and under the supervision of the registered nursing staff.

One of the reasons why tuberculosis hospitals have special need of practical nurses is the lack of volunteer service. Only a very few Red Cross Volunteer Nurses' Aides have assisted in tuberculosis hospitals. Girls and boys of high school age are not wanted as messengers be-

---

* A few special tuberculosis hospitals still give a basic course in professional nursing with outside affiliations in general and maternity hospitals. These basic programs of study have been decreasing in recent years, and only about a dozen are functioning now.

cause of the risk to them; workers over thirty-five are preferred. Red Cross Gray Ladies are helping considerably, but they have no direct contact with patients.

DUTIES OF PRACTICAL NURSES

A careful review was made following visits in 1943–1945 to 13 tuberculosis hospitals or divisions for tuberculosis in general hospitals where practical nurses (licensed and unlicensed) were employed, in order to size up the type of duty assigned to them. The hospitals were located in six states and their capacity ranged from 60 to 2,000 beds; state, county, municipal, and private institutions were included. In three of the hospitals pupil practical nurses were having their training. As "graduates" were serving on a level with registered nurses in many of these hospitals, their duties are not included here.

As in general hospitals, it was rare to find practical nurses in charge of wards or alone at night in charge of acutely ill patients. The ratio of practical to professional nurses on duty at night drops, just as in general hospitals.

Duties forbidden to practical nurses, except in very real emergency, were catheterizations; oxygen therapy; care of postoperative patients; care of patients (until convalescent) with extensive surgery, especially thorocoplasty and lobectomy; transfusions; intramuscular injections; health advice and education except of the most elementary sort. Practical nurses were not assisting in the operating rooms, but were in treatment rooms, in some of the clinics, and in one x-ray department.

In 1938, a study of professional nursing procedures in six tuberculosis hospitals listed the following routine nursing procedures reported by hospitals as "good nursing practice" for each bed patient in every twenty-four hours (12).

Morning care without full bath
†Morning back rub
Toilet and oral hygiene before breakfast and dinner
Toilet before meals and before sleeping
Bedpan 6 times
Evening care—back rub
*Sputum collection and disposal

* Frequently assigned to non-nurses.
† Not daily events for patients out of danger.

*Meals and between-meal nourishment
†T.P.R.
†Bed bath

All the procedures on this list are now being carried out by practical nurses or aides in tuberculosis wards, except for critically ill patients. Following is a list of other duties recorded in this study, which are ordinarily carried out only by registered nurses but are now frequently assigned to practical nurses.

Admission of patients—weighing, etc.
Collection of specimens
Gastric contents to laboratory
‡Spinal puncture
Enema
Douche
Blood pressure
‡Medications
‡Aspiration of fluid
Application of hot compresses
Application of cold compresses
Shampoo
Sitzbath
Foot soak, hand soak
Transfer of patient
Care after death
‡Oxygen tent
‡Carbon dioxide inhalation
‡Postural drainage
Heat lamp treatment

‡Pneumothorax
Intravenous injection
Major surgical dressings
Minor surgical dressings
Throat irrigation
Hypodermic injection
Installation of drops in eye
Nose spray, throat spray
‡Preparation for operation
Changing position of patient
Feeding helpless patient
Preparation for x-ray
Transportation, wheel chair
Rectal irrigation
‡Bladder irrigation
Benzoin inhalation
Special care of mouth
Application of ointment or lotion
Throat gargle
Analgesic rub
Wintergreen rub

As recorded in this study, the total time spent by nurses during each twenty-four hours in the care of semi-ambulant patients was 1.5 hours; ambulant patients, 30 minutes; bed patients for medical care, 2.7 hours, and for surgical care, 3.3 hours (13). This was in peacetime; during the war many hospitals had to cut nursing time in half. In all six hospitals, an increase in staff was recommended to give adequate

* Frequently assigned to non-nurses.
† Not daily events for patients out of danger.
‡ Ordinarily done only by registered nurses, but with assistance from nonprofessional worker.

care. No study was made of the work that could be assigned to subsidiary workers, but this was one of the recommendations of the committee (14).

It does not take a "study" to see the many places in the large tuberculosis hospitals where practical nurses can be used to advantage after special instruction and under continued professional nursing supervision. A few of the duties they might perform are charge of ambulatory patients, night duty in convalescent wards, charge of supply rooms, assisting in treatment rooms (pneumothorax, etc.), assisting in clinics, assisting in wards of acutely ill patients, always under registered nurse direction, most of the work in children's wards, depending somewhat on the type of case.

In a great many tuberculosis hospitals since the war, registered nurses have not had time to instruct patients in their own care, in future adjustment to home and work, and in the protection of others. An efficient corps of well trained practical nurses, whose duties have been sharply defined and restricted to those safe for them to perform, would relieve the professional nurse so that time could be given to these "lessons." To make the excuse that "We have no time to teach and supervise practical nurses" is like saying that an army should be made up of officers to save time in training privates. Eventually, a head or "charge" practical nurse should be developed who would share with the professional nurse the responsibility of teaching and supervising this group.

THE DANGER OF WORKING IN A TUBERCULOSIS HOSPITAL

That there is danger to the nurse, be she professional or practical, in working with patients with active tuberculosis goes without saying. Unfortunately there is no proof, at least no definite study has been made, to indicate for which group the work is safer. There are hospitals with good and bad records for both groups. One of the best reports comes from Fairmount Hospital in Kalamazoo, Michigan, where only one practical nurse has broken down in twenty years of their employment, and her condition was discovered at the early minimal stage, she recovered and was back on duty within a year (15). The Municipal Tuberculosis Sanitarium in Peoria, Illinois, has a similar enviable record among professional nurses (16).

Supervisors are agreed regarding certain rules for all workers. They must receive orientation to the hospital no matter how thorough has been their experience elsewhere, and practical nurses will take a longer time to learn procedures than the professionals. Neither professional nor practical nurses should care for positive sputum cases until they have given absolute evidence of having mastered and understood the routines and the reasons for them. Observing good technique and obeying the rules must become second nature, and supervision must be maintained throughout the entire period of the affiliation.

According to Dr. Pollak, a well conducted tuberculosis sanatorium, where tuberculosis preventive measures are insisted upon for both patients and nursing staff, is a much safer place in which to work than the average general hospital, where the problem of tuberculosis is entirely neglected (16).

SALARIES AND PERSONNEL POLICIES

In the hospitals visited, practical nurses, trained attendants, and ward aides received from $60 to $130 a month with maintenance.* In all situations the base salaries of the professional nurses were higher by $5 or more than the maximum for the practical nurses. In one institution there was a difference of $25.

It was usual to find the same personnel practices applying to both groups of nurses, except that vacation periods were frequently one week less for practical nurses.

Practical nurse students were allowed from $30 to $75 a month and maintenance. The higher allowance went to those being trained within the hospital for continued work there, and reached its maximum in the second year—fairly good evidence that the hospital felt it was getting service from the student, not just teaching her.

"WE LIKE PRACTICAL NURSES"

Throughout the tuberculosis hospitals general approbation of the service of practical nurses from superintendents, doctors, patients, and other nurses was expressed to the writer. Several stated that practical nurses have a personality well adapted to the emotional problems of chronic illness. As a director of nurses in a tuberculosis hospital wrote:

During the depression I tried employing graduate nurses, but it was

---

* Civil Service usually classes these workers as trained attendants, and their salaries usually carried overtime pay and a war bonus.

not entirely satisfactory as they stayed only until they could find other work. Nursing chronically ill and convalescent patients did not especially attract them. Other fields of nursing were more attractive. Following this experience we expanded our practical nurse program, giving them more general work and responsibilities, so when this crisis came we rode the tide very well until about a year and a half ago. Then we too began to feel the shortage, but we still retained quality nursing even though we had to reorganize our work.

All administrators expressed a wish to secure more well trained and licensed practical nurses. To this end, there would seem to be four essential steps:

Assurance of sound health in all students and prospective graduate employees, and continued health supervision as long as they are employed

Sound grounding in practical nursing in an approved school before orientation to the tuberculosis hospital, unless the tuberculosis hospital is itself running an approved school of practical nursing

State licensure of practical nurses now practicing in tuberculosis hospitals, if necessary offering affiliations in general services to qualify for state recognition and examination

Instruction and continued supervision by professional nurses of both student and graduate practical nurses, and in-service programs to maintain interest.

REFERENCES

1 "Hospital service in the United States, 1945," *Journal of the American Medical Association* 127:777, 779, 781, March 31, 1945.
2 Louise Tattershall and Margaret D. West, "Wartime nursing care in 604 general hospitals," *American Journal of Nursing* 44:211–214, March 1944; Louise M. Tattershall and Marion E. Altenderfer, "Paid auxiliary nursing workers employed in general hospitals," *ibid.* 44:752–756, August 1944; Tattershall and Altenderfer, "Nursing personnel in general hospitals," *ibid.* 44:853–858, September 1944; Tattershall and Altenderfer, "Hours of nursing service in general hospitals," *ibid.* 44:963–966, October 1944.
3 Dorothy Deming, "Nursing in tuberculosis hospitals," *American Journal of Nursing* 43:1101–1108, December 1943, at p. 1102.
4 Information from Viktor O. Wilson, M.D., Director, Division of Child Hygiene, Minnesota Department of Health.

5 American Trudeau Society, "Minimal medical and administrative standards for tuberculosis hospitals and sanatoria; a report of the Committee on Sanatorium Standards," *American Review of Tuberculosis* 51:481–487, May 1945.

6 *Personnel problems of sanatoria resulting from war conditions;* report of a study made by the Committee on Sanatorium Standards of the American Trudeau Society, New York, National Tuberculosis Association, 1943, p. 18. See also the rating form for appraising sanatoria of the American Sanatorium Association and the National Tuberculosis Association, 1932, Nos. 71–73; Philip P. Jacobs, *Control of tuberculosis in the United States,* rev. ed., New York, National Tuberculosis Association, 1940, p. 126.

7 "A study of the nursing care of tuberculosis patients," *American Journal of Nursing* 38:1021–1037, September 1938, at p. 1037.

8 Deming (note 3), pp. 1102–1103.

9 *Personnel problems* (note 6), pp. 25, 26, 27, 28, 29, 31.

10 See also comment made by Dr. J. L. Moorman, Oklahoma City, to the effect that girls trained in his hospital "more nearly meet our needs than the graduate nurse called in from outside," *Southern Medical Journal* 24:902, October 1931.

11 *Personnel problems* (note 6), p. 10.

12 "A study of nursing care" (note 7), pp. 1027–1030, 1037.

13 "A study of nursing care" (note 7), pp. 1030–1031.

14 "A study of nursing care" (note 7), p. 1026.

15 Personal letter to the writer from the director of nurses, Fairmount Hospital, Kalamazoo, Michigan, February 28, 1945.

16 M. Pollak, "Don't neglect tuberculosis," *American Journal of Nursing* 44:1133–1134, December 1944, at p. 1134.

CHAPTER EIGHT

The Chronically Ill and the Aged;
Convalescents

THE CARE OF THE CHRONICALLY ILL AND THE AGED

OVER THE years, ever since professional nurses first won recognition through state registration, there has been one group of patients for whom all are agreed practical nursing is needed—the chronically ill. Federal, national, and state agencies have supported this contention time and again. Surveys and studies have proved it to everyone's satisfaction (1), and the laws in all the states licensing practical nurses specifically mention the care of the chronically sick as a legitimate field in which practical nurses may function. This is the type of case that private-duty professional nurses are usually willing to share with practical nurses, and there can be no doubt about the joyful reception families accord the practical nurse when she takes over the burden of a bedfast invalid.

The care of the chronically ill is a growing problem. We have an aging population who are surviving the hazards of childhood, adolescence, and child-bearing to fall victims of the so-called degenerative diseases usually developing in middle or later life. "Most of us, instead of dying incontinently of communicable disease, may now expect to live to run the gantlet of diseases which seem not to be communicable" (2). The three leading causes of death in the United States are heart disease, cancer, and cerebral hemorrhage, with nephritis and diabetes following closely. We have not conquered any one of them to the degree that we have routed pneumonia. One has only to look down the long reaches of the "day room" in any of our mental institutions filled with two or three hundred victims hopelessly afflicted with the various forms of senile psychoses to know that there are still rather dreadful penalties for living long.

Estimates indicate that by 1980—to look ahead less than thirty-five years—persons in middle and old age, that is over forty-five, will constitute a group 120 per cent larger than in 1930—assuming no outside influences (3). The records of cases cared for by practical nurses in homes reveal that much of their service is to people over forty-five with the familiar diseases of old age. There will be more and more of the same experience (4). Already visiting nurse associations report an increasing number of visits to bedridden patients of this age group.

Another addition—a tragic one—to those long-time case loads are the returning war wounded, some of them incapacitated for life, who will be entitled to medical and nursing care, including rehabilitation, "surpassing what was formerly available to the civilian long-term patients" (5). Plans of our government to see that these veterans are well served include the future provision of some 300,000 beds—at this writing there are about 80,000 (6). Many of the occupants of these beds will be lifetime charges, others will come and go, for example, veterans suffering from the remittent types of tropical diseases. All are entitled to free care from Uncle Sam and will form a considerable group of patients who fall under the classification of the chronically ill. Here again, however, a distinction will have to be made between those needing either practical or professional nursing and those for whom both types of nursing must be provided.

Statistical studies show that the average duration of illness increases with age (7), and older persons seem to suffer more illnesses requiring nursing care (8). We definitely face the growing problem of supplying long-term nursing service to this group, some of whom will need periods of hospital treatment as well as continued care at home. Many cannot afford professional nurses. Even moderately well-to-do families find some diseases a decided drain on family resources (9). It is hardly fair to jeopardize a talented young man's education to pay for three months of professional nursing service for an eighty-year-old grandfather in the terminal stages of paraplegia. "Is life or death more important?" the harassed mother demanded of the public health nurse. "Eighty years against eighteen. Tell me what to do!" Obviously, a less costly practical nurse giving care under professional supervision would help the budget materially.

Indeed, the greatest change in nursing as the result of the aging population, authorities agree, will be a reduction in the demand for private-duty professional nursing (10). In the report of the Committee on the Costs of Medical Care, the average nursing service given by practical nurses, in or outside hospitals, amounted to 19.3 days per case, as against 12.3 days per case by professional nurses. One may deduce from this that the practical nurse was already being used after the acute conditions had subsided (11).

The nursing care given the aged and chronically ill has never been anything to be proud of. We think of England's almshouses, of Bedlam Asylum, of early conditions in our own state and county poorhouses. In 1844, Dorothea Dix reported county poorhouses "in deplorable condition" (12). As late as 1928, Helen W. Munson, writing of nursing care for the inmates of almshouses said, "Nursing—skilled nursing—hardly touches the inmates of almshouses [the poor, the aged, the chronically sick] at all." In 1928–1929, of 10,072 inmates of almshouses, 6,291 were sick or infirm and 20 to 30 per cent were in need of nursing care—not just physical, custodial care. Almshouses employed few registered nurses; in New York state only 3 out of 27 employed them. Care was frequently given by inmates; often the matron had to do all the nursing. In some cities at this period visiting nurse associations had refused to add the care of any more "chronics." Unspeakable conditions have been reported through the years (13).

Conditions are but slightly improved in some of our county homes today. The situation has been eased in some states by the withdrawal to state institutions of patients suffering from special conditions, such as tuberculosis, cancer, and mental disease, but up-to-date, properly equipped, comfortable institutions where adequate medical supervision and skilled nursing care are available are still only blueprints in many states. A well trained corps of practical nurses could handle most of the care so badly needed by the inmates in the infirmaries of our present-day almshouses (14).

Although the writer is in entire agreement with the general statement that the chronically ill need practical nurses, she is equally convinced they need professional nursing also and in greater amount than they are now receiving it. There are many reasons why this is so. Even superficial observation and study of this group of patients and their nursing care at home and in hospitals shows that the whole situation surrounding longtime illness has changed, and it will change even more in the next decade. Sweeping statements as to who should give care and where are no longer safe; conclusions lightly drawn ten years ago no longer fit the facts, and professional nurses are becoming acutely aware that the turn of events is making the nursing of the chronically ill a specialty in itself.

In the minds of many nurses and laymen, a chronic patient is still pictured as an elderly, infirm person, probably bedridden, certainly housebound, who has no hope of improvement and every likelihood of being a helpless invalid for the rest of his days. Arthritis, paralysis, unhealed fractures, heart disease, cancer, and old age are thought of as the usually crippling conditions. Actually, there is no age limit for those who may suffer from prolonged illness or injury, no line of demarcation between what may be called acute and chronic stages, and no typical disease which can be, strictly speaking, classified as "chronic." An illness of normally short duration may leave a condition which will incapacitate an individual for years, a "chronic" illness may clear up in short order. During chronicity a condition may develop which is acute in the extreme. Babies under six months are in our general and orthopedic hospitals today starting successive surgical repairs or medical treatments which will drag on for years (15).

Today, authorities dealing with prolonged illness do not admit that a chronic condition exists unless "the disease is progressive and the prognosis indefinite" (16). Even then, there will be periods in the course of a chronic illness during which the patient must be considered as acutely ill, given treatments appropriate to the new or intensified condition (frequently available only in hospitals), and attended by nurses equipped to give the highest degree of skillful care. A simple example of such a situation is that of a mentally ill patient who develops lobar pneumonia with cardiac distress and spends a week in an oxygen tent. There are, of course, diseases which are normally of long duration; diabetes is typical of the group. Tuberculosis, mental disease, and orthopedic conditions are apt to incapacitate for many months, but need not or may not.

The point to be emphasized, therefore, is that, regardless of whether the patient is cared for at home or in an institution, there may be periods when professional nursing care is essential. We cannot say that the care of the chronically ill belongs solely in the hands of practical nurses.

The present-day attitude toward the afflictions of old age is a hopeful one. It attacks the former negative psychology that accepted old age almost as a disease and substitutes a picture of quiet enjoyment of all that has gone before. The concept of preventing deterioration and subacute infirmities by a rational adjustment to decreased physical strength under medical supervision is taking away much of the dread of old age. Even when inevitable handicaps overtake a person, the doctor still holds a trump card—restoration through modern medical care or surgery of sufficient activity to be satisfying even though limited. In effect the doctor says, "This condition need not be so 'chronic' as you think; we can better the situation. Come into the hospital for a few weeks and let us show you."

The problem of nursing the chronic sick has also been brought forcibly to the attention of the English authorities. Before the war the College of Nursing in Great Britain preferred to have "attendants" trained on the job in each institution and were opposed to the training of practical nurses (17). Discussions as to proper individual care for the growing case load of chronically ill were widespread and vigorous. Hospitals had great difficulty in attracting a well qualified staff, "partly because of the nature of the nursing itself, and partly because of the conditions under which it is carried out. The employment of an 'assistant nurse' (not registered) is often thoroughly unsatisfactory. . . . The establishment and recognition of a second grade of nurse . . . would be likely to meet with keen opposition from a certain section of the nursing profession" (18). However, by 1942, through a reorganization of nursing, not only had a second level of nursing been recognized as appropriate for the care of this group of patients, but the registered professional nurses had accepted a plan which gives the assistant nurse legal status. Their major function will be the care, under professional supervision, of the aged ill and the mentally afflicted.

Studies of Chronic Illness

Our most reliable sources of information on the prevalence and costs of chronic disease in this country are the reports from the National Health Survey (1935–1936) made by the United States Public Health Service (18) and those from the Committee on the Costs of Medical Care (19). In the former survey, of those reported to have chronic disease, 30 per cent were under thirty-five years of age and 15 per cent were over sixty-five, leaving 55 per cent in the productive age group. Unfortunately, this study did not differentiate between care given by registered and nonprofessional nurses, or between licensed and unlicensed practical nurses.

Studies of chronic illness in New York city have shown that nursing care of the home cases was seriously inadequate. On the other hand, it is too costly to keep these patients in general hospitals and the atmosphere is "inappropriate" (20). It was suggested that small well regulated nursing homes were needed.*

In 1931, a study of 78 private homes for the care of the aged in New York city, housing 8,300 inmates, revealed equally inadequate nursing care. In 67 homes, 64 professional nurses and 165 attendants were employed for 2,822 persons. Infirmaries supplied 1,541 beds in these homes. Some of these homes used visiting nurse service (23). Many of the patients had been in the homes ten years or more. Homes without infirmaries sent their sick to hospitals. One of the recommendations resulting from this study was the setting of a standard for medical and nursing care in private homes: at least one registered nurse and a complement of practical nurses and attendants in all homes for the aged in which the city of New York paid for the care of dependent chronically ill patients, the ratio being one registered nurse to every 100 patients, assisted by practical nurses and attendants in the ratio of one to 25 patients (24). It is not known whether this standard was attained or is held to now in times of shortages.

In 1937, 62 per cent of the welfare institutions and the homes for the indigent of the state of New Jersey employed subsidiary workers (25). A sampling of 24 hospitals of all types in Pennsylvania in 1939 showed 20 employing some form of nurses' aides, but only 4 reported these as practical nurses. The physicians who reported that they were using the service of practical nurses in homes said that one-half the nurses were serving chronically ill (medical) cases (26).

One of the most recent studies of the chronically ill was undertaken on a state-wide basis by the Research Division of the Public Welfare Council in Connecticut. In 1944 the population of the state was 1,760,-000, about half urban. The study concerned mainly the indigent recipients of public assistance, but a few hospitals and private agencies sup-

* In 1933, of 1,935 cases visited, 805 were physically ill or disabled, 151 were mentally ill, 201 were both physically and mentally ill, leaving 778 who showed no disability (21). The diagnoses in 27,507 cases over sixty-five years of age discharged from New York city hospitals were diseases of the cardio-vascular system, alcoholism, arteriosclerosis, cataract, fractures, traumatic conditions, and cancer. Of 746 cases, 44 were bedridden and 149 were homebound. In the study of chronic patients made in connection with the Visiting Housekeeper project, 600 patients were divided into two groups: 388 needing custodial care and 212 needing nursing only; of the latter, 93 were bedridden, 84 homebound, 35 up and about (22).

plied data. No record was made of the type of nursing service being rendered. The diseases reported were typical of those found in previous studies. The age distribution of patients was wide, but the distribution within the age groups was of interest, showing that 76 per cent (of 26,000 persons) were adults, 29 per cent over 75 years of age. Of 19,858 patients, 1,899 were bedridden, 5,691 partially ambulatory, and 9,601 ambulatory; the condition of 2,667 was unknown (27).

Recommendations growing out of this study take into consideration the need for more public health nurses, more bedside nursing care in families, more institutional and clinical facilities and beds to serve the chronically ill, and a "housekeepers-aide corps" to be established, "probably under the supervision and pay of the nursing agency" (28). If by this "corps" is meant merely housekeepers, the public health nurses will be doing many of the simpler nursing jobs more economically performed by practical nurses; if a housekeeper-nursing service is intended, the licensed practical nurses in Connecticut (the legal title is trained attendant) may question where the line can be drawn between their functions and those of the nursing housekeepers (29). The five recommended state boarding homes for the aged are to have the service of resident professional nurses, but nothing is said about the use of licensed practical nurses.

This study shows vividly the conditions surrounding chronic illness which concern nurses. Undoubtedly, questions as to who is to do what and how more professional supervision will be provided will be solved as the further steps in studying ways and means are developed.

In November 1944, the Chicago Council of Social Agencies reported on its Central Service for the Chronically Ill, now conducted by the Institute of Medicine and financed by the Community Fund:

> . . . There are between 45,000 and 50,000 chronic invalids in Cook County, of whom about 15,000 must have care outside their own homes. The Service takes care of about 5,000 of the invalids, in the Home for Incurables, in the hospital section at Oak Forest, in general hospitals and in the better nursing homes. However, "two-thirds of the invalids who need care away from home are scattered over the city and county in inadequate boarding houses and so-called nursing homes. . . ."
> . . . The good Lord Himself couldn't give $100 worth of care for $40 a month. The main trouble with the homes I have seen is lack of money and know-how. Most of them don't know the first thing about business.

They don't even include their own salaries in the cost of the homes. We've had one meeting for these operators; about 30 of them came. It's awfully hard for them to get away. . . .

While the medical profession is dealing with the alleviation and prevention of chronic illness and welfare forces are planning care for those who are already disabled, advice and leadership are needed by the agencies already serving the community and the patients (as well as their families) who need help. This is the present job of the Central Service—and while it may never be finished, it is certainly well begun (30).

It is evident from the scattered and incomplete statistics cited above that no nation-wide, comprehensive data exist showing the amount of demand for practical nursing care of the chronically ill, nor do we have reports on the number of practical nurses, licensed or unlicensed, now employed in such care in homes or institutions throughout the United States. The irrefutable evidence of the need for more practical nurses in this field can be found in the rising case load, the fact that professional nurses' time is being taken by complicated treatments, and the demand on the part of families, and now of hospitals, for practical nurses.

Types of Care Needed by the Chronically Ill

Roughly, chronically ill patients fall into three classes: those requiring rather intensive professional nursing care with or without the help of practical nurses, those needing practical nursing care under professional supervision, and those who can get along with custodial care (31), not necessarily by a practical nurse. The first group usually makes use of special and general hospitals and outpatient services; the second is usually at home, in nursing homes, foster homes, or homes for the aged; and the last group may be almost anywhere, except in general and special hospitals. In all these situations, except the last, the licensed practical nurse has a place, and in all the agencies caring for the aged the case load of long-term illness is growing heavier.

There is another small group of patients who do not need or who refuse care in an institution, yet who cannot maintain their own homes. Most of these patients cannot be cared for by relatives for one reason or another. They usually have a chronic condition which may be progressing slowly, but they are not completely incapacitated. Usually they are able to pay something for care which approximates what they would secure in their own homes. Such patients usually do well in small nursing homes or foster nursing homes. Practical nurses are ideal in caring for this group, under professional nursing supervision. Such service might be on a part-time basis. The New York City Department of Public Welfare has recently added an experimental program of foster home care for the aged and chronically ill (32).

Old people who are not ill or in need of nursing treatments, but are feeble, easily tired and confused, partially incapacitated, and frequently incontinent, need mainly custodial care. Some responsible, friendly person must keep these people warm, dry, fed, clothed, and protected from accident. Someone must supervise their meals, their use of wheel chairs, elevators, and stairs, and see that they are kept busy with whatever light duties they are able to do. Someone must be on hand at night in case of emergency. Their care resembles that needed by little children. Visiting or continual housekeeper service by an individual who knows a little home nursing is a possible solution to this problem for those at home.

In 1935, the Housekeeping Service for Chronic Patients at Home, a W.P.A. project instituted in New York city and elsewhere, went a long way toward serving the group of dependent old-age clients with illness, of whom 97 per cent were found to be handicapped by some chronic infirmity (33). Nursing care and supervision were usually given by the visiting nurse service. The housekeeping aides were trained to care for the aged and infirm, to provide occupations for them, and to care for children. If necessary, the visiting nurse taught the housekeeper to give certain simple nursing care, such as she would teach a member of the family. In New York city, about 20 per cent of the families did not need professional nursing services; those who did were visited as often as four times a week, as infrequently as once a month. The charge for the housekeeper's service in these projects was $2.75 a day (34).

While the line between housekeeper service and practical nursing is now indefinite, it is clear that, if the presence of an invalid needing nursing is the reason for calling in outside help, that assistance should be from someone qualified to care for the patient, the household being secondary. If, however, the care of the patient is only incidental to the need of homemaking, a housekeeper is the more suitable worker. In deciding who shall care for these patients, the experience in New York showed that as much depended on the family situation as on the physical condition of the invalid. Joint conferences of all those concerned with the case—doctor, nurse, practical nurse, social worker, and family —may be needed to decide the best adjustment of service in a given family (35).

In institutions, custodial care also includes assisting patients to take part in the activities of the group, escorting them to chapel, to occupational therapy rooms, and to parties. The custodian or attendant should know how to take temperature, give bed baths, and prepare invalid diets. She must be able to give conservative advice regarding the common cold, sore throat, constipation, and other "household" emergencies.

There are typical housekeeping duties on the wards of all institutions—including the special hospitals—which do not call for nursing training of any type, yet which all too frequently are assigned to professional or practical nurses.* Such are supervision of heavy cleaning (walls, floors, windows, units, diet kitchens, rugs, drapes, etc.) ; care of linen closet; serving; mending; care of patients' clothes, lockers, beds; disinfection of units; care of ward plants and flowers. Responsibility for these duties could be assigned to the housekeeping department of the hospital, which in many institutions is under the charge of the director of nurses. A good housekeeping department with an experienced supervising housekeeper would lift an immense burden from the shoulders of many a weary professional nurse. Reassignment of the duties suitable for a non-nursing staff would result in more nursing time for the patients.

Duties of Practical Nurses

The physical care of aged and chronic patients, aside from special treatments ordered to suit each case, is much the same day in and day out wherever the patient may be, and the duties assigned to practical nurses in institutions are also much the same everywhere.

Routine physical care includes bathing, feeding, toilet, special care

---

* During wartime visits to some fifty institutions of from 50 to 7,000 beds, registered nurses were seen dusting lockers, spraying mattresses, polishing glass doors, and were usually responsible for supervising all the ward cleaning.

of back, care of bed, dressing and undressing, assistance with wheel chair, crutches, etc., and diversions for the patient. Special care is given as needed: temperature, pulse, respiration; care of the helpless, unconscious, or dying; restraint; simple dressings; irrigations, poultices, enemas; preoperative and postoperative care; simple medications.

Practical nurses in hospitals are usually asked to care for specimens, supplies, equipment, linen, flowers, water pitchers, medicine cabinets, and beds, and to make beds and do cleaning of ward units and lavatories. They take patients to and from treatment rooms, admit and dismiss cases. Postmortem care is their responsibility.

In all institutions, the practical nurse assists the registered nurse in any way requested, the registered nurse taking the responsibility when she assigns a task. Such duties as watching an unconscious patient, checking on the ice supply for oxygen tents, observing the rate of an intravenous injection are typical assignments.

In a hospital of approximately 100 beds for chronically ill men, women, and adolescents, in Hamilton, Ontario, the students from the school for practical nurses take considerable responsibility for all bed care, under close supervision of registered nurses.

Usually the policy of the hospital dictates the assignment of more difficult duties, such as the giving of "single order" medications. Here again we find the greatest variation in the treatments a practical nurse may give. In a large home for the aged, practical nurses were limited to giving general care, giving enemas, taking temperatures, and reinforcing dressings. In a hospital, practical nurses gave all medications, including all types of hypodermics, colostomy irrigations, and dressings. Rules about hypodermics were found to differ under certain conditions. In one hospital, practical nurses who are "graduates of a course in practical nursing" may give hypodermics. In another, practical nurses may give hypodermics, but not of narcotics. In another, pupil practical nurses were taught in class to give hypodermics but the hospital did not allow them to administer them to hospital patients. In still another, practical nurses were forbidden to give medications of any kind.

It is pertinent to ask at this point: What is the objection to teaching practical nurses to administer medications in undivided doses by hypodermic? Patients, families, even children are being taught to give their own insulin injections. What is there so difficult or dangerous about giving a hypodermic? The only answer the writer could elicit was, "We do not think it is safe."*

In addition to the routine physical care of chronically ill patients, housekeeping and home-making duties vary all the way from almost no responsibility in either institution or home to the point where three-quarters of the practical nurse's time is occupied by nonpatient service. In most private homes about half of her time is given to home duties, but that division may vary greatly with each day. Saturday, for example, when the children are home and the weekend shopping and planning must be finished, is devoted largely to housekeeping. If the patient is restless, has a bad night, or is in pain, much of the twenty-four hours goes into her care. The practical nurse is taught during her training to schedule the invalid's day, week, and even month, covering such activities as shampoos, turning mattresses, rearranging room, and so forth, leaving time to run the house, prepare meals, and take care of the children. Professional nurses receive very little instruction in these household matters and no practice. "I'd be floored," a professional nurse told the writer, "if in addition to caring for my patient, I had to take on the running of the house, planning rationed meals, and caring for the children—all on a budget. I'd hate it because I would not do it well."

Special Problems in Hospitals and Homes

At Montifiore Hospital in New York city, a large voluntary hospital that accepts all types of "chronic illness" except mental cases, the lists of treatments and departments rendering service to patients read like those in a general hospital for acute illness. A careful survey made by the hospital itself disclosed that these patients needed more medication by mouth and rectum and hypodermically than most patients in general hospitals. Treatments comprised a wide range: irrigations of the bladder, colon, stomach, eye, ear, and throat; protoclysis; paracentesis of abdomen and thorax; artificial pneumothorax; douches; massage; lumbar punctures; intravenous injections—to say nothing of emergencies such as cerebral hemorrhage, heart failure, and fractures. Many patients were in casts. Special diets included those for diabetes, peptic

---

* This is reminiscent of the experience of professional nurses. In 1887, it was routine in Old Blockley Hospital in Philadelphia to call a doctor to give a hypodermic at night (36).

ulcer, pernicious anemia, malnutrition, and nephritis. Patients were receiving service from such departments as x-ray, fluoroscopy, cystoscopy, physiotherapy, dental hygiene, and, of course, the operating rooms for major and minor surgery. Quantitatively, the chronic patient in a hospital needs as much care as an acutely ill patient (37).

The average length of stay of the so-called chronic patient at Montifiore was six weeks (few stayed longer than three months), proving that patients are hospitalized for treatment. The aim is to send them home improved. Indeed, Dr. E. M. Bluestone, Medical Director of Montefiore Hospital, looks forward to the time when "no distinction will be made between [long-term and short-term] patients when we plan for their care, so long as they require intensive medical care in a hospital" (38). Some patients return to the care of practical nurses at home, some to a custodial type of care at home or in another institution, while many report to hospital outpatient services or go to their doctor's offices.

On the day of the writer's visit to Montefiore, nearly 95 per cent of the beds were occupied. It was very evident that the type of treatment being given called for the skill and knowledge of a professional nurse supplemented by efficient practical nursing under supervision. Indeed, the service of the practical nurses there is really built around the central professional nursing staff and supports it at points designated by the professional nursing supervisor.* It appeared to be a smoothly functioning plan which could be copied in giving service in the home.

Dr. Boas stresses a point about hospital service to the chronically ill which applies also to home care: the supervisor must know and study the chronic patient. "Nursing technique is not made simpler by the fact that illness is protracted in its course" (39). An analysis of the treatments and procedures, and of the patient's temperament—and, in the home, of the family situation—must be made before a division of responsibilities between professional and practical nurses can be made.

Nurses must learn to appreciate the difference in attitude of hospital patients ill a long time and those under care for a brief period who confidently look forward to a return to normal life shortly. "A conscientious nurse is challenged by the various types of patients and their acceptance or rejection of their handicaps. Complete acceptance of help-

---

* There is a school for practical nurses at Montefiore Hospital. Graduate practical nurses are also employed.

lessness may be worse than constant fretting against fate. Stimulation is needed by one, comfort and calm acceptance by the other, while both need interests in which to forget themselves. Not twice will the need or the handling of the need be the same." She cites preparing vegetables for dinner (40).

There are complicating factors in chronic illness cared for at home that make such cases difficult for practical nurses working alone. The most socially significant distinction between acute and chronic illness from the home standpoint, and therefore the home nurse's viewpoint, is its effect on family situations. Almost any family can cope with a week or two of acute illness; a bedfast or housebound patient demanding care for months or even years is a different problem entirely, and one that calls for varied adjustments. "The presence of an invalid whose physical and mental suffering, whose needs, desires, whims and fancies are always in the foreground determines the work, the recreation and the development of the lives of other members of the family. . . . Among the poor these difficulties are accentuated" (41). The attitude of the family toward the invalid, their ability to pay for care to relieve the homemaker of the nursing burden, their efforts to continue normal family social life, are all typical problems posed by prolonged illness in the home.

Some of these problems become too great for the practical nurse to handle without help from outside sources. The physician calling once or twice a month may not even be aware of the difficulties. The advantages to the practical nurse and the family of supervisory and consultant service from a professional nurse, preferably a public health nurse, in such situations cannot be overestimated (42). She will know what other kinds of workers and community resources to draw upon.

The practical nurse should not be expected to take full responsibility of a home case if a chronic condition is likely to shift rapidly to an acute stage. Such responsibility is not only fraught with danger to the patient but is definitely unfair to the nurse. There is no better illustration of this than the care of a cardiac patient.

Heart disease calls for many highly scientific tests, procedures, and medications during diagnosis and treatment, most of which are carried out in hospitals or doctors' offices. Professional nurses assist with many procedures in which a thorough understanding of the principles of physics and chemistry and experience in taking extremely accurate measurements are needed. The physician relies on the nurse for close observation and interpretation of symptoms—especially variations in pulse and respiration—and expects her to adjust her nursing care and supervision of the case to suit these changes. The nurse must understand the implication of new symptoms and must use her judgment in carrying out the doctor's orders until he can be reached. The practical nurse does not receive this sort of grounding in her school, she does not have the background of even elementary science or the experience to enable her to judge these conditions. She has never handled and dissected a heart, probably never attended an autopsy, never seen the irregular, wavering peaks of the heartbeats made in sphygmographic tracings of the pulse, never listened with a stethoscope to a fluttering, racing heart, never taken blood pressure. Her knowledge of the heart and its function is elementary in the extreme—about that of a high school senior. Yet the complete home care of a cardiac patient is frequently put into her hands.

If the cardiac patient is at home in the sole care of a practical nurse, the doctor must take time to explain fully just what may be expected, what symptoms to watch for, what activities may be allowed. In heart conditions there is frequently a difference between the amount of activity a patient can undertake and the amount he should undertake in order to prevent further damage and assure recovery (43). Unless the doctor makes it absolutely clear what he wants the patient to do and not to do, the practical nurse may easily be persuaded to let her patient do more than he should. It is so much a question of judgment and she has so little by which to judge. She may not even understand the full meaning of the terms the doctor uses so glibly. Furthermore, discriminating judgment in the care of the cardiac goes far beyond the doctor's written orders, and that is where the practical nurse's understanding cannot follow.

An example of a near catastrophe in a Michigan home demonstrates this point. The doctor thought he had stated clearly that the patient might be allowed only moderate activity, no strain, no excitement, no stair climbing; he should have eight hours' sleep at night, two hours' daytime rest, a short walk on the level in fine weather. There came a day when the patient's bowels had not moved in thirty-six hours. About an hour after an unusually large and rich meal he offered to help his wife move some books from one low shelf to another, involving stooping and lifting several books at a time. He did this for some ten minutes. The practical nurse was "just about to stop him" when he gasped, clutched his side, and sank into a chair struggling for breath. The attack was not fatal, but the nurse admitted she had not realized there was any danger in what her patient was doing.

There are, of course, cardiac conditions so serious that professional nursing only should be considered for them: congestive heart failure, angina pectoris when recurrent, coronary thrombosis or occlusion, and many others. The doctor should be the one to decide, but the registered nurse (at the registry, the visiting nurse association, or in the hospital) may have to decide on the assignment of duties. Again, the vital importance of shared responsibilities and close supervision of the practical nurse is apparent.

The care of long-time illness in young or old is not easy. Doctors and nurses agree heartily with the families of these patients—that the invalid is nearly always "difficult" or has his difficult days. Depression, discouragement, irritability, loss of appetite, sleeplessness, whining, rebellion, being sorry for himself, seeking attention, refusing to obey orders, and relapsing into sulky silences, are all moods through which the average person passes while he learns to live a restricted life. Nurses soon discover that an invalid of any age reverts to the behavior and attitudes, often the interests, of a lower age level: men become boys, boys become children, children become babies. These changes are not easy to handle. It takes considerable personal resourcefulness, infinite patience, maturity of judgment, and insight on the part of the nurse to work out happy solutions of the problems.

"Those caring for the chronically ill at home," writes Dr. Boas, "have at times been undisciplined, unresourceful, often irresponsible and lazy and at times cruel and neglectful. . . . Older women make more satisfactory attendants for the chronically ill than do the younger ones" (44). A young woman is apt to find the case unexciting; she lacks the necessary patience and tolerance.

Dr. Zeman writes, "The important emotion which dominates the attitude of old people in illness is fear, fear of suffering, fear of death and the bitter realization of increasing uselessness." The second fear usually decreases with age, the third may grow and be accompanied by the despair of becoming economically dependent (45). Fundamental to all treatment of these patients—indeed to all patients—is the basic realization that one is dealing with an individual and not a disease (46). No matter how commonplace or desperate the conditions or outlook may appear to the nurse, the invalid believes his case to be exceptional. Nurses must learn to foster and share this optimism and to build on it.

Many trivial things become more important to a chronic invalid than to the acutely ill patient. An attendant with a creative imagination can do much to relieve the monotony of the invalid's life. Sunshine, a view, visitors, rearrangement of the room, plants, pets, games, light handiwork, colorful dressing gowns, attractive trays, variations in food, attention to comfortable posture, something to read, to hear, to talk about—these are only a few of the mental "boosts" all nurses must learn to give their patients. Schools for practical nurses are doing a better job every year in enriching the practical nurses' armamentarium in this field of simple occupational therapy. As a result, many practical nurses are far better equipped now in this respect than are professional nurses.

In looking at the function of the practical nurse serving in homes where there is chronic illness, we must not lose sight of one of her greatest assets, that of holding the home together. Two actual cases will illustrate this contribution.

Mrs. Eves was eighty, her sister, Miss Olds, seventy-eight. They had lived together for forty years. They owned a small five-room house. One night Mrs. Eves fell down the cellar stairs and broke her hip. She refused to go to the hospital. Her doctor immobilized the hip as best he could. Miss Olds was too feeble to lift her sister. The third day after the accident the doctor came with papers for Miss Olds to sign, admitting her sister to a hospital and herself to an old ladies' home. Miss Olds tore up the papers. The doctor called the visiting nurse who in turn secured a practical nurse next day. For six weeks the elderly sisters—well fed, well nursed, clean, comfortable, resigned to facing the coming separation as long as they were together—were really happy. After the funeral, Miss Olds still had enough money to pay her admission fees to the old ladies' home.

Mrs. Hunt's husband was in the Marines, her two children in grade school. Her mother, nearing ninety, was bedridden, paralyzed on the left side. She was an unusually heavy woman for her years, being tall and large boned. She spoke with great difficulty. She had to be fed, bathed, clothed and diapered like a baby, and Mrs. Hunt did it all in spite of being frail herself. She weighed 115 pounds and had had one kidney removed. Then she caught flu. The doctor was getting ready to send both women to the hospital and the children to the city shelter when a neighbor suggested a practical nurse. She was still there after five months. Mrs. Hunt had gained five pounds, she could get outdoors every day, and the children were better cared for in every way.

"No one will ever know," a young working woman said to the writer in a Boston home, "what it meant to have Miss Blank come in and take care of my father. It wasn't just the nursing care, it was the way she made a home for us."

A pertinent observation was made by another user of this type of service: A public health nurse can easily meet the skilled nursing needs of the aged ill at home, "but if the floor is dirty, the dishes piled in the sink, and the patient in need of clean linen, fresh clothing or properly cooked meals, no one will expect the visiting nurse to drop her profession and become a houseworker" (47). Yet the comfort of the patient and the encouragement to recovery depend on just such practical, everyday matters as clean clothes, good food, and an orderly house.

Those studying the visiting housekeeper project in New York concluded, ". . . it is a public benefit to keep people [chronically ill] in their homes where possible, instead of assigning them to occupy hospital beds sorely needed for serious and emergency illness" (48). People—especially elderly people—are usually happier and more cheerful in the surroundings and normal atmosphere of a home. There are today hundreds of homes where practical nurses are preventing the breakup of family ties, the separation of children, and the loss of the home as a home.

Planning for the Future

As Dr. Bluestone truly states, "There is no denying the priority of the claim of the short-term patient, but our plan for the long-term patient is the measure of our philanthropy in the last analysis" (49). All the foregoing statements regarding nursing service to long-term invalids boils down to the conclusion that the complexity of the problem, the increasing number of chronically ill, and our expanding knowledge of the field of geriatrics call for:

Special emphasis on the care of the chronically ill during the training of all nurses, both professional and practical

A survey of the amount and kind of nursing service needed by these patients at home and in institutions

A study of the problems peculiar to the case before dividing the care of a patient between professional and practical nurses

Provision for professional nursing supervision wherever practical nurses are serving

We may also conclude that because the majority of chronically ill patients have only brief periods when professional nursing service alone is needed, and the happiness of the patient and family depend so greatly on receiving practical nursing care, the most valuable contribution practical nurses can make to the medical care program is in this field, while the professional nurse may regard her contribution as the supervision of practical nursing care wherever it is rendered.

THE CARE OF CANCER PATIENTS

Inasmuch as cancer, the second ranking cause of death in the United States, has become of outstanding interest to public health authorities, scientists, and the medical and nursing professions, an effort was made to see nursing services for cancer patients at home, in general hospitals, and in special institutions for the care of malignant diseases. Needless to say, many of the patients seen in the homes for the aged or in the subacute wards of hospitals were cancer patients.

Patients in the special cancer hospitals are all receiving treatments which must be in the hands or under the very close supervision of registered nurses. Except, however, for those critically ill or needing special treatments, cancer patients may be and are very efficiently and safely nursed by practical nurses. Many patients are up and about, needing the same sort of general supervision as convalescents. Many patients are staying in the hospital for massive doses of x-ray or the insertion of radium. Many surgical patients are ambulatory after the first few days and many hundreds go home as soon as possible, relying on visiting nurse service at first, later returning for follow-up treatment or supervision in the outpatient clinics.

In addition to caring for the patients who are currently under treatment for malignant disease and who are for the most part up and about, the practical nurses assist the professional nurses in the care of seriously ill bedridden patients and those for whom very complicated treatments or dressings are necessary. The care of the terminal case can be largely in the hands of a practical nurse, with continuous watchful supervision from the professional.

In the special cancer hospitals, all dressings, irrigations, special douches, and medications are assigned to professional nurses. Practical nurses give baths, make beds, reinforce dressings, feed helpless patients, give enemas, and assist in the treatment, x-ray* clinic, and examining rooms. On the day of the writer's visit to one special cancer hospital there were 195 patients, 67 full time professional nurses (the normal peacetime staff was 132), 12 licensed practical nurses, and two or three Red Cross Volunteer Nurses' Aides on duty on each floor during the day. Cadet student nurses were expected for six months' service in the near future. Many parttime professional nurses were also helping out. No practical nurses were serving in the operating rooms, though they assisted in the supply room.

This hospital had made a very detailed study of the jobs which could be assigned to workers other than nurses. Practical nurses no longer carried messages, left their floors for supplies, or handled food trays. As soon as it was found that a total of eight hours of nursing time a week went into answering telephone calls, all calls were routed through a special receptionist. In this hospital, one gained the impression that practical nurses were being used to their best capacity, but for no service that a non-nurse could do. Similarly, no professional nurse was doing practical nursing or an aide's job. "We could use many more practical nurses if we could get them. There is always need for their service in this type of hospital," said the director of nurses.

In another special cancer hospital of 64 beds, 42 professional nurses and 5 practical nurses were employed. Red Cross Grey Ladies were assisting in the dispensary. More practical nurses could be used if available, but "not many more."

Practical nurses were not on night duty in any of the special hospitals visited.

In observing the situations in these hospitals where almost without exception 50 per cent of the nursing care given cancer patients was or could have been given by practical nurses—with the probable exception of patients having extensive surgery whose care might be restricted to professional nursing for four or five days before and after

---

* In one special hospital, however, the practical nurses had been taken out of the high power x-ray treatment rooms.

operation—one could not help questioning whether in the future ratios of practical nurses to professional staff might not be reversed. Instead of one or two practical nurses and five or six professional nurses assigned to each ward or floor of chronically ill patients, might not six or seven licensed practical nurses working under the supervision of three professionals (one for each shift) result in as good service to the patient?

Such a suggestion is predicated on the assumption that the practical nurses would be graduates of a state approved course in practical nursing, licensèd to practice, and under expert, continual professional supervision.

Salaries and Personnel Policies

The salaries for practical nurses in special cancer hospitals came within the same range as in general institutions: in private hospitals, $75 to $110 a month with full maintenance (laundry and all meals); in public (civil service) hospitals, $100 to $125 plus 20 per cent bonus for the duration of the war (no meals or maintenance).

The same personnel policies applied to both practical and professional nursing groups. The practical nurses were included in staff activities, shared the dining room, observed new treatments, and attended lectures that interested them. They were given orientation to their work by the director of nursing education.

The ages of practical nurses in these institutions were slightly higher —thirty to forty-five—than in general hospitals.

Home Care

The nursing care of the cancer patient at home is a greater responsibility for the practical nurse than in the hospital. There are many such cases, ranging from the convalescent who keeps the practical nurse a few days or weeks to tide over recovery from surgical procedures, to the patient who has returned home to die. As institutions prefer to send moribund patients home, visiting nurses and practical nurses care for many of these distressing cases. To the practical nurse on full time home duty they present a special problem, for their care nearly always calls for procedures practical nurses have not been taught in the schools and are not allowed to do in the hospitals. These include catheterization of both men and women patients, colostomy and other internal irrigations, difficult deep dressings where there is profuse discharge, hypodermic injections of narcotics, medications dangerous to have about the house, and caring for the quite frequent emergency of hemorrhage. Yet, as the doctors invariably point out when a visiting nurse worries about leaving the evening catheterization of a patient to a practical nurse, the treatment is essential to a good night's rest for the patient. Since the patient is beyond help, the only thing that matters is to make him comfortable, and there is no one else to do it.

CARE IN CONVALESCENCE

Like the chronic state, convalescence has no recognizable boundaries. To the physician, it may appear to start when the red blood count rises, the temperature falls, or congestion clears; to the patient, it is the day he sits up, gets out of bed, or eats solid food; while to the nurse, the signs take the form of irritability, boredom, and fretfulness in her patient. If the illness has been acute or long drawn out, convalescence is accompanied by easy fatigue, lack of interest in anything calling for effort, and a finicky appetite (50). "With nervous energy diminished, all the organs are below their normal degree of functional activity" (51), and the state may present "organic, psychogenic or even purely imaginary phenomena about which we know far too little" (52).

Convalescence—again like chronic disease—is no longer shoved aside as less interesting or less important than acute illness. In the light of present-day therapeutic measures, convalescent care and rehabilitation present a field of ever widening interest (53). Rest, good food, fresh air, and sunshine—once considered the only essentials to recovery—are but the basis on which to build such accompaniments as occupational and physical therapies, special diets, supervised diversions and vocational re-training programs. The emotional factors in evidence during convalescence from various types of illness and injuries are being studied, especially in the armed forces, and it would appear that the hospital of the future will not consider its service complete or the patient cured without a carefully planned period of supervised convalescence, either in a special division or building set aside for the purpose or in a country branch where medical and nursing care are supplied. Seven hospitals in New York city maintained convalescent homes of the latter type in 1944 (54). Satisfactory and complete convalescence is a preventive against relapse, reinfection, or decline into a state of chronic illness (55).

Home convalescent care is an ideal field for the service of the licensed practical nurse, provided the patient does not need continuous skilled treatments. For the occasional skilled service, a professional nurse from the Visiting Nurse Association is usually available—though this is not true in rural areas, of course. Registries report a constant demand from convalescent patients, and practical nurses like this type of case.

The duties of the practical nurse in the care of the home convalescent differ little from those described in the nursing of chronic illness except that more attention may have to be given to preparing dainty, nourishing, and suitable meals to tempt a lagging appetite, to suggesting diversions, and to keeping the home quiet and running smoothly. One of the nurse's greatest problems will be to teach the patient to adjust to his limitations of strength and at the same time not permit him to lapse into coddled enjoyment of invalidism. The elderly convalescent patient is especially hard to deal with, frequently not wishing to leave his bed or, going to the other extreme, resenting all protection.

Home is the natural and most frequently used haven of convalescence, but it is not always the best place for the patient. Overcrowding, the presence of children, household or business cares and worries, stairs to climb, absence of assistance, or lack of proper meals may make home undesirable even if part time nursing service can be secured. Early dismissal from the hospital to make room for sicker patients, after such treatments as the sulfa drugs and high-powered x-ray exposures which leave an exaggerated state of depression or discomfort, may make continued care away from home desirable. Often patients assigned to the outpatient service live too far from the hospital to make frequent trips. They, too, would do better in a convalescent institution where the same treatments are available.

Convalescent institutions may also be used as places in which to rest and build up reserves preparatory to surgical operations or between stages of surgery. Occasionally they are visited for purely preventive purposes and should undoubtedly be used more frequently in this way. They should never be employed, however, as homes for the chronically ill (56).

If the patient does not recuperate at home or with relatives, he may go to a resort, a hotel, a nursing home, or to a bona fide convalescent institution. Day camps, summer camps, and preventoria may receive the children. There may be no nursing care of any description needed or available or there may be all sorts of skilled nursing treatments, special diets, and continued medical supervision ordered and provided. Undoubtedly, thousands of patients who never receive it would benefit by a period of convalescence away from home, under the watchful eye of a doctor or nurse.* The American Public Health Association has suggested a standard of 7.5 beds for convalescence for each 10,000 population (58), in addition to the beds for tuberculosis cases. It is not known how many communities reach this standard.

There are no statistics for the country as a whole showing the number of nonprofessional nurses employed in convalescent homes. This is partly because convalescent homes may be anything from Mrs. Jones' Nursing Home, a six-room cottage accommodating two patients, to a two-hundred-acre estate caring for three or four hundred, with a complete professional staff. In the New York Survey a convalescent home was defined as "An institution for the care of patients during a period of recovery after a period of illness, giving some health supervision, and incorporated not for profit under the management of a responsible board of public spirited citizens. The institution may charge a fee for its services but does not attempt to maintain itself entirely from fees" (59).

In Minnesota in 1944, chronic and convalescent homes licensed by the State Department of Health employed 317 nonregistered and 57 registered nurses (60). In the New York Metropolitan area, in 1940, 42 homes employed sufficient nurses and "subsidiary workers," including practical nurses, to provide one nurse for each 9.4 beds on the average, but some homes could report only one nurse to 76 beds. One home accommodating 15 adults had no nursing personnel. In four, the only registered nurse was the administrator. The homes for children were better staffed than were those for adults (61).

In 1944, the census of registered hospitals in the United States showed that there were 109 institutions for "rest and convalescence,"

---

* In New York city in 1940, 37 hospitals referred only 14,642 ward patients to convalescent homes out of 314,899 ward discharges (57).

representing 13,825 beds and 34 bassinets. The average census was 7,993 patients, and these homes were only 57.8 per cent occupied (62). Authorities have not agreed upon a desirable ratio of convalescent patients to professional or practical nurses. The New York Committee suggested a ratio of one nurse of any type to each 9 beds (63). Studies in this field are needed.

In a study of nursing time in Neustadter Home, Yonkers, which is a branch of Mt. Sinai Hospital in New York city, sixty minutes was the minimum care required by each patient in twenty-four hours (64). Most of the patients were up and about each day, but many required special treatments because they came directly from the hospital wards. In this home (capacity 56 beds), six registered nurses (including the administrator) and two unlicensed attendants cared for the patients. Special diets, medications, treatments, and constant oversight were needed by the convalescents, who presented such conditions as cardiac decompensation, rheumatic fever, diabetes, draining wounds, osteomyelitis, cholesistectomy, thyroidectomy, mastectomy, and gastric ulcers of various types—to name but a few. Emergencies were not uncommon. A visiting physician was in charge of the patients and was always on call. The nurses had standing orders, and there was a well equipped treatment room. The trip from the suburban institution to the parent hospital in the city could be made by automobile in thirty minutes.

The attendants in this convalescent home have been taught "on the job." They are taught only the type of care nurses' aides would give: temperature, pulse, and respiration, feeding, baths, soapsuds enemas, night care, and the general supervision of "up" patients. Medications are all given by the professional nurses. The home has a qualified occupational therapist and supervised recreation.

Some convalescent homes conduct training courses for children's nurses or practical nurses. In the New York area "these homes had a high standard of medical service" (65).

The director of a private convalescent home of 48 patients told the writer she believed a registered nurse should be on duty at all times, one to cover each of the eight-hour shifts. This home had two professional nurses and three licensed practical nurses in January 1945. Many of the patients came directly from the hospitals and needed considerable care, special diets, and supervision.

A large convalescent home (capacity 250) had 165 patients in January 1945 (the census is much higher in summer) and employed five registered nurses and two experienced practical nurses with two "night helpers." A doctor was in residence. Certain types of care could not be given—colostomy irrigations, for example—and patients must be able to look out for themselves and to go to meals in the dining room. Nurses had a twelve-hour day with two hours off duty.

Among the qualifications required of the practical nurses serving in convalescent homes, in addition to skill in simple nursing procedures, directors of nurses mentioned ability to handle fractious or homesick people, awareness of the neurotic tendencies of those debilitated by long or serious illness, willingness to play games, take walks, or plan diversions for bored patients, and close observation for signs of fatigue or unfavorable symptoms among the guests.

If patients are being sent directly from hospitals to convalescent homes, it is evident that a professional nurse should be in charge of their care, although she may delegate nearly all services to practical nurses. The number of practical nurses needed will undoubtedly depend on the condition of the patients, the types of treatments ordered, the services provided in the home—even the layout of the building may be a factor. Most convalescent homes do not accept bed patients, some accept only patients able to take entire care of themselves. A licensed practical nurse with wide experience in meeting emergencies would be quite capable of handling this latter type of home under close medical supervision if few patients were accepted. If, however, there were many patients in need of continued nursing care and treatments and only one nurse could be employed, authorities would agree that she should be a professional nurse (66).

Much more needs to be known by medical science about the nursing requirements of patients convalescing in institutions, because the stage of their recovery and the treatments ordered by the doctors are the deciding factors in assigning professional or practical nurses. Much better and more economical service could probably be rendered in all hospitals if there were earlier separation of the convalescents from the acute cases, with care rendered to the former by licensed practical nurses under professional supervision.

It has been announced that the Army plans to increase its capacity for convalescent cases to some 100,000 beds. (In 1944 there were 9 convalescent hospitals with a total of 30,000 beds [67]). The Veterans Administration plans for the expansion of permanent service to veterans, much of which will be of convalescent type. All signs point to a growing demand in this field for licensed practical nurses of both sexes.

Salaries found in convalescent homes where some nursing care is expected of the nonprofessional attendants ranged from $60 a month with full maintenance for unlicensed attendants to $5.50 a day for trained and licensed practical nurses who lived out. Registered nurses' salaries ranged from $130 a month with full maintenance to $7.50 a day, living out.

REFERENCES

1 See especially Josephine Goldmark, *Nursing and nursing education in the United States;* report of the Committee for the Study of Nursing Education, New York, Macmillan, 1923; May Ayres Burgess, *Nurses, patients and pocketbooks;* report of study of the economics of nursing by the Committee on the Grading of Nursing Schools, New York, the Committee, 1928; I. S. Falk, C. Rufus Rorem, and Martha D. Ring, *The costs of medical care;* a summary of investigations on the economic aspects of the prevention and care of illness, Chicago, University of Chicago Press, 1933 (Committee on the Costs of Medical Care No. 27); Ernst P. Boas, *The unseen plague; chronic disease,* New York, Augustin, 1940, p. 14. For a recent statement, see Morris Hinenberg, "The acid test of practical nursing," *Modern Hospital* 64:63–64, January 1945.

2 Geddes Smith, *Plague on us,* New York, Commonwealth Fund, 1941, p. 250.

3 George St. J. Perrott and Dorothy F. Holland, "Population trends and problems of public health," *Milbank Memorial Fund Quarterly* 18:359–392, October 1940, p. 361.

4 Perrott and Holland (note 3), p. 361. "Deaths of persons 45 years of age and over constituted over two-thirds of all deaths in this country in 1935: in the Registration States of 1900, the proportion was approximately two-fifths."

5 Mary G. O'Connell, "Facilities for chronically ill and convalescent patients," *Hospital Progress* 25:281–282, October 1944.

6 "War veterans will require 300,000 hospital beds in 20 years," *Hospital Management* 58:31, August 1944.

7 Perrott and Holland (note 3), p. 366.

8 Selwyn D. Collins, "Frequency and volume of nursing service in relation to all illnesses among 9,000 families; based on nation-wide periodic canvasses, 1928–1931," *Milbank Memorial Fund Quarterly* 21:5–36, January 1943.

9 Eight long-time nonsurgical cases had practical nurses for an aggregate of 1,708 days. Diagnoses were mental illness, cardiac disease, tuberculosis of the spine, hypertension, paralysis, cancer, accident, and premature twins. In the last case, both professional and practical nurses were on duty as the other children in the family developed whooping cough. The practical nurse remained 56 days on the case. Collins (note 8), p. 11.

10 Perrott and Holland (note 3), p. 383.

11 Collins (note 8), p. 12.

12 State Charities Aid Association, *Report of Committee on Hospitals, 1872*, "Training school for nurses," New York, Putnam, 1877, p. 3.

13 Helen W. Munson, "The care of the sick in almshouses," *American Journal of Nursing* 30:1226, 1227, 1230, October 1930. See also *Some American almshouses;* report of the Women's Department, New York, National Civic Federation, 1927.

14 An example of what may be done is the Monroe County Home and Infirmary at Rochester, N.Y. See also Karl F. Heiser, "Chronic illness in Connecticut in 1944," *Public Health Nursing* 37:85–92, February 1945.

15 For information on chronic conditions among persons less than eighteen years of age, see Ernst P. Boas, "A community program for the care of the chronic sick," *Hospitals* 10:18–25, February 1936.

16 Mary C. Jarrett, *The care of the chronic sick in private homes for the aged in and near New York city*, New York, Welfare Council, 1931.

17 National Institute of Health, *The magnitude of the chronic disease problem in the United States*, United States Public Health Service, 1938 (Sickness and Medical Care Series, Bulletin 6).

18 Editorial, "Nursing problems; report by British Medical Association on questions raised by the College of Nursing," *British Medical Journal*, supplement, June 26, 1937, pp. 410–413.

19 Falk, Rorem, and Ring (note 1).

20 Mary C. Jarrett, *Chronic illness in New York city*, New York, Columbia University Press, 1933, vol. 1, p. 17.

21 O'Connell (note 5), p. 282; Jarrett (note 16), pp. 43, 44, 47; and Jarrett (note 20), p. 17.

22 Mary C. Jarrett, Housekeeping service for home care of chronic pa-

tients, W.P.A. Project 165–97–7002, December 1938, appendix, p. 62, table 9.

23 Jarrett (note 22), pp. 57–60, 65.

24 Marie de Montalvo, "When age and illness meet; New York's home care of dependents," *Trained Nurse and Hospital Review* 102:315–321, April 1939.

25 Ella Hasenjaeger, "The subsidiary worker," *American Journal of Nursing* 38:772–776, July 1938.

26 State Nurses' Association, *Study of the subsidiary worker in nursing service in Pennsylvania, 1939–1940,* pp. 17, 41.

27 Heiser (note 14). See also another recent study by Jean Downes, "Findings of the study of chronic disease in the Eastern Health District of Baltimore," IN *New steps in public health;* report of the 22nd annual conference of the Milbank Memorial Fund, New York, 1945, pp. 3, 6–7. This study does not analyze the nursing service available to these patients.

28 Heiser (note 14), p. 91.

29 Compare Ernst P. Boas, "The chronically sick; the social and mental aspects of their nursing care," *American Journal of Nursing* 37:137–143, February 1937, at pp. 142–143. "There is no clear distinction between the duties of these two types of worker."

30 News note, "Chicago care of chronic invalids," *Public Health Nursing* 37:221–222, April 1945.

31 Boas (note 29), p. 137.

32 O'Connell (note 5), p. 282.

33 Montalvo (note 24), p. 315.

34 Jarrett (note 22), table 7, pp. 60, 22, 35.

35 Boas (note 29), pp. 142–143.

36 Netta Ford, "Subsidiary worker and her place, if any, in nursing," *Hospitals* 11:91–94, November 1937, at p. 92.

37 Boas (note 29), pp. 141–143.

38 E. M. Bluestone, "The chronics; they belong in general hospitals," *Trained Nurse and Hospital Review* 114:17–20, January 1945, at p. 17.

39 Boas (note 29), p. 141.

40 Mary M. A. Weiss, "The chronically ill," *American Journal of Nursing* 38:399–401, April 1938, at pp. 399–400.

41 Boas (note 1), p. 14.

42 For examples of the type of wise counsel available to practical nurses from outside sources, see Jarrett (note 22), appendix, p. 51. Excellent illustrations of the way in which public health nurses have helped to

solve the problems created by chronic illness at home will be found in Marguerite A. Wales, *The public health nurse in action,* New York, Macmillan, 1941, chapter VIII, "The chronically ill patient," pp. 330–377.

43 Evelyn M. Crowley, "Convalescent care in heart disease," *American Journal of Nursing* 44:1124–1128, December 1944.

44 Boas (note 29), p. 142.

45 Family Welfare Association of America, *Mental hygiene in old age,* New York, the Association, 1937, p. 39. See also A. W. Worcester, *The care of the aged, the dying and the dead,* Springfield, Ill., Thomas, 1935.

46 Boas (note 29), p. 143.

47 Montalvo (note 24), p. 315.

48 Montalvo (note 24), p. 316. See also Helen Hardy Brunot, *Old age in New York city;* an analysis of some problems of the aged, based on 3,106 requests for information about health and welfare services, New York, Welfare Council, 1944.

49 Bluestone (note 38), p. 17.

50 Part of a definition formulated by Drs. Charles C. Treud and James A. Halsted, Research Bureau, Boston, for the Council of Agencies; it appears on page 12 of *Facilities for convalescent care in Boston,* published by the Council, June 1938.

51 From a definition by Brochin (1877) quoted by John Bryant, *Convalescence,* New York, Burke Foundation, 1927, p. 171.

52 Elizabeth G. Gardiner and Francisca K. Thomas, *The road to recovery from illness;* a study of convalescent homes serving New York city, New York, Hospital Council of Greater New York, 1945, p. 12.

53 In 1860 Florence Nightingale wrote, "The reparative process has been hindered by some want of knowledge or attention." Nurses, she added, should assist in this process. *Notes on nursing,* Boston, William Carter, 1860.

54 Gardiner and Thomas (note 52), pp. 33–35.

55 Boas (note 1), p. 87. See also O'Connell (note 5), p. 282.

56 Gardiner and Thomas (note 52), pp. 76–77.

57 Gardiner and Thomas (note 52), p. 68.

58 Isadore Rosenfield, "What hospital facilities are needed for proper convalescent care and rehabilitation?" *Hospital Management* 58:24–26, December 1944.

59 Gardiner and Thomas (note 52), p. 40. See also Elizabeth G. Gardiner, *Convalescent homes in Philadelphia,* Council of Social Agencies, 1939.

60 *Report on nursing service in hospitals and related institutions,* Minnesota State Department of Health, 1944 (leaflet).

61 Gardiner and Thomas (note 52), p. 88.

62 "Hospital service in the United States, 1945," *Journal of the American Medical Association* 127:778–779, March 13, 1945.

63 Gardiner and Thomas (note 52), p. 131.

64 Gardiner and Thomas (note 52), p. 131.

65 Gardiner and Thomas (note 52), pp. 131–132.

66 Gardiner and Thomas (note 52), p. 132.

67 News note, "70,000 more beds for Army wounded," *American Journal of Nursing* 45:240, March 1945.

CHAPTER NINE

Industry

PREVENTIVE medicine in industry as elsewhere, quite apart from social considerations, has been found to pay. It is vastly cheaper to prevent an accident or illness than to pay for reparative treatment. The United States Public Health Service has shown that an expenditure by a company of $8 per year per worker for a health program should yield the company a return of $12 per year per worker, or 15 per cent, while the yearly loss to a company employing 500 workers that operates without a health program is $30,900 or about $60 per worker. Reports from a study of small plants showed that when a health program was instituted, the reduction in illness, accidents, absenteeism, and turnover ranged from 27.3 to 62.8 per cent, to say nothing of the good will and happier relationships promoted. "No plant however small can afford to be without a health program" (1).

In all industrial health programs, both registered and nonprofessional nurses have had an established place, the former since 1895, the latter for as long as there has been need for someone to give first aid or help to sick employees—which means for as long as people have worked together. Whether an industrial establishment has a formal medical department or not, it always has some "first aider," volunteer or paid, trained or amateur, who steps into the breach when there is an accident or illness among the workers. These first aid men were the forerunners of the modern medical department staff and still continue to be a mainstay in small plants, in first aid stations in large plants at a distance from the central medical department, and on the night shifts in thousands of industries both large and small. It is now customary to designate the workers who are to give first aid and to require of them the satisfactory completion of a standard course in first aid, that of either the American Red Cross or the United States Bureau of Mines.

The boom interest in industrial health and nursing between 1941 and 1945 was clearly the result of expanding war production. A survey showed that 2,450 full time registered nurses began their service to industry in 1942, and in more than 100 plants industrial nursing was added for the first time in that year (2). In all, there were in January

1945 nearly 14,000 industrial nurses at work as compared with 6,000 in 1940 (3). The United States Public Health Service predicts the need for 20,000 industrial nurses within a few years—or when our population reaches 138,000,000 (4). No one knows how many practical nurses are employed in industry today, and no estimate has been ventured as to the future demands.

Some 39 hospitals connected with industries provided 2,893 beds and 6 bassinets in 1944. There were 55,974 admissions, and the average census was 1,789 (5). Presumably all the nurses serving in these hospitals were registered, but no report is available as to their number.

TYPES OF NURSING SERVICE

Roughly, there are three groups who have some responsibility for the nursing care of employees who are injured or become ill while at work: registered professional nurses; licensed practical nurses or other trained technicians; and nonprofessional, usually unlicensed, semi-trained workers, such as first aiders, medical secretaries, matrons, and the like. Usually they function under the direction of a licensed physician, full time, part time, or on call.

Many years ago, Florence Swift Wright pointed out that the function of the industrial (registered) nurse was not confined to finger wrapping, first aid, and the keeping of correct records for the medical director. "The growth of her work was only limited by time, by strength and vision and by the initiative allowed her by her employer" (6). The National Organization for Public Health Nursing, recognizing the need for better service to industrial workers, organized the first national section for industrial nurses in 1920 and studied the whole situation in 1929 (7). Both registered and nonprofessional workers were found in industry then.

The United States Public Health Service has for some years been deeply concerned with the responsibility of the nursing profession in the field of industrial hygiene. The industrial nurse, J. J. Bloomfield believes, must "first of all be a good nurse, thoroughly acquainted with industry and industrial processes, be well trained in public health, and have some knowledge of labor legislation, social problems, community welfare, and industrial hygiene practice . . . in short, industrial nursing is as highly specialized a profession as are industrial medicine, public health administration, or similar branches of the profession requiring post graduate education" (8).

The registered industrial nurse needs to know something of the labor conditions in her plant, compensation and insurance regulations, rehabilitation policies, industrial hazards, diseases and poisons peculiar to the plant processes; she must have some knowledge of the principles of nutrition, and be up to date in first aid and surgical procedures, health teaching methods and materials. She should be thoroughly grounded in the principles of public health. She will be expected to qualify as a teacher of Red Cross home nursing classes (9). In communities where there is no visiting nurse service, some plants find it profitable to have a plant nurse visit sick employees or members of their families at home. Here again is a field primarily for the professional nurse, preferably one with public health nursing experience, for she must be able to give skilled bedside nursing care and be a good health teacher as well. She must understand the use of community resources and interpret to the employer the social and health conditions which may affect the productive capacity of the worker (10).

During the war, the replacement of men by women in such large numbers added appreciably to the responsibilities of the registered nurses in industry. Women present all kinds of special problems—their muscular strength is not half that of men, their average height is less, calling for adjustments in work processes, their home cares and schedules interrupt their attention and slow up production. Environment, recreation, refreshment, and adequate rest rooms mean more to them than to men (11). Safe work clothing must be worn. Industrial nurses who have accepted the problems connected with these developments as their concern have been busy indeed. Few, however, have actually the time to step outside the medical department, and women's advisers, counsellors, and matrons have taken over these opportunities for service.

THE PLACE OF THE PRACTICAL NURSE

Comparatively few industries have recognized the value of the trained and licensed practical nurse as an assistant to the professional staff. Rather—and unfortunately—several industries under the pressure of war production and the scarcity of registered nurses have employed unlicensed practical nurses in place of registered nurses. In rare cases, a practical nurse is skillful enough, experienced enough, and astute enough to swing the job to the satisfaction of the employer and medical director without the supervision of a registered nurse. If she is wise she protects herself by constant referral to the doctor, by obtaining written "standing orders" from him covering all emergencies and common complaints—and she learns when to stop. Experience (and most practical nurses employed prior to 1941 in industry had been a long time on the job), trial and error, familiarity with the doctor's ways and with the problems of the industry have sometimes produced an acceptable substitute for a registered nurse. In other plants, management is only waiting for peacetime conditions to replace the practical staff with professional nurses. "Industry has no place for the half-trained woman unless she is to be confined within the four walls of a first-aid room and even there she is a potential source of danger" (12). Plants employing only practical nurses will be fewer, it is believed, as more professional nurses become available and as industrial physicians accept and adopt the preventive aspects of the industrial hygiene program which call so insistently for prepared and informed nurses.

Occasionally, a practical nurse of many years' experience will be in charge of registered nurses in industry. To the writer's knowledge, this was true in 1944 in two industries in New York state and at least one in California. Some half dozen establishments in New York state employ practical nurses only, and five employ licensed practical nurses under registered nurses. This type of information cannot always be secured from state files, although the number of registered nurses employed in industry is now always obtainable.*

In 1944 in the state of Washington, which does not license practical nurses, only one plant had attempted to train and employ practical nurses. Two other establishments had employed a practical nurse as their only nurse for a year (13).

In 1942, 868 establishments employing nurses were surveyed by the Committee to Study the Duties of Nurses in Industry (Public Health Nursing Section of the American Public Health Association) with the help of the Industrial Hygiene Division of the National Institute of

---

* Six states, with and without laws to license practical nurses, were asked for these figures. No recent industrial surveys have included the group as differentiated from other nonprofessional workers in medical departments.

Health. There were 3,027 full time registered nurses and 785 nonprofessional workers employed in the establishments surveyed. Twenty-two per cent of the plants employed the latter group, which included first aid workers, practical nurses, pharmacists' mates, and medical corpsmen. No distinction was made between licensed and unlicensed practical nurses or practical nurses who had previously completed a course of any kind in nursing (14).

The Committee reported on the nonprofessional attendant situation as follows:

The employment of nonprofessional attendants in the plant medical department is another factor influencing the scope of nurses' activities. Although a well-organized plan for the use of nonprofessional attendants should serve to release the nurse's time for duties requiring her professional skill, it was not always possible to determine from the schedules wherein the functions of nonprofessional attendants differed from those of nurses.

According to the recommendation of the advisory committee, the nonprofessional attendant relieves the nurse whenever possible of routine duties not requiring nursing skills. *In some plants these attendants, in addition to assisting with physical examinations and making home calls, assumed full responsibility in first-aid substations in larger plants or on night shifts.* In 123, or 14 per cent, of the plants working extra shifts . . . nonprofessional and other attendants were on duty on one or both shifts. This number includes 18 plants which employed medical students and 12 plants which employed both nurses and attendants for duty on one or both extra shifts, the attendants supposedly working in an auxiliary capacity. Otherwise, the attendants were alone on one or both extra shifts with responsibility for emergency treatment and care of injured and ill workers. In three plants which employed full-time registered nurses as well, it was reported that first-aid attendants were in charge of the dispensary.

Of the 753 nonprofessional attendants employed in the plants, 30 per cent were reported as supervised by nurses. This number includes practical nurses, first-aid attendants and medical corpsmen, but excludes medical students and technicians who were not reported as coming under the nurse's supervision. *Occasionally the attendants had the same status as registered nurses, and, in a few instances, drew larger salaries. Sometimes they were designated as the supervisors.*

It is questioned how much the use of nonprofessional attendants is in conformity with standards unless they are functioning under specific orders. [The italics are mine.]

From the italicized statements two facts are clear: many of the attendant duties described should be carried by professional nurses—home calls, for example—while others could very well be assigned to well trained and supervised practical nurses. On the other hand, it is not clear who is to do the "routine duties not requiring nursing skills." Practical nurses, unless they nurse, should be replaced by medical secretaries, clerical workers, and matrons.

Thirty-four plants reported that their service was carried solely by practical nurses and first-aid workers, the total employed being 30 female and 20 male workers. The plants, located in 16 states, ranged in size from less than 500 to 5,000 employees.

It was found that the activities of nonprofessional nursing personnel did not differ in scope from those of full-time and part-time graduate registered nurses. However, limitations in the character as well as in the extent of participation in plant health services were implied.

Although a physician was on call in 25 plants and served part time in 9 plants, written standing orders and procedures were provided in only 2 plants, and these were for practical nurses. In only one establishment was any specific activity reported in the field of health education and supervision. The keynote was definitely on safety. . . .

The character of nursing treatment and care, which comprised the sole activity of the attendants in 13 plants, was necessarily limited. Assistance with physical examinations was reported in eight of the 16 plants with physical examination programs, and, in 4 of these, the attendants did the urinalyses. In 1 plant the first-aid worker made "screening inspections" of employees which included a complete health history, the measurement tests, and urinalyses; workers with gross abnormalities were sent to the physician's office. In 2 plants some home visiting was done, and, in a third establishment, the attendant functioned as a welfare visitor with activities including physical inspections and history taking on each new female employee, visits to their homes, and periodic visits to substations in branch offices. In 10 plants the attendants were reported as performing clerical and unskilled work.

It is evident from this review that nonprofessional nursing personnel have responsibilities commensurate with those of graduate registered nurses. Certain industries apparently found this type of service satisfactory, since 15 attendants have been with their present companies for more than 10 years.

Licensed practical nurses, under the supervision of a registered nurse, might have been safer workers than the semi-trained, unsupervised, and heterogeneous group revealed by the survey. On the other hand the Committee especially emphasized the gravity of using professional nursing time for non-nursing duties. Fourteen per cent of the plants were found to be guilty of this mistake.

It is questioned whether nursing time should be available for non-nursing service duties, particularly as the survey showed that some of the responsibilities of the medical personnel were being carried by personnel in other plant departments, for example, follow-up of defects by the personnel department.

There needs to be a more widespread understanding of what constitutes a sound industrial health program, and an understanding of the nurses' participation in that program. The present-day program in industrial hygiene, in which management, labor, and the medical profession participate, should help to meet the need, but in addition, nurses and representatives of their respective plant managements need to make a thorough study of the needs of the individual plant and how the nursing activities may be planned to meet these needs. . . .

The use of nonprofessional attendants is important in industry today, as elsewhere, because of the shortage of nurses. However, it does not appear that the same safeguards in the use of nonprofessional attendants have been followed in industry as have been followed, for example, in the preparation and use of volunteer nurses' aides in the hospitals.

According to the survey findings, the first-aid workers were frequently used in place of a nurse on the additional shifts and in first-aid substations. A clear differentiation between the duties of the professional and nonprofessional personnel was not found owing in part, perhaps, to the manner in which the data were obtained in the survey.

. . . Further study of the uses of nonprofessional attendants is indicated, with an attempt to assign duties which may safely be assumed by nonprofessional workers, thus conserving nursing time for activities requiring nursing skill.

The Committee concluded by recommending that during the war emergency

. . . it is essential that careful consideration be given to the utilization of nonprofessional clinic assistants under supervision of a nurse to keep at a minimum the number of nurses needed, and that the activities of the nurse be limited to essential nursing functions.

The United States Public Health Service recommends one registered nurse for 300 workers, two or more for 600 workers, three for 1,000 (16). No mention is made of practical nurse quotas. It would seem when three or more registered nurses are employed in plants of 1,000 or more, a practical nurse could assist in the duties described on pages 154–155. She would be an asset to the department in releasing professional service to employees and plant activities. It is desirable to have enough nonprofessional nursing duties to keep a full time practical nurse busy, although she might give part time to the health service if employed elsewhere in the plant. It is interesting that Miss Wright also made the point that the registered nurse should have clerical assistance from the start, but that the second person employed should be another registered nurse to relieve the first for lunch periods, vacations, sick leave, etc., or to serve when the nurse in charge is out in the plant (17). While the practical nurse would be expected to assist in record-keeping, and it is well for her to know how to type, her time should not be taken up with clerical duties which are better performed by a medical secretary. She is there as an assistant nurse, when there are enough supplementary duties of this type.

DUTIES

Opportunities in professional service for which the practical nurse could release the registered nurse in industry include the following (18).

Individual conferences with workers: when reporting, injured or sick, to the health service; after examination or treatment; when presenting personal or family problems; when returning for dressings or after illness; when in need of health education; when referred to community service agencies; when followed up after preplacement examinations, correction of defects, or changing health habits

Contacts with plant personnel: foremen, personnel department, cafeteria director, safety personnel, etc.

Attendance at meetings: plant, community, professional

Visits to plant

Writing reports, analyzing work, administration of service, review of accomplishments (19)

The professional nurse should retain all the duties that involve giving health advice other than very elementary suggestions approved by the doctor and the registered nurse and should handle all problems relating to working and home conditions, personal adjustments, referrals to community agencies, and administrative problems as they relate to nursing or medical policies. She is entirely responsible for the work, assignment of duties, and supervision of the practical nurse and other auxiliary help (20).

One reason why instruction and advice in health education should come from the professional nurse is the need for discriminating judgment in the amount and character of information given to each employee. The wise distribution of printed pamphlets is part of this duty, after medical approval of them has been given. Aside from the variations in individuals' ability to absorb and use this type of advice and help, there is always the question of authoritativeness of information given orally. We do not suffer so much these days from old forms of quackery—snake oil and magic herbs—but there are still over-sold popular "essentials to health" such as vitamins in capsule form. Without a background of knowledge in nutrition, chemistry, materia medica, and physiology, the practical nurse finds it difficult not to believe what she reads and hears and not to share her own or friends' experience with a "sovereign remedy." A professional nurse reported to the writer that a practical nurse (unlicensed) was overheard saying, out of the kindness of her heart, to an elderly worker: "If I were you, I'd use a hot cooked onion when your ear aches. I find there's nothing like it. Tie it over your ear as hot as you can stand it."

Other responsibilities which are solely those of the registered nurse in charge of a department are, in the absence of the doctor, answering questions regarding a patient's condition, the release of diagnosis, making arrangements for home care or for transportation of an injured worker, initiation with doctor's consent of campaigns of various kinds (better lunches, use of snack bar, early report of colds, etc.), and problems presented by home contacts with communicable disease. The registered nurse is expected to be on the alert for maladjusted employees showing such problems as personality clashes, overfatigue, eyestrain, malnutrition, home anxieties, all of which can be smoothed over by tactful handling if taken in time.

As the job of the professional nurse in industry develops into a more highly specialized field, there is more room left for the practical nurse.

"It has been proven," writes an industrial nurse, "that, under adequate supervision, many duties previously performed by nurses in hospitals as well as industry can be successfully accomplished by nonprofessional personnel" (21).

Considerable space has been given here to the functions of the registered professional nurse in industry to make clear these points:

Work of this calibre is definitely beyond the capacities (education, training, and experience) of the practical nurse. *If only one nurse can be employed, she should be a registered professional nurse,* even if part of her time is taken up in elementary nursing procedures. These she can do, but a practical nurse cannot do professional nursing.

Work of this nature, calling for the professional nurse's service outside the first aid room, cannot be adequately undertaken and properly pursued by her unless she has assistance with the routine duties which can be delegated to auxiliary workers. In a small plant, this may take the form of clerical and matron service; in a large plant, practical nursing, clerical, and matron services.

Many of the duties expected of the practical nurse assisting the professional staff in industry are similar to those carried on in clinics and outpatient services (see pages 176–178). They are listed here for greater clarity:

Admission routine: temperature, pulse, respiration; weighing; measuring; records; chaperoning female patients; care of specimens

Setting up clinic and examining and treatment rooms

Care and cleaning of equipment

Preparation and sterilizing supplies, ordering supplies

Care of medicine cabinet, care of bulletin board

Care of rest rooms and cots if connected with medical department

Supervision of patients in rest rooms

Keeping and filing records, day sheets. If there is no clerical assistance, copying schedules, lists, filling out reports, posting routines, typing, other clerical work as registered nurse directs

Simple dressings, redressings, reinforcement of dressings

Application of hot water bags, ice caps, compresses, protective ointments, light treatments (as ordered)

Simple treatments as ordered: painting throats, rubbing backs, removal of splinters, soaks

Assistance to the registered nurse in all difficult treatments and in emer-
gencies
First aid according to standing orders
First advice according to standing orders
Answering telephones, assisting patients to undress and dress, keeping
order in waiting room, etc.

A matron, maid, or janitor is usually in charge of the toilets connected with the medical department and of the rest and locker rooms
in the plant. The training and supervision of matrons may be the practical nurse's responsibility.

Other duties peculiar to each industry could doubtless be found by
the professional nurse and assigned, in whole or in part, to the practical nurse.

All duties should be outlined, written, posted, revised, taught, and
supervised by the registered nurse. If the registered nurse has not the
ability to give such instruction and supervision, then it would be better
not to delegate these duties to nonprofessional staff (22).

It is vitally important that the practical nurse be trained in the detail
of record-keeping. Compensation laws and accident insurance policies
demand complete, accurate, and on-the-spot descriptions of injuries
(23). It is not enough to report "crushed finger, hammering tacks,"
but rather "contusion, left first finger, anterior surface and nail involved. Was hammering tacks in crates on floor of shipping room."
The time, the date, and treatment given should be recorded.

The written standing orders which the practical nurse may follow
need to be particularly clear and comprehensive and must cover not
only first aid in the usual sense, but the first advice which a practical
nurse may offer until supplemented by other. "Backache" or "back
strain" suggests a dozen possible causes such as postural defect, injury,
strain, dislocation, wrong height of work bench or machine, arthritis,
kidney trouble, displaced uterus, too high heels, etc., and "first advice" offered must be of very limited nature and must stress medical attention. Four or five routine measures, however, may be safely suggested to an employee at the beginning of a common cold.

The professional nurse is responsible for seeing that the practical
nurse knows what first aid steps to take in case of emergencies when
both she and the doctor are absent. Such first aid should relate directly
to the hazards peculiar to that industry. Many practical nurses will

have had the Red Cross first aid course; others, if licensed, will have received first aid lessons at their schools. Even then, industrial accidents may call for first aid measures that are quite different from anything they have learned; for example, chemical burns requiring a specially developed reagent applied promptly in a certain way. Or their lessons may have taught them to do too much for the patient from the point of view of industry and the insurance carrier. First aid to injured eyes and foreign body in the eye are examples. Special aseptic techniques have been developed for the handling of various eye injuries which require considerable skill. If the practical nurse is to perform any of these, she needs extremely thorough instruction and repeated practice. She may have to forget what she has previously learned.

Fractures present another typical situation. First aid courses teach emergency splinting and removal of the patient to a hospital or home, warmly wrapped. In the plant, the slogan is "let 'em lie," wrap warmly, and send for the doctor.

The question of relieving the professional nurse is always a matter to plan carefully. If the night shift is light and the practical nurse is well trained in her work, understands procedures, and knows which cases to report immediately to the doctor and which personal problems to refer later to her nurse supervisor, her employment at night can be made safe, but much will depend on guidance and instruction from a professional nurse on day duty in the department.

One of the suitable jobs for the practical nurse in industry where many women are employed is that of matron or women's adviser. The woman who has poise and good judgment and who can recognize worry, fatigue, unhappiness, and illness when she sees them fits well into this position. She in no sense takes the place of the nurse; all cases of illness and minor injury which may turn up in the rest room or lounge over which she has supervision she refers to the registered nurse in the medical department. Her knowledge of sickness and experience in handling patients, however, stand her in good stead. This is an especially desirable job for an older practical nurse of good educational background who is unable to carry a heavy program of bedside nursing and who is looking for security in later life. Approachableness, common sense, friendliness, and quiet self-confidence are assets in persuading employees to come freely for advice or help. A licensed practical nurse of proved ability could probably combine her work with relieving or assisting the professional nurse in emergencies in the medical department.

THE NEED IN A SMALL PLANT—A PROFESSIONAL NURSE

Nursing service to small plants may seem of minor significance until we realize that small plants (those of less than 500 workers) employ about 60 per cent of all the industrial workers in the United States, comprising the bulk of our man and woman power—20,000,000 workers (24). Their health is of paramount importance. It must also be remembered that if there are three shifts, three nurses will be required to cover the twenty-four-hour period, unless the "graveyard shift" is covered by a qualified first aid worker.

In these small plants it is more than ever important that the one nurse (full or part time) be fully qualified. For one thing, the doctor is apt to be only on call, or at most on a part time schedule (25); unlike a hospital ward, there is no supervising nurse to whom to turn in an emergency, and the responsibilities in health, supervision, personnel problems, and plant relationships are far beyond the practical nurse's experience.

The increasing use of group medical services by small plants, whereby medical and nursing care is purchased from outside, points even more strongly to the need for a professionally qualified nurse, since she is in the plant only at stated intervals and must be keenly aware of all the problems in her job. A professional nurse will need to spend at least two hours a week in the plant for each 100 employees, and her program must be carefully outlined and backed by standing orders and the approval of the doctor (26). The advantage to a small industry of part time professional nursing service purchased and supervised from visiting nurse associations on a contract basis becomes evident as we consider these factors (27).

Except in the newer plants, in the additions for wartime expansion, and in a handful of large, well established industries, the "first aid" medical departments are crowded into small space, quite often grubby, dark, noisy, and furnished with makeshift equipment. In some cases, space, light, and quiet have to be sacrificed to locate the first aid room close to the workers. Working conditions for doctors and nurses are far from ideal and privacy for the injured worker is seldom possible. The writer has seen 300 employees a day coming to a space 10 by 15 feet in area in which two nurses were working. This high pressure program adds just another strain to which the practical nurse is not always equal, even when working with a registered nurse. It also presents a handicap to professional supervision.

For all these reasons, registered nurses should be the first nurses employed and practical nurses should be added only when the time arrives for a supervised program of subsidiary nursing duties. In a light, nonhazardous job in a small plant, there may never be a place for a licensed practical nurse, but a busy medical department in a heavy industry employing many unskilled workers can use a licensed practical nurse full time just as soon as each shift is headed by a professional nurse. Every situation, however, will be a rule unto itself.

SALARIES

There has been no study of this subject. Questions by the writer in some half dozen plants, two in Michigan, three in New York, one in Massachusetts, received widely varied answers, and no conclusions can be drawn. The range was from $75 a month for a part time first aider to $2,500 a year for a "supervising" practical nurse who had been on the job many years and was receiving a war bonus.* Where practical nurses were newly employed and no professional nurse was on duty a salary of $1,700 was paid; where there was a professional nursing staff, $1,500. The largest amount reported paid to a licensed practical nurse under professional supervision was $1,750.

In California in 1944 registered nurses in industry were receiving a minimum of 75 cents an hour, while in Ohio staff nurses received an average of $155.25 a month, supervisors $189.75 to $281.75 (28).

ATTITUDES TOWARD PRACTICAL NURSES IN INDUSTRY

Registered nurses in industry are not very favorably inclined just now to the use of practical nurses for supplementary nursing service. Their reasons run the gamut of all those cited elsewhere in this book, with some new and special ones. Enough plants employ only practical nurses to make competition real. Many industrial nurses have never seen the work of licensed practical nurses and what they know of so-

---

* Reported by a registered nurse outside the industry.

called practical nursing is bad, so they have no wish to open the door to them. They do not want to be responsible for untrained, unlicensed workers. Also, occasional experience with nonprofessional workers— not necessarily trained practical nurses—has shown them to be too willing to attempt procedures for which they are not prepared but not willing to accept the routine changes in shifts of duty necessary today. Also, the turnover among them is high.

Some registered nurses make the point that even the simple first aid dressing or brief check-up visit from the employee gives the professional nurse a chance to talk with the worker, to know him, and to offer a word of health advice, a chance which she would not want to hand over to a practical nurse. If these opportunities were used, there would be no arguing this point, but most employees are run through as fast as possible, not even sitting down for care, and conversation is reduced to a minimum. This speed is especially noticeable when the employee is on piece work and every minute away from his job means lost money to him.

Another argument against practical nurses is based on the crying need for a different type of worker. "If we must use nonprofessional staff, give us clerical service. We need that more than nursing help." This is undoubtedly true of even a small staff. Clerical help should be assigned from the start to the nursing service, and practical nurses added only when the nursing load grows too heavy.

Registered nurses also feel that their struggle to win a place in the plant might be jeopardized by the addition of nonprofessional helpers. Many doctors do not yet understand the function of the professional nurse in industry, so they might not make a clear distinction in practical nursing duties.

In Detroit, a registered nurse reported that untrained "nurses" have been placed in the medical department of an industry under a supervisor with limited training. Some of the unregistered nurses are receiving higher salaries than the professional staff (29). This type of experience has naturally turned registered nurses against the employment of practical nurses.

Where licensed and trained practical nurses are functioning under the supervision of registered nurses, however, their service is acceptable and liked.

The best evidence the writer has that practical nurses can be trained to give reliable and efficient service to sick and injured employees under the supervision of registered nurses comes from the United States Navy Shipyard at Mare Island, California. In 1944, sixteen Navy corpsmen under the supervision of three Navy (registered) nurses cared for about 300 patients daily in the Navy Medical Department. Care included preemployment examinations as well as all types of illness and injuries suffered on the job. Within a few miles, three other shipyards with the same hazards, caring for just about the same number of patients daily and not conducting preemployment examinations, were hiring registered nurses only. These professional nurses were so busy giving soaks, bandaging fingers, and keeping the routine work of the department going that they had no time to talk to patients.

At present, state industrial departments do not have a published policy with regard to the use of practical nurses, but they cooperate in promoting better service and training for them and extend any help they can to schools for practical nurses which wish their students to see industrial health activities. The consultant (professional) nurses on state department staffs have promoted the employment of well qualified industrial nurses and done much to interpret their service to management. The function and place of the qualified practical nurse in industry needs to be explored much further, however, and interpretation and promotion are needed among both doctors and nurses, with stress laid on the service as supplementary to professional nursing and always carried on under registered nurse supervision.

THE FUTURE FIELD

Dr. James A. Townsend, Chief of the Division of Industrial Hygiene, National Institute of Health, wrote in 1943: "There can be no doubt that the war has set the stage for a new industrial era in the United States." He pointed out that the training of subprofessional workers for the new industrial hygiene program offers a challenge to professional leaders (30). The plans for intensive training should start now. He believed a vigorous plan of education in industrial hygiene should be written, with the help of federal funds if needed, into our public health training programs, not forgetting the needs of small industrial plants.

Whether the licensed practical nurse can measure up to the responsibilities expected of her in industry, whether the opportunity for special training will be opened to her, or him—for this is an appropriate field for male practical nurses in plants employing only men—and, most significant of all, whether the medical and nursing professions will recognize the place of this subsidiary worker in industry rest with the turn of future events. At present the field lies fallow, awaiting the courage and foresight of a leader in industry, medicine, nursing, or all three.

REFERENCES

1 Victor G. Heiser, *Health on the production front*, New York, National Association of Manufacturers, 1944, pp. 45, 47, 49. See also Comments, *Illinois State Medical Journal* 85:203, April 1944.
2 "Duties of nurses in industry," *Public Health Nursing* 35:383–398, July 1943, at p. 392.
3 American Nurses' Association, Nursing Information Bureau, cooperating with the National League of Nursing Education and the National Organization for Public Health Nursing, *Facts about nursing, 1945,* p. 67.
4 Joseph W. Mountin, "Suggestions to nurses on postwar adjustments," *American Journal of Nursing* 44:321–325, April 1944.
5 "Hospital service in the United States, 1945," *Journal of the American Medical Association* 127:777, March 31, 1945.
6 Florence Swift Wright, *Industrial nursing*, New York, Macmillan, 1919, p. 7.
7 Louise M. Tattershall, "Nurses in commerce and industry," *Public Health Nursing* 22:147–148, March 1930; and Louise M. Tattershall, "Public health nursing in industry," *Public Health Nursing* 24:550, October 1932. More than a thousand establishments participated in this study.
8 J. J. Bloomfield, "The responsibility of the nursing profession in industrial hygiene," *Public Health Reports* 56:1131–1141, May 1941 (Reprint 2286), at pp. 1134–1135.
9 See Bethel J. McGrath, *Nursing in commerce and industry*, New York, Commonwealth Fund, 1946.
10 Heiser (note 1), p. 33.
11 Heiser (note 1), p. 58.
12 Wright (note 6), p. 11.
13 Letters to the writer from the Industrial Advisory Public Health

Nurse, State Department of Health, Washington, November 6, 1944.

14 Olive M. Whitlock, Victoria M. Trasko, F. Ruth Kahl, *Nursing practices in industry*, Washington, Government Printing Office, 1944, (Public Health Bulletin 283), pp. 3, 9.

15 Whitlock et al. (note 14), pp. 36, 39, 43–44, 50.

16 Whitlock et al. (note 14), p. 37.

17 Wright (note 6), p. 68. See also Olive Whitlock, "Nursing service," IN *Manual of industrial hygiene*, edited by William M. Gafafer, Philadelphia, Saunders, 1943, p. 70.

18 Whitlock (note 17), pp. 69–73. See also F. Clare Sykes, "Factory nursing in wartime Britain," *American Journal of Nursing* 44:938–939, October 1944.

19 For example, see Anna M. Fillmore, "Nursing records in industry," *American Journal of Public Health* 35:221–227, March 1945, especially p. 227.

20 A satisfactory division of duties has been worked out by the Visiting Nurse Service of New York in an industry of 600 employees where a registered nurse and a practical nurse are working together, covering two shifts with an overlap of service. See also Mary Jane Nickerson, "The public health nurse in a small industry," *Public Health Nursing* 37:343–347, July 1945.

21 Alice J. Patrinic, "The industrial nurse supervisor," *Public Health Nursing* 36:533–535, October 1944.

22 Whitlock (note 17), p. 81.

23 Whitlock et al. (note 14), p. 37.

24 Heiser (note 1), p. iv.

25 Heiser (note 1), pp. 11–12.

26 Heiser (note 1), p. 11. See also "A place for the assistant nurse," *Lancet* 243:374–375, September 26, 1942. "Not to be employed alone in small industries"; Sykes (note 18).

27 Anna M. Fillmore, "Part-time nursing service to the small plant," *Public Health Nursing* 37:130–137, March 1945, at pp. 130–131, 135.

28 American Nurses' Association, Nursing Information Bureau, cooperating with the National League of Nursing Education and the National Organization for Public Health Nursing, *Facts about nursing, 1944*, pp. 76–77.

29 Letter to the editor, *R.N.—A Journal for Nurses* 8:14, March 1945.

30 James G. Townsend, "Industrial hygiene in the post-war world," *American Journal of Public Health* 34:739–745, July 1944, at pp. 739, 742.

CHAPTER TEN

The Newest Field—Public Health

VISITING NURSE ASSOCIATIONS

ALTHOUGH practical nurses were employed on the staffs of visiting nurse associations at the time of the 1918–1919 influenza epidemics and have been associated as visiting housekeepers in various experiments (see page 47), it is only within the last ten years that any appreciable number of agencies in the field of public health have made definite and permanent positions for them in home visiting and clinic service.

The first home visitors to the sick in this country, as in Europe, were untrained but "reliable" women employed by private agencies, usually for a specific group rather than for anyone in the community in need of home care (1). By the time concerted effort was made to establish visiting nursing service, patterned more or less on William Rathbone's experiment in Liverpool, England, in 1859, it was possible to secure graduates of the early schools of nursing, and we are told that the first visiting nurse employed by the Women's Board of the New York City Mission in 1877 was a Bellevue Hospital graduate (2).

Between 1885 and 1912, during the adolescent years of the public health nursing movement, there was a continual struggle to raise the level of service to that given by trained and registered nurses. One of the most pressing reasons for the establishment of the National Organization for Public Health Nursing in 1912 was to set standards for the employment of visiting nurses. In that year there were ten types of agencies employing visiting nurses, among them 28 churches for service to parish members and 108 clubs and societies (3). Nursing care at home was frequently provided by totally untrained women. It is not surprising, then, that all the emphasis in initiating this new service was put on employing the best prepared staffs that could be found and that consternation among the some 600 agencies employing visiting nurses (probably about 2,000 nurses [4]) was created by the announcement, early in 1912, that the Metropolitan Life Insurance Company (engaged, since 1909, in a plan to pay visiting nurse associations for visits to sick policy holders) was about to send out a group of untrained women to do nursing in the homes of chronic patients under the supervision of the regular trained nurse.

At the same time, the New York State Department of Education advocated training nurse attendants in hospitals too small for professional nursing schools. "Nursing service for all the people must come from some source," comments the editor of the *American Journal of Nursing* wisely, so "it is evident we will have a 'second grade woman' in the field" (5). As evidenced by articles and letters to the *Journal* at this time, agitation centered on the training and supervision of this group, and considerable misgiving was felt as to their legal status. A questionnaire sent to eight of the largest visiting nurse associations returned six approving replies, the other two expressing fear that the service could not be controlled and that "false standards of efficiency" would be set up in the minds of the public. Five of six registries questioned were already placing attendants, but they reported that they were unsatisfactory, incompetent, and officious, and that they tried to charge too much. The salaries proposed at this time were from $17 to $25 a week (6). Apparently the Metropolitan Life Insurance Company plan was dropped, not to be taken up again until requests to recognize licensed practical nursing service came from the visiting nurse associations themselves in 1940–1944.

During the influenza epidemics of 1918 and 1919, so great was the demand for home nurses and so willing was the public to pay anything for help that maids, housekeepers, hairdressers, and laundresses left their own work, donned white, and hired out as graduate nurses, or enrolled at the commercial registries as nurses. Even with the return of thousands of nurses from military service, Cecilia A. Evans wrote, "there seems to be a growing demand for a type of woman with much less training than that which the graduate has" (7).

Pressed by the demand, the Cleveland Visiting Nurse Association in 1919 embarked upon a plan for the training of attendants which sounds very like our courses for practical nurses of today. It consisted of two months of theory followed by four of practice in homes under supervision. "We feel very strongly that our idea should be to train these attendants for the care of convalescents and chronics only, so as not in any way to infringe on the province of the private duty nurse" (8). Yet in three years this "determined effort" was abandoned, because it was found that attendants were answering calls on their own initiative and exceeding their prescribed duties.

The same year found the Visiting Nurse Association of Springfield, Mass., busy with a group of attendants, "women of tact and common sense," who were hired to help the graduate nurse with difficult cases in homes where there was more than one patient and to give care to chronics and convalescents. Full time service was offered certain families, all under close supervision (9).

Apparently, the possibility of both training and employing attendants in visiting nurse associations interested administrators during the months following World War I, for not only did Cleveland, Springfield, and Boston experiment with staffs but the Visiting Nurse Association of Orange, N.J., proposed that visiting nurse associations assume full responsibility for recruiting, conducting a course, and employing and supervising the graduates (10). Much of the April and May 1919 issues of *The Public Health Nurse* was devoted to the problem of the attendant. Katharine Shepard described the work of the attendants in the Household Nursing Association of Boston (11), and Grace Bentley summarized what she felt had been learned from the Cleveland experiment (12).

As many of the conclusions drawn from these early experiments are corroborated by the experiences of agencies now employing practical nurses and others suggest ideas for future trial, they are briefly cited here:

The practical nurse should not accompany the public health nurse on visits just to perform minor duties, because these frequently present opportunities for the latter to teach health to the patient and family.

It is not safe to send the practical nurse alone to a new case, because the condition of the patient is unknown and the visiting nurse association is responsible.

Adjustments in the home are too difficult for the practiced nurse who tries to carry a case alone.

The full time of a supervisor is necessary to select, train, and supervise these workers.

The less previous experience in sickness a trainee has had the better. She has less to unlearn if she has not been in situations where she has been taught badly or not at all yet thinks she knows it all.

Older women make better practical nurses than young women.

The practical nurse should be assigned to full time service in the home when needed.

Attendants trained in hospitals only are not so satisfactory for home service, as they do not know enough about housekeeping.

Training these women in hospitals where there is a professional nursing school creates unrest and dissatisfaction.

Miss Evans did not feel it wise to train attendants in visiting nurse associations, as it is important to keep the distinction between them and the graduate nurses. The central school is just as sound for training attendants as for training professional nurses, wrote Miss Evans, anticipating developments by twenty-five years. She pointed out that such a school provides improved teaching equipment and experienced faculty, lends dignity to the program, and does much to inform the public about qualified practical nurses; it also attracts a better class of candidates: the result is better service to patients, and the group has greater self-respect and is protected from the influx of untrained workers (13).

In 1923–1924 the first study of the cost of visiting nursing recognized the employment of paid nonprofessional assistants in clinics and supplied a method for estimating the cost of their service. The study referred to the plan as "a complicated system to incorporate into the work of an organization, but where the nursing of chronics is an appreciable part of an agency's program, it is a resource worthy of consideration" (14).

In 1933, the Community Health Association in Boston employed practical nurses for the care of chronic patients. The service was found to be prohibitive in travel time, as the cases were scattered, and in the amount of supervision necessary. The plan was tried again in 1941, however, and is now functioning successfully.

As late as 1936, Miss Gardner wrote that the administrative difficulties in adding practical nurses to a visiting nurse staff were so great that "no noteworthy development in this much needed type of service had taken place" (15).

Most of these programs for the use of trained practical nurses under the supervision of public health nurses functioned in urban centers. A few rural areas, however, had attempted to study the situation and the local town and county nurses were developing more or less formal ways of securing practical nursing assistance for patients needing bed-side care (16). In Cattaraugus County, N.Y., in 1931, a survey of 120 home cases revealed that 22 were under the care of a practical nurse who was not a member of the family or a neighbor. About a third of the cases were not receiving adequate care of any kind. Dr. Winslow pointed out that there was no reason to think that a plan could not be worked out to provide supervision by the county nurse of the practical nurses giving bedside care in rural families—"an inspiring example of what may be done in carrying health to the farm dweller" (17).

The Maternity Center Association of New York has been concerned for years in seeing that expectant mothers receive help from qualified practical nurses at home during the "lying-in" period or on the mother's return from the hospital. The Association's survey of community resources for maternity care includes such questions as: Are there subsidiary workers on the staff to work under the supervision of the visiting nurses? How many practical nurses cared for obstetric patients during the year? Are they registered and licensed by the state? Does their training fit them to care for obstetric patients? How are they secured? Are their credentials examined? Are they supervised? How? (18)

Our entrance into the second world war brought an immediate realization that nonprofessional assistance would be needed at a hundred points in the public health program and that this assistance would be volunteer and paid, trained and untrained, full time and part time, men, women, boys, and girls (19). Health departments and visiting nurse associations welcomed the services of Red Cross workers and Red Cross Volunteer Nurses' Aides and began a tentative exploration of the employment of paid practical nurses. By 1943, the National Organization for Public Health Nursing reported that sixteen of 584 public health nursing agencies were employing full time practical nurses; twelve had initiated the service between 1940 and 1943. Among the sixteen, there were eleven nonofficial agencies, three county health departments, a municipal health department, and a "combination" official-nonofficial agency (20).

So far as could be determined, these sixteen public health nursing agencies were in January 1945 employing 55 practical nurses, not all of whom were licensed in states without a law. The Visiting Nurse Service of New York led in size of staff with 18 nurses, who made 6 per cent of the bedside care visits for the Service in 1944. For the writer's list of public health nursing agencies employing practical nurses as of March 1945, see Appendix, page 351.

Problems Related to the Service of Practical Nurses

In general, administrators agree that service from practical nurses cannot be safely installed without providing adequate and continuous supervision. Selection and oversight of cases and planning of the service takes more time than for the professional staff. Nearly all patients require full bedside care, frequently taking two or three hours, and many patients have to be lifted, so the time devoted to each case is high and the physical strain heavier than in the usual visit schedule. Practical nurses, therefore, cannot carry as many cases as the professional public health staff and they must be watched for overfatigue and back strains. The supervisor or the staff nurse in whose district the practical nurse is working takes the responsibility for assigning and following the progress of each case. All health teaching and the handling of social problems and instruction of other members of the family in the care of the patient are the responsibility of the professional nurse. Practical nurses cannot be expected to detect significant changes in their patients' condition and are not prepared to cope with social problems. The public health nurse must visit often enough to be satisfied that practical nursing service is suitable and effective and that no chance for health instruction is being missed. With the newer developments in the care of the chronic patient, it is specially important for the public health nurse to make routine visits to all elderly people under the care of practical nurses (21).

Occasionally, both the family and the doctor need to have this type of service explained to them by the supervisor. In a personal communication to the writer, the director of the family nursing service in a midwestern city wrote:

This experiment has indicated that we need to do a great deal in educating the public as to the difference between graduate and practical nurses, and that the nurses themselves aren't certain how to proceed. It is the responsibility of the graduate nurse to explain to the patient or family that the practical nurse will be coming in, but patients ask the practical nurse what hospital she came from and when she graduated, and then the confusion begins. The practical nurse does not always follow through with the explanation as to length of course, etc. Difference in uniform does not help much because we have student nurses in the state public health nurses' uniform, students in their hospital uniforms, and students in the Cadet Corps uniform.

In February 1944, the Metropolitan Life Insurance Company established policies for the use of practical nurses and auxiliary workers in public health nursing agencies holding contracts for service to Metropolitan policyholders. A rider is given to an affiliated agency upon request, provided the following conditions are met (22).

That the plan for the use of practical nurses have the approval of the agency's medical advisory committee

That the practical nurse be well selected and be a graduate of a recognized school of practical nurses or have had satisfactory experience

That the agency have a carefully worked out plan for the introduction of the practical nurse and a schedule of field supervisory visits

That the public health nurse continue to give care between the visits of the practical nurse and supervise the care given by the practical nurse

That the practical nurse be assigned only to cases that have already been seen by the public health nurse, and to those patients who are not acutely ill

That the usual fee for visits be charged whether the visit is made by a public health nurse or a practical nurse

That such riders be reviewed at the end of one year

This agreement was originally for the duration of the war only. The John Hancock Mutual Life Insurance Company offers the same arrangement.

The policies of most visiting nurse associations that offer practical nursing service are:

New cases are visited by public health nurses and dismissal visits are usually made by them.

Families in which there are social problems or need of health supervision are not assigned to practical nurses.

The same charge per visit is made regardless of which nurse makes the visit. This is because bedside care visits take longer, and there is the same overhead for both workers. Travel time is higher for practical nurses because their cases are more widely scattered and they require more supervisory time. These two items offset the saving in salary.

All referrals to community resources and reports to doctors go through the professional nurse.

Nursing procedures permitted practical nurses are limited; they correspond to those allowed on hospital duty. Some agencies do not assign maternity cases to practical nurses.

If a new treatment is ordered, the practical nurse must secure office permission to carry it out. Any change in the patient's condition must be reported at once.

In a few agencies, the practical nurse is allowed to stay to prepare a simple meal, or to arrange her visit so as to help with some household routines. The question of permitting the nurse to remain longer comes up fairly frequently. It would appear that visiting nurse associations could run a full time (eight hour) practical nursing service in addition to the part time service if they wanted to and if they could get enough well prepared practical nurses.

Patients with communicable disease are never assigned to practical nurses unless convalescent, with the possible exception of patients mildly ill with grippe (23). In explanation of this policy, administrators emphasize that it is one thing to ask a member of the household to learn certain procedures for his own safety and that of the others in the household, and quite another to risk the health of an untrained outsider. Doctors and registered nurses agree that the fewer people in contact with the source of infection, the better for all concerned. Furthermore, in communicable disease more than in most home illnesses, circumstances alter procedures. The same rigid routine cannot always be adhered to. Besides familiarity with aseptic techniques, the nurse must have fundamental knowledge of each type of communicable disease, its mode of spread, complications, and sequelae. An estimate must be made of the family's ability, intelligence, time, and physical means to carry out routines before they are taught. Interpretation of the doctor's orders to Mrs. Smith in a case of scarlet fever may be couched in college classroom phraseology, while the nurse may have to say to Mrs. Brown, "The bugs are in his spit." Teaching and procedures will also vary in homes with and without children, with and without bathrooms and running water, with and without food handlers caring for the patient, with and without members of the family going to school or to work. Knowledge of local and sometimes state health department regulations is essential. One of the most important functions of the public health nurse is to assist in determining the original source of infection. This may call for specialized knowledge, to say nothing of skill in interviewing and consumate tact. Immunization procedures and facilities must be known. Safety for all counsels professional nursing service in the home care of communicable disease.

There are, of course, stages in the communicable disease when a practical nurse may function safely and be of great assistance in hastening recovery, as for example in caring for an arrested case of tuberculosis, in helping the mother of a family adjust to her housework, or, in emergencies, helping out with specific steps in care. In Rhode Island, for example, in the 1943 epidemic of poliomyelitis, some of the practical nurses assisted with hot packs. In January 1945, a practical nurse, under the supervision of both a registered nurse and a physical therapist, was in charge of all the "packers" at Harper Hospital, Detroit, in a ward of 12 polio patients, victims of the 1944 epidemic.

The Case Load

Typical cases carried by practical nurses in eight agencies were surprisingly alike. In fact, eight conditions appeared on every list sent to the author: arthritis, arteriosclerosis, paralysis, cardiac conditions, cancer, diabetes, senility, and "debility due to old age." Other conditions frequently reported were fractures, anemias, nephritis, sciatica, cardiorenal conditions, and chronic bronchitis.

Five or six visits per day per nurse were usual, but several agencies reported only 4.6. Travel time everywhere was high—20 to 25 per cent of the total time on duty (24).

Division of Duties

Just as the practical nurse in the hospital frees the professional nurse for more difficult skills, treatments, tests, and procedures, so in the public health field, whenever a visit or a case can be turned over to a practical nurse, the public health nurse uses the time for the special teaching and preventive function for which she has been prepared. For besides thorough knowledge of her own professional nursing field, its progress and application, besides her knowledge of community resources, the well prepared public health nurse is expected to be alive to the trends in current events and to place her rich experience at the service of those who are striving for improvement in all the fields related to health. Take, for example, the subject of housing. No one knows better than the public health nurse who visits seven or eight families a day, many in substandard houses or even hovels, how much

our cities, towns, and villages need housing reform. She sees the bene-
ficial effects of decent, clean, sunny homes in the new housing projects.
She feels a responsibility for these conditions. She is expected to have
—and she has—a social conscience informed by study, observation,
and firsthand experience. Hers is the responsibility of sharing in the
larger aspects of such movements. The practical nurse, on the other
hand, observes and reports conditions and tries to teach families to
adapt in practical ways to whatever situations surround them. The
public health nurse goes much further. She helps instigate action,
serves on housing committees, speaks to citizen groups, joins in planning projects. Other areas of interest may be recreation, fire prevention, safety, or delinquency.

The public health nurse is expected to know from her preparation
in the field of sociology and social problems, not only the responsible
agencies to whom to report conditions but how to report them, how to
discriminate between the serious and the trivial, to know enough of the
local ordinances or laws to understand where individual effort stops
and legal responsibility begins. Schools of professional nursing attempt to give their students an appreciation of the development of
society (25). The urban community, the rural community, the functions of modern government, the social problems needing reform are
covered for the student nurse in lectures, classroom discussions, observation, and outside reading, in all approximately thirty hours of lectures. The public health nursing student goes into this field even more
intensively after graduation from the school of nursing. She usually
adds, as a part of her basic preparation for public health, a full course
in sociology—two to four university credits. Compare this with the
eight to twenty pages devoted to all such subjects in the textbooks for
practical nurses, or the hour or so of discussion following an occasional
lecture or visit to a home.

Teaching good health habits may sound easy—all a nurse has to do
is explain a set of "keep well" rules, some behavior "don't's," and some
warnings against catching diseases, and leave lists of balanced diets.
But it is not so simple. Not only does the public health nurse have to be
thoroughly grounded in up-to-date subject matter, but she has to know
how to teach and how to adapt her teaching to old, young, rich, poor,
handicapped, college bred, and illiterate, and be able to select appropriate printed material which will impress her message on those who

can read or see, and she must make the family want to follow her suggestions. Only a well educated nurse can do this type of teaching successfully.

Salaries and Personnel Policies

The range of salaries paid practical nurses in public health work (most of whom are licensed and all of whom are trained*) is $90 to $150 a month. In only one agency do the maximum salaries of the practical nurses overlap the minimum salaries of the professional nurses, but only for those without public health preparation. There is usually a difference of $5 to $10 a month, in some cases as much as $40. Nearly all the agencies have at least two salary rates, the beginners' and the maximum. The former may be paid for three, six, or twelve months, the latter is usually reached in two years. In six agencies employing one to eighteen practical nurses, the average maximum salary was $125 in 1945.

In the agencies employing practical nurses, personnel policies usually apply to the whole staff, including medical supervision, vacations, sick leave, etc. Group insurance plans (health, hospital, and annuity) cover the whole staff.

The uniforms of the practical nurses are usually distinctly different from those of the public health staff. They may be blue (not the public health blue, however), tan, grey, or white. One of the most attractive is that worn by the practical nurses in New Britain, Connecticut: tan tailored one or two piece dress similar to that worn by the Army Nurse Corps; brown coat sweater or hip-length tailored cloth jacket; tan or brown tailored hat or beret; dark brown tailored top coat; yellow silk scarf; tan or brown gloves; brown plain leather Cuban or flat heeled oxfords, with harmonizing stockings (suede leather, cutwork, two-tone effects, or strap pumps are not acceptable); plain dark brown socks (to be worn for warmth only); watch with second hand; fountain pen with brown ink; no jewelry except school pin and watch (wearing of wedding ring is optional).

Practical nurses over fifty years of age find public health nursing very strenuous, so the younger group is preferred.

---

* If by "training" in two agencies we can accept years of successful private duty experience.

Attitudes Toward the Service

Every agency reported that doctors, families, and patients were enthusiastic about the service. Five agencies had some difficulty at first in convincing the professional staff that it was wise to employ practical nurses. At present there is general acceptance and in most instances warm appreciation of their help. All the agencies are exceedingly careful not to permit the practical nurses to care for patients who need private duty professional nursing.

No public health nursing association had given the service special publicity.

As for the practical nurses themselves, they love their work, genuinely and devotedly. Either the visiting nurse associations have been unusually lucky or skillful in picking their staffs or the work really is ideally suited to the capacities and tastes of practical nurses, for they are a happy group. A professional nurse wondered why a practical nurse was not bored with caring for five chronic patients a day, every day. The practical nurse answered for herself: "I can see why you feel that way. You are trained to do many other things. My training was with chronic patients. It's what I want to do and what I prepared myself to do." Supervisors assist, of course, in seeing that the practical nurses do not get bored. A change of district, new cases, or the development of a specialty stimulate a fresh point of view. Most practical nurses actually dislike change, however. They like their patients too well.

As Mildred Hatton, Educational Director of the Providence, R.I., District Nurse Association, points out, the most important factor in using nonprofessional staff is that each person's work "should be so clearly defined that she will instantly recognize any deviation and seek professional help" (26).

CLINICS

Public health nurses have always depended to some extent upon nonprofessional help in the clinics and health conferences under their supervision. Usually, except in well organized, large urban clinics, this help has taken the form of volunteer service from local groups of women, sometimes high school girls or Red Cross aides. It has ranged from sporadic, rather undependable interest to the most loyal, efficient, practical help in equipping and running the clinic, assisting with patients, and rallying other citizens to its support. Many a clinic and preschool or infant conference owes its continuance to volunteer help. Most public health nurses would feel that the value of such willing service in promoting community understanding of the health program is inestimable (27). Hence it would be unfortunate to take any of these responsibilities out of the hands of volunteers for the sake of keeping practical nurses busy or of securing slightly better technically trained help.

However, when volunteer help fails or is undependable or the clinic becomes so large that a multitude of subprofessional duties accumulate and professional nursing time is being taken from the patients by routines which a practical nurse could do, then good management dictates the employment of nonprofessional assistance. During the present emergency, many health department clinics have employed as "clinic nurse" a registered nurse without public health training, whose duties are confined to clinic activities. She makes few if any home calls but is responsible for assisting with treatments and for record-keeping and office work, with some duties in the actual administration of vaccines and the like. These nurses may be on full or part time. Georgia, for example, had on January 1, 1944, 17 full time and 101 part time clinic nurses (28). "Non-public health nurses ['clinic nurses'] seem to be needed the most, in addition to well-qualified public health nurses and volunteer or paid auxiliary workers, in large clinics where numerous technical procedures are involved in diagnosis, tests, and treatments" (29). Venereal disease, tuberculosis, and maternity clinics offer opportunities of this kind.

In 1942–1943, partly as a means of discovering which duties performed by public health nurses in clinics could be assigned to nonprofessional workers, the Committee on Nursing Administration of the National Organization for Public Health Nursing surveyed and evaluated 212 clinics and health conferences of various types (child health, crippled children, maternity, tuberculosis, and venereal disease) in 38 states and the District of Columbia. A list of activities was drawn up and an attempt was made to indicate the primary task of the public health nurse. It was particularly important to relate these to direct personal contact with patients and opportunities for extending health education since these are the two points where the public health nurse is most effective. It was clear at once that many of the desirable opportunities for using the public health nurses' abilities were either not being realized at all or were being assigned to less competent personnel, while at the same time—and often in the same clinic—her valuable professional contribution was not being made because she was too busy with routine, even clerical jobs. Above all, this study brought out the value of careful analysis of all the routine duties in every type of clinic or conference to determine which duties are appropriate for public health nurses, practical nurses, and clerical help, and for which and when volunteers may serve (30). From the list of the procedures reviewed in that study the present writer has selected—arbitrarily—those duties which she has seen practical nurses carry out or knows that they are taught in the approved schools. (See also the list of duties recommended for "auxiliary workers" as stated by the surveyors, pp. 11–15 of the study.)

A. ACTIVITIES IN PREPARATION FOR THE CLINIC SESSION

    Registration or admission to clinic service*
    Assigning patients to physicians**
    Selection and placement of stationery*
    Supervision of ventilation, heating, and lighting of clinic rooms
    Preparation of play space for children
    Preparation of dressing rooms and/or cubicles
    Distribution and care of linen
    Setting up examination tables and/or trays
    Setting up treatment tables and/or trays
    Setting up equipment for urine and hemoglobin tests
    Setting up equipment for taking temperature, pulse, and respiration
    Preparation for sterilization of solutions, instruments, syringes, and gloves
    Placing in and removal of above materials from sterilizer
    Preparation of equipment for cleaning instruments and syringes
    Preparation of equipment for heating baby bottles
    Supervision of toilet facilities
    Supervision of facilities for taking specimens

B. ACTIVITIES DURING CLINIC SESSION

    1. *Items Common to All Types of Clinics*
    Registration or admission of patients**
    Removal of records from files*
    Checking appointment cards and schedules*

* Can be performed by medical secretary or clerk.
** Limited, means that a part of this service must be performed by the public health nurse.

Giving serial numbers to patients*
Ushering patients through clinic
Transferring records from one clinic worker to another*
Directing patients to dressing, weighing, conference, medical examination, treatment, x-ray rooms, and to laboratory
Preparing patients for medical examination
Taking dictation from physicians*
Preparing examination table between patients
Giving return appointments for clinics if not accompanied by other instructions*

2. *Additional Items for Each Type of Clinic*
  a. Child health conferences
  Supervision of children's play
  Arrangement for care of baby carriages
  Attaching forms for immunization or vaccination to case record*
  Assisting parents in preparation of children for medical examination
  Supervising procedures in dressing and weighing rooms
  Keeping rooms and/or cubicles in order
  Taking and recording weight and height
  Taking and recording temperature, pulse, and respiration
  Making out certificates for immunizing treatments*
  Recording treatments on patients' records*
  b. Crippled children's clinics
  Care of patients' needs while waiting
  Accompanying patients to lavatory, to dressing, examining, and treatment rooms
  Special care of stretcher patients
  Preparing patients for medical examination
  c. Maternity clinics
  Making out forms for Wassermann tests and for vaginal smears*
  Weighing patients
  Taking temperature, pulse, and respiration
  Testing urine
  Testing hemoglobin (simple tests)
  Recording tests on patients' case records*
  Resterilizing gloves and instruments while the clinic is in session
  d. Tuberculosis clinics

* Can be performed by medical secretary or clerk.

Taking and recording temperature
Taking and recording weight
Remaining with patients in x-ray room
Preparing patients for Mantoux and patch tests
Resterilizing syringes and needles while the clinic is in session
Making out forms for sputum tests*
  e. Venereal disease clinics
Taking and recording weight
Testing urine
Assisting with Wassermann tests
Cleaning syringes and needles and sterilizing them between treatments
Entering treatments on patients' case records*
Completion of Wassermann specimen data for mailing*

C. ACTIVITIES AFTER THE CLINIC SESSION
Checking appointment cards*
Filing cards and records*
Making out reports of clinic*
Putting clinic rooms in order
Disposing of soiled linen
Disposing of exhibit and teaching materials*
Cleaning examining and treatment tables and trays; also urinalysis, hemoglobin, and thermometer trays
Cleaning syringes, needles, gloves, and instruments
Refilling containers with solutions
Preparing materials for sterilization
Preparing supplies, such as gauze dressings, cotton balls, and applicators
Ordering supplies**

This survey indicates that if the public health nurse is really fulfilling her proper function in clinics, her time before and after the session can be cut two-thirds by proper allocation of duties to nonprofessional workers. During the clinic session, the surveyors felt, a reallocation of duties was needed rather than any effort to cut down on time now spent (31).

The professional duties with their implied opportunities for better

---

* Can be performed by medical secretary or clerk.
** Limited, means that a part of this service must be performed by the public health nurse.

service are a challenge to any clinic administrator. At the same time they form a sound reason for considering the use of other nurses as relief to the public health nurses. Incidentally, such relief would give the public health nurses more time for developing the clinic as a teaching center for student practice of various types and more time for home visiting (32).

Practical nurses are used as assistants in some clinics and health conferences conducted by visiting nurse associations. In one agency in the Middle West, the practical nurse spends half her time in taking juvenile court wards to clinics for examination and treatment. In a visiting nurse service in New York city, practical nurses are assigned to assist the public health nurse in part time service to industries. "Nurses' aides"—one of the Civil Service titles for practical nurses—are employed in the rapid treatment clinics for venereal disease, and increasingly in health and welfare departments the problem of nursing care for dependent chronic patients who wish to remain at home and use outpatient services when they can suggests the employment of practical nurses who might serve in giving nursing care at home as well as in assisting in such clinics. We have probably only touched the edge of the field of usefulness of the well prepared practical nurse in combined and shared services in home and clinic visits.

In clinic situations, as elsewhere, provision must be made for adequate teaching and supervision of the practical nurses.

SCHOOL NURSING

So far as is known there are no full time, full paid practical nurses working in the primary and secondary schools, either in charge of service or as assistants to the school nurse, although they may help on a voluntary basis. The reason for this is fourfold:

The registered nurse can find all the assistance she needs among the teachers, older pupils, and parents

Nearly all the school nurses' responsibilities call for a high degree of training, no part of which should be in the hands of a semi-prepared person other than the assistants mentioned above

Much of school nursing service is part time, especially in rural areas

No continuous bedside nursing is given by the school medical department; children sick at home are referred to community agencies or the parents are taught to give care

The school nurse cooperates with available nursing services in the community and when necessary assists a family to find a qualified practical nurse, even offering to supervise her care, but all the school health services either relate to conditions which the teachers, parents, and pupils themselves should handle or are strictly professional procedures. Except in very large city school systems, there is virtually no in-between job for a practical nurse assistant. The trend is to place more and more responsibility on teachers and parents, and the employment of a practical nurse would defeat this purpose (33). In a real sense, the school health program is an educational activity in which the personnel participates; it does not deal with illness or the bedside nursing of illness. Even the routine duties of weighing, measuring, filing health records, keeping the first aid equipment clean, etc., are more profitably done by the students as part of their experience in learning about health (34).

THE FUTURE OF THE PRACTICAL NURSE IN PUBLIC HEALTH

The experience of the score or more agencies over the last twenty years in employing practical nurses in public health programs of all types would seem to indicate a few essential safeguards and needed studies. It is important to:

Survey the case load and the patients' needs to see if there is enough work suitable for practical nurses and to determine the suitable duties in clinic services

Prepare for the employment of practical nurses through group discussions with all members of the staff (it is assumed that the board and medical advisers have endorsed the plan)

Select trained—if possible licensed—practical nurses with some experience in home situations as well as basic training on hospital wards

Differentiate these workers in the minds of the public from the public health nursing staff by a distinctive uniform of different color as well as an emblem

Provide an abundance of supervision to introduce and teach the staff routines, to select and oversee cases, and to assist in developing skills and aptitudes

Secure the doctor's approval before turning over a case to a practical nurse

Reduce and simplify the record work, as practical nurses find record-keeping difficult

If several practical nurses are employed, plan in-service educational programs especially for them and arrange for them to share any professional staff conferences that they would find useful

Provide cars for practical nurses who cover a wide territory in order to
reduce travel time

As experience with the service develops, study the nature of the demand
and need for it with a view to adjusting the amount of time the
practical nurses are permitted to stay in the homes. If licensed
practical nurses are not available from other sources for private
duty in homes, their provision on other than a visit basis is the
responsibility of the visiting nurse association

For many years, public health nurses and private duty nurses have
been reluctant to leave the bedside care of really sick people in the
hands of incompetent, sketchily taught amateurs, yet because of the
impossibility of finding competent practical nurses they have been
forced to do so. Families and neighbors can be taught to do a great
deal, sometimes all that is needed, especially if the patient is a child,
but there are situations in which the conscientious nurse worries about
her patient in her absence and would welcome a trained helping hand.

The fact that several agencies have steadily added to their staffs of
practical nurses and plan to retain this group permanently is convincing
evidence that here is a new field for the well prepared practical nurse.
In a personal communication to the writer, the director and educational
director of the Community Health Service of Minneapolis, which em-
ploys four full time practical nurses, summarizes the conclusion of its
staff thus:

The staff are wholeheartedly in favor of the use of practical nurses to
assist them with the district work. We are now caring for more chronically
ill patients—perhaps because we have the practical nurses and because
hospitals and rest home facilities are limited for the chronically ill patient
who needs care. Our public health nurses feel we are meeting the needs of
the chronically ill in the community more effectively. They also are relieved
of many visits which they know are necessary but do not require their more
technical skills. I think we have been very fortunate in finding very suitable personnel in the practical nurse group.

The 1944 Census of Public Health Nurses in the United States revealed 845 counties (more than one-fourth the total number) without
public health nursing service of any type. The ratio of public health

nurses to population (estimated population for November 1943) was one to more than 5,000 in 39 states, whereas the recommended ratio is one nurse to 2,000 population. Some states in New England came closest to the recommended ratio with one to 3,000. If cities which have the most abundant supply of public health nurses could add competent licensed practical nurses to the professional staff, would it not be possible to release one or more public health nurses qualified to participate in a county public health program? Pearl McIver, chief of the Office of Public Health Nursing, Bureau of State Services, United States Public Health Service, looking at postwar needs, has suggested that not every nurse employed in a public health nursing agency needs to have completed an approved program of study in public health nursing. She poses the question: "Could an area be served by a team of nurses consisting of a fully prepared public health nurse who might have as assistant a senior cadet [student] nurse; a returned veteran nurse who has not had special training or experience in public health nursing; or a competent practical nurse?" (35)

In 1943 in 600 communities with populations of 10,000, there was no form of public health nursing service for the sick at home. Many of these communities were in states without legal control of practical nursing. The National Organization for Public Health Nursing is helping to promote visiting nursing services in some of these places (36). An over-all study of the types of nursing services needed in a given community is much to be desired.

Bedside nursing care under the supervision of health departments is increasing in some areas. It is not known how much of this service would be suitable for practical nurses. It is known that the case load of chronic patients is increasing in both official and nonofficial agencies.

Inasmuch as practical nursing service in the field of public health is in its infancy—one might almost say embryo form except in visiting nurse associations—it would be unwise to hold out great hope for an immediate expansion or demand for their services in all health agencies. That there is a place for them, the writer believes, is incontrovertible. How many we will need, how they should be prepared for the specialty of public health—if at all except on the job—and what combinations of agencies might join in using their services are mere speculations. The United States Public Health Service is already entering a great postwar expansion in public health activities, including a widespread development in hospital, clinic, and outpatient facilities. No less than 65,000 public health nurses are needed for a population of 135,000,000 if one public health nurse is provided for each 2,000 people. In what ratio licensed practical nurses should be supplied is not known. Of two things we can be assured from the history and present practices in public health nursing agencies: administrators will demand basic training and recognized status in candidates for positions in this field, and professional supervision will be supplied from the first to the last day of their service.

REFERENCES

1 For example, in 1812 the Women's Benevolent Society in Charleston, S.C., engaged a "nurse" to visit sick, wounded, or incapacitated sailors returning from the War of 1812. Mary S. Gardner, *Public health nursing*, 3d ed., rev., New York, Macmillan, 1936, p. 26.
2 Gardner (note 1), pp. 26–27.
3 Gardner (note 1), pp. 40–41.
4 Gardner (note 1), p. 463. See also statistics gathered by Ysabella G. Waters, *Visiting nurse in the United States*, New York, Charities Publication Committee, 1909, pp. 368–378.
5 Editorial, *American Journal of Nursing* 12:277, April 1912.
6 Editorial (ref. 5), p. 278. See also Grace Allison, "Shall attendants be trained and registered?" *American Journal of Nursing* 12:928–931, August 1912.
7 Cecelia A. Evans, "How shall the attendants be trained?" *Public Health Nurse* 11:340–342, May 1919.
8 Emma Mandery, "A suggestive plan for training attendants in Cleveland," *Public Health Nurse* 11:256–257, April 1919.
9 Florence M. Caldwell, "The attendant as an assistant to public health nurses," *Public Health Nurse* 11:346, May 1919.
10 Margaret N. Pierson, "Supervised home nursing," *Public Health Nurse* 11:343–344, May 1919.
11 Katharine Shepard, "The attendant in the home," *Public Health Nurse* 11:258–260, April 1919.
12 Grace Bentley, "The supervised attendant service in Cleveland," *Public Health Nurse* 11:251–256, April 1919.
13 Evans (note 7), pp. 340–342.
14 National Organization for Public Health Nursing, *Report of the Committee to Study Visiting Nursing*, New York, Metropolitan Life

Insurance Company, 1924, pp. 30–31, 148. See also the comment on page 29 of the report: "Some agencies have a more liberal policy toward the care of chronic patients . . . an average load of 56–60 chronics is usual for a staff of 41 nurses." For up-to-date suggestions on record-keeping and counting visits, see "Auxiliary workers in public health nursing agencies," *Public Health Nursing* 35:103, February 1943.

15 Gardner (note 1), p. 36.

16 See such developments as that in Tioga County, New York, under the auspices of the Maternity Center Association (*Public Health Nurse* 19:599–601, December 1927) and the extension of the Red Cross Nursing Classes in rural areas.

17 C.-E. A. Winslow, *Health on the farm and in the village; a review and evaluation of the Cattaraugus County health demonstration,* New York, Macmillan, 1931, pp. 182–183. For a discussion of the use of practical nurses in home confinement cases in Cattaraugus County, New York, see Henry R. O'Brien, "Nursing study in a home delivery area," *Public Health Nursing* 36:554–561, November 1944, at p. 555. Of 2,179 deliveries, 120, or 5.5 per cent, were attended by practical nurses; 87 of these families were in fair or good economic circumstances, 33 were poor.

18 Maternity Center Association, *Public health nursing in obstetrics,* New York, the Association, 1940, part I, pp. 68, 74. See also, for use of practical nurses in obstetric cases, Caroline C. Van Blarcom, *Getting ready to be a mother,* rev. by Hazel Corbin, 4th ed., New York, Macmillan, 1940, pp. 65–66.

19 For evidence of this realization, see the index for *Public Health Nursing* for 1940–1945 under headings Subsidiary workers, Volunteer workers, Auxiliary workers, especially March 1940, p. 142; December 1942, pp. 659–662; March 1944, pp. 137, 142; April 1944, p. 206. See also Dorothy Carter, *Volunteers and other auxiliary workers,* New York, National Organization for Public Health Nursing, 1943, especially sections on selection of personnel, pp. 14–15.

20 Dorothy E. Wiesner and Margaret M. Murphy, "Inactive nurses and auxiliary workers," *Public Health Nursing* 36:142–143, March 1944.

21 C.-E. A. Winslow, "Has public health nursing reached its destination?" *Public Health Nursing* 36:609–616, December 1944, at pp. 610, 615. Approximately a third of the visits of rural public health nurses in New York state are now for bedside care. In New Orleans, a staff of about ten nurses is engaged in a demonstration of care in the field of geriatrics. P. 611.

22 Personal communication to the writer from the Director of Nursing Bureau, Welfare Division, Metropolitan Life Insurance Company, February 1945.

23 The importance of professional nursing supervision of tuberculosis cases cared for at home is shown in the series of leaflets entitled *Home care of tuberculosis* published by the National Tuberculosis Association, New York, 1943.

24 The most complete report to date of practical nursing service describes the Visiting Nurse Service of New York. Elisabeth Cogswell Phillips, "Practical nurses in a public health agency," *Public Health Nursing* 36:516–519, October 1944; *American Journal of Nursing*, 44:974–975, October 1944.

25 See, for example, Gladys Sellew, *Sociology and social problems in nursing service*, Philadelphia, Saunders, 1941, chapters 1–4.

26 "Guidance for today and tomorrow," *Public Health Nursing* 36:426–429, August 1944, at p. 427. For selection of duties for subsidiary workers, see Ruth B. Freeman, *Techniques in supervision in public health nursing*, Philadelphia, Saunders, 1944, pp. 69–70.

27 For ways of using various kinds of personnel in official agencies, see Alberta B. Wilson, "Using emergency personnel," *Public Health Nursing* 36:137–141, March 1944.

28 Abbie R. Weaver, "A statewide immunization program," *Public Health Nursing* 36:575–578, November 1944.

29 Hortense Hilbert, "Public health nursing services in clinics," *Public Health Nursing* 36:209–220, May 1944; 36:287–293, June 1944 (reprint, p. 7).

30 Hilbert (note 29), reprint, pp. 5–6, 21–22. Copies of the clinic schedule employed in this survey are available from the National Organization for Public Health Nursing.

31 Hilbert (note 29), reprint, pp. 7–9.

32 Hilbert (note 29), reprint, p. 20.

33 Ruth E. Grout, "Nurse in wartime school health program," *Public Health Nursing* 34:477–481, September 1942.

34 Bosse B. Randle, "Wartime essentials in school nursing," *Public Health Nursing* 35:482–483, September 1943. See also Editorials, "School nurse and community" and "School nursing: what is its future?" *Public Health Nursing* 36:441–442, September 1944.

35 Pearl McIver, "The 1944 census of public health nurses," *Public Health Nursing* 36:498–501, October 1944.

36 News note, "AWCS project," *Public Health Nursing* 36:541–542, October 1944.

CHAPTER ELEVEN

Uncle Sam Needs Practical Nurses

FEDERAL institutions using attendants* for nursing service are administered by the following departments:

Veterans Administration, Nursing Service, Washington, D.C.
Public Health Service, Washington, D.C.
  Bureau of Medical Services, Office of Nursing
  Bureau of State Services, Office of Public Health Nursing
Office of Indian Affairs, Nursing Service, Chicago, Illinois
Army Nurse Corps, Washington, D.C.
Navy Nurse Corps, Washington, D.C.

With the exception of the Army and Navy, all the appointments open to attendants in federal institutions are classified by the United States Civil Service Commission (there is a nursing consultant to the Medical Division), and the Appointees have Civil Service status, including retirement benefits.

Coming also under Civil Service appointment are the positions in the municipal hospitals of the District of Columbia (general medical, surgical, tuberculosis, and mental), the Home for the Aged, and the Department of Health. Attendants of various types must meet the same qualifications as in other federal institutions.

There is no class under Civil Service designated as "practical nurse." The classified positions (subprofessional) that call for duties corresponding to those of a practical nurse are hospital attendant, trained

Note. The material for this chapter was gathered mainly through visits to and correspondence with the various federal departments. Appreciation is here expressed to the superintendents and directors of nurses who supplied figures and arranged visits to hospitals with typical attendant problems.

* The term "attendants" as used in this chapter designates any one of the classes of workers listed on page 187 who perform duties similar or equivalent to those of a practical nurse.

No attempt has been made to describe the services in all types of federally supported institutions but only those where the greatest number of attendants are employed. The Tennessee Valley Authority, War Relocation Centers, emergency services in departmental agencies, and the executive nursing staffs (for example, the Children's Bureau) are not included.

attendant, nurses' aide, and nursing assistant. There is also a medical guard attendant in the federal prison hospitals with some nursing duties. The CPC-18 attendant classification has included a few simple nursing duties such as alcohol rubs, preoperative shaving, and enemas. Some of the positions are being reclassified and call for men graduate nurses.

In 1945 salaries ranged from $1,200 (SP-1) to $2,000 (SP-6) without overtime allowances (with overtime, $1,560 to $2,600) (1). The highest class, SP-6, is for a type of supervising or charge attendant who must work up to the position through the lower classes, SP-1 to SP-5. There are comparatively few attendants holding the SP-6 rating. The position is secured by years of service and evidence of satisfactory performance of duties and dependability, rather than by the addition of new skills or further formal training.

Of these positions the one entitled "nursing attendant," which was a war emergency appointment, most nearly corresponds in description of duties to a licensed practical nurse who is a graduate of an approved school of practical nursing (2). However, the requirement of two full years of high school differs, as the majority of the schools of practical nursing require only grammar school graduation. The applicant for the position of nursing assistant who cannot present evidence of two years of high school is given a two-hour written examination with a required passing mark of 70 for nonpreference candidates, 65 for those with military preference, and 60 for candidates with veterans disability preference.

An applicant must show a minimum of six months as a student nurse in a recognized school of nursing or one year of satisfactory experience as a trained attendant or practical nurse.

The description of the duties of the nursing assistant follows.

Under immediate supervision of a Graduate Nurse on a ward to administer light body massage, to give baths and to take and record temperatures of other than seriously and critically ill patients; to serve prescribed between meal nourishments; to clean medicine cabinets, medicine trays and glasses; maintain Nurse's Office in orderly condition; maintain ward roster of patients; answer telephone; direct and supervise ward visitors; receive and distribute mail to patients; collect and dispatch patients' outgoing mail; perform such other related duties as will enable Nurses to render greater professional service to patients (3).

It will be seen that several of the duties listed here would be carried by ward maids, medical secretaries, volunteers, or clerks in many non-governmental hospitals. Revision of this job description is planned, however.

All attendants, nurses' aides, and nursing assistants who apply to federal institutions for employment, besides meeting minimum qualifications in education and training, must be citizens of the United States and at least twenty-one years of age and must pass a physical examination that is far more complete than that given attendants in most private hospitals. There is no maximum age limit at present. Before the war, eligibles who had not reached their thirtieth birthday were not considered for appointment to positions involving the care of tuberculous patients, but this regulation was waived for the duration. Many of the requirements were not observed during the war emergency but are now again in effect.

DUTIES IN FEDERAL INSTITUTIONS

The duties of attendants in federal institutions show the same variation as in all hospitals. They depend usually upon the degree of responsibility that the individual nurse in charge of a ward decides the attendant may assume, the competence the attendant displays, and the amount of formal teaching the institution has time for. For example, in hospital No. 1 attendants were not permitted to take the temperature of any patient at any time; in hospital No. 2 an attendant was left alone during the lunch period in a ward of 30 acutely ill surgical patients; in hospital No. 3 a male attendant had to be reminded to wash bed pans after use. All three situations sound unreasonable, but investigation revealed what might be called extenuating circumstances in all. In hospital No. 1, government compensation regulations require very close supervision of all patients at all times by registered nurses. In hospital No. 2 the shortage of registered nurses was so acute that if the attendant did not take over the ward either there would be no one in charge or the registered nurse would go lunchless. The attendant had a Red Cross Volunteer Nurses' Aide who could telephone or go for help if it was needed. In hospital No. 3 the supply of applicants for the job was so meager the hospital was forced to employ anyone it could get.

With variable ward conditions, rapid turnover, and differing degrees of preparation among attendants, there is really little wonder that the duties actually assigned to workers do not tally with the Civil Service job descriptions (4). Frequently, also, an institution develops its own colloquial name for the worker as a means of clarifyng his or her place on the ward. For example, for the sake of definiteness a woman worker on the ward classified by Civil Service as an attendant may be called a nurses' aide, a man worker may be called an orderly. An attendant may be designated by the service to which she is attached: orthopedic ward attendant, operating room attendant, etc. (Some of the latter have a SP-3 or SP-4 rating.) Under wartime emergency conditions in many hospitals, these positions involved nursing duties ranging from the simplest procedures to those usually considered only within the province of the registered nurse.*

Many hospital wards employ all or only two or three of the following types of workers: registered nurse (not always one on duty on each ward at night but always one for every two wards), student nurse, nursing assistant, trained attendant, nurses' aide, attendant, orderly, ward maid or ward man, janitor. The fewer the classes represented, the further removed they were from the duties outlined in the Civil Service job description—but the simpler it seemed to be to tell the visitor what each person did. Nursing assistants, nurses' aides, and trained attendants did not appear together on the same ward, but any one of these could be working on a ward where orderlies, ward maids, ward men, or janitors were helping. Cleaning and related nonpatient duties took about half the time of most attendants, nearly all the time of the orderlies and ward maids, all the time of the janitor unless, due to scarcity of male attendants, the janitor was pinch-hitting as an orderly. In many hospitals, both public and private, nurses are still carrying out the duties of orderlies.

Some of the jobs being carried by attendants in these public hospitals were of special interest in showing what can be done to develop a particular ability or aptitude in an attendant. Four such positions are described here.

Clinic Attendant: Assistance in the daily treatment clinic in a home for

---

* It is quite possible to have these duties shift from registered nurse to attendant for a week and back again the next. In one institution visited by the writer, an order—the ink still wet—permitted attendants "until further notice" to feed helpless patients. They had been forbidden to do this the previous week.

the aged consisted in helping the patients down to the clinic if necessary, getting them ready and into position for treatment, applying dressings under the doctor's supervision (as for leg ulcers), keeping clinic room in order, cleaning up after treatments, filing records, maintaining supplies, taking a monthly inventory, and occasionally handing out routine medications from stock, again under the doctor's supervision. This was a part time job, the balance being spent in ward duties.

Orthopedic Assistant: A male attendant trained to assist in an orthopedic clinic to help with heavy lifting of patients in casts had considerable responsibility for assisting the doctor and for moving, weighing, and adjusting patients, handling materials, preparing and applying plaster bandages or casts; caring for equipment including minor repairs on braces; cleaning and preparing the clinic quarters; keeping appointment schedules for patients; and answering the telephone. Although this job represented a promotion over the duties of a ward attendant with nursing duties, very little nursing care was involved.

Charge Attendant: In a large institution for mental cases, a few attendants have reached the "charge attendant" status, SP-6. Their duties are supervisory in nature and great responsibility is placed upon them for maintaining continual attendant service over the hospital. The present turnover in labor prevents the normal rate of promotion to the supervisory level.

Supply Room Attendant: An attendant had been trained to assist in the supply room serving the delivery rooms and large maternity division of a general public hospital. The job was similar to that in a central supply room in a general hospital except that it was largely preparing, checking, sterilizing, cleaning, and repairing equipment used solely in the obstetrical service, including, however, solutions, gloves, etc., used in the delivery room. It seemed to call for an excellent memory, meticulous attention to caring for and keeping track of materials, and manual dexterity in handling utensils. A thorough drilling in method had been given by a registered nurse. The wall was plastered with lists, routines, and schedules as reminders to the attendant, and judgment was seldom needed. There was no contact with patients or the delivery rooms proper.

It would seem as if many of the jobs in supply and stock rooms, especially those where the attendant has the responsibility of making up solutions, assembling sets, care of needles, tubing, instruments, sterilization, etc., were similar to a laboratory technician's job. It is questionable whether the procedures need to be carried out by a worker with nurse's training.

In actual practice, the trained attendant's duties in many institutions varied only slightly from those described for the nursing assistant and are very like those assigned to practical nurses in nongovernmental hospitals of all types. The same rule of placing responsibility on the registered nurse-in-charge for the instruction, supervision, and delegation of duties holds in both public and private institution.

SALARIES

The salary of nursing assistants (SP-3), as announced in 1943 began at $1,440 (base), plus overtime, making a total of $1,752 a year. A 15 per cent increase in basic pay rates covered these classes in July 1945.

The classification has not attracted many applicants. Those who stepped into it were mostly the trained attendants in SP-1 and SP-2 classes (salary around $1,300). Now that the war is over, there will probably be some new analyses of these positions and reclassification of the present incumbents. Licensed practical nurses might, when legislation becomes nationwide, be graded in the upper subprofessional grades.*

VETERANS ADMINISTRATION

Most of the patients in the general and special hospitals of the Veterans Administration are men. There have been units for women patients in some of the institutions (for nurse veterans of previous wars) and it is anticipated that the women's services of World War II will discharge many female veterans in need of care, which will in turn call for more women attendants.

In February 1945 there were 75,320 beds in the hospitals under the Veterans Administration served by 4,150 registered nurses and some 8,000 attendants. In November 1942 there were 62,650 beds, 4,044 registered nurses, and 10,000 attendants. It can be understood from these comparisons why the shortage in nursing service has been of genuine concern to administrators in the veterans facilities (5). During the next five years 114,539 beds are to be made available.

* It will be remembered that registered nurses of staff level have been classed as SP-6 to SP-10. As of July 1, 1945, registered nurses employed in the hospitals of the Veterans Administration were reclassified as P-1. A general scaling upward has been recommended by the American Nurses' Association, placing all registered nurses in the professional grades.

In January 1945 Brigadier General Frank T. Hines estimated the shortage of registered nurses for psychiatric cases alone as 750 to 1,000. An additional 3,000 nurses were needed by July 1, 1945 (6). There would be an even greater shortage in attendant service were it not for soldiers on limited service assigned to Veterans Administration hospitals. With the close of the war, the problems of assuring veterans of adequate nursing service, including attendant service, is being considered as of equal importance to the need of nursing care for soldiers and sailors still in Army and Navy hospitals. By 1976, 300,000 patients are expected in these hospitals (7).

In the Veterans Administration hospitals the desired ratio of registered nurses to patients (general medical, surgical, and tuberculosis hospitals) has been one to 6.5 to one to 7.5; in mental hospitals, one to 25. The ratio of attendants to patients has been one to 1.5 to one to 6.5 in general hospitals; one to 5 to one to 5.5 in neuropsychiatric hospitals. It should be remembered that most of the patients are males in these hospitals and most of the registered nurses are females, so comparisons cannot be drawn too closely with nonfederal hospitals.

A handbook of information and instruction is given every attendant entering upon work in the Veterans Administration hospitals (8). This booklet gives the rules and the personnel policies of the institution, and has a special section devoted to the regulations for the care of mentally ill patients. When a new hospital is opened, it has been customary to transfer a nucleus of experienced attendants from another service, thus assuring the patients of acceptable care while the new attendant staff is learning the work.

Ever since 1928 the Veterans Administration has made special effort to train its attendants. A suggested outline for the training course is provided by the superintendent of nurses of the Administration and each hospital adapts the material to meet its own needs (9). In 1945 the course consisted of 30 hours of formal classroom work—an hour a week—with orientation to the hospital and all its departments, supervised work on the wards (at first in housekeeping duties, later with patients), demonstrations, and quizzes. The chief nurse is responsible for all the class arrangements and for the correlation of teaching and practice. There is an examination at the completion of the period. The course is conducted at least twice a year. Credit for passing the course is given in the efficiency ratings under Civil Service regulations.

Some of the lectures are presented by the chief nurse, some by a medical officer. The chief topics covered, aside from introductory talks and observation of the plant, are (10):

Hospital rules and etiquette
Hygiene and sanitation
Anatomy and physiology
Care of various types of mental patients
Emergencies
First aid
Care of government property
Symptoms of mental disease: typical cases and how to deal with them; dangers and precautions
Tuberculosis
Elementary nursing
Nursing care of special diseases
Social hygiene practice for employees
Mental hygiene for employees

Under "elementary nursing" attendants are taught:

Ethics and deportment
Hospital housekeeping and ward management
Ward diet kitchen
Laundry and linen room
Admission of patients
General care of patient in bed: beds and bed making; undressing; bed baths; wheel chairs; moving; carrying; toilet needs (A.M. and P.M. care, etc.); care of hair, nails, etc.
Bedsores
Simple dressings
Counterirritants: hot and cold applications
Enemata, irrigation
Preoperative and postoperative care
Serving food to bed patients and to restive patients
Use of disinfectants and other poisonous solutions
Method of disinfecting rooms, linen, dishes, sputum, etc.
Care of body after death

A recent supplementary outline (9) to the course adds taking of temperature, pulse, and respiration; symptoms to observe in patients; preparation for tube feeding; physical therapy; occupational therapy and diversions; shock, fever, and malaria therapies. The attendant's duties in relation to these last-named therapies and an explanation of their purpose are given in these classes.

The list of attendants' duties has been given here at considerable length to show how closely they resemble the duties usually assigned to practical nurses in private hospitals (see pages 67–68).

To attract and retain attendants, Miss Pedersen wrote in 1930, it is necessary to offer attractive, comfortable living quarters, systematic increase in salary, and definite course of instruction. There must be provision for recreation, smoking rooms, radio connections in bedrooms, and good reading lights. Quiet bedrooms for those on night duty are essential. A study of turnover showed a drop to 60.26 per cent from 101.24 per cent after such changes were instituted. Clean uniforms, provided and laundered by the hospital, not only make a better impression on the public and patients but build up the attendants' morale (11).

The veterans hospitals as a whole have not made very wide use of Red Cross Volunteer Nurses' Aides, although a few hospitals not too far removed from cities have good sized groups. Very few, if any, of these aides have sought paid status, and it is not expected that many will.

The positions for attendants will in all probability be closed to non-veterans until the supply of veterans of World War II needing or seeking this type of job is exhausted. This ruling will affect all federal hospitals under Civil Service. It is anticipated that there will be a generous supply of professional, subprofessional, and custodial workers for these hospitals; veteran corpsmen and corpswomen from the women's services, the Army, and the Navy, pharmacist's mates, and medical and surgical technicians are likely to seek these positions, as well as convalescent veterans, both men and women, who may remain to serve in various capacities in the hospitals. Therefore, while the jobs for attendants are many, the applicants who are veterans with preference will also be many.

PUBLIC HEALTH SERVICE

Bureau of Medical Services, Office of Nursing

The United States Public Health Service has one of the oldest hospital services in the United States, established by Act of Congress in

1798. Originally vested with responsibility for the care of sick and disabled seamen, the Service now administers the nursing care in marine hospitals; federal prisons; hospitals for those suffering from drug addiction; Freedmen's Hospital at Washington, D.C.; the National Leprosarium at Carville, Louisiana; during the war the hospitals connected with the relocation centers (enemy aliens rounded up in 1941); hospitals for the Coast Guard and the War Shipping Administration (training stations to teach nursing arts to pharmacist's mates and station hospitals); and the infirmaries and first aid stations for the residents and workers in government living quarters in Washington—in all, hospital beds requiring the service of some 1,150 registered nurses as of February 1945.* The bed capacity of the marine hospitals alone was 6,630. They were filled to capacity and new hospitals are being planned.

The list of federal employees entitled to care in all these institutions includes seven types of merchant seamen, three classes of coast guards (including SPARS), and nine other groups. The function of the nursing service is to "provide nursing care to all service beneficiaries in the hospitals and dispensaries and to instruct trainees of the Maritime Service and Coast Guard in the Nursing Arts" (12). Over 600,000 persons applied for treatment at marine hospitals in 1943–44.

Attendants are on duty in nearly all the institutions under the Bureau of Medical Services. They do not, however, carry all the duties considered the equivalent of those performed by practical nurses or highly trained attendants. The Service plans to publish a training manual, but at present each institution prepares its own outline of instruction and the attendant learns on the job. Previous experience or training is unnecessary. These attendants are recruited locally and are given a CPC grade by Civil Service.

The absence of a group corresponding to licensed practical nurses does not mean that the Bureau of Medical Service does not approve the use of the subsidiary workers. Quite the opposite. Full time nurses' aides are employed, and Red Cross Volunteer Nurses' Aides have been functioning satisfactorily in several marine hospitals, while the ques-

---

* In 1922 nursing care of veterans was transferred to the newly created Veterans Bureau. In 1934 all questions regarding public health nursing were referred to the States Relations Division of the Public Health Service, now the Bureau of State Services, Office of Public Health Nursing.

tion of using SPARS as nurses' aides was being considered as this book was prepared (February 1945). The fact that the Service has for several years supplied registered nurse instructors for the training of pharmacist's mates, and had a large school for training them at Sheepshead Bay, Brooklyn,* indicates the Service's appreciation of this type of worker.

The reservoir of veterans trained as corpsmen and pharmacist's mates may supply the Service many of the attendants, practical nurses, and nursing assistants it needs. Most of the marine hospitals take care of acutely ill patients for whom registered nurses must perform most of the nursing duties.

Bureau of State Services, Office of Public Health Nursing

Under the Office of Public Health Nursing, besides the executive and district consultant staffs and the registered nurses assigned to some of the special projects of the Service (for example, the rapid-treatment centers for venereal diseases), there is a class of nursing assistants or nurses' aides who are employed under direct supervision of registered nurses in the infirmaries connected with the Federal Public Housing projects (13). The Federal Housing Authority reimburses the Public Health Service for the salary of these nursing staffs. Such developments have usually been near the centers of war industries and military camps —Marin City, California, was typical† (14). Although nurses are recruited locally through Civil Service, the appointments receive final approval from and the aides are supervised by the staff of the Public Health Service.

The duties of these nursing assistants in the infirmaries consist in carrying out simple nursing procedures, always under the direction of a registered nurse, for patients with mild illness or during convalescence. Acutely ill patients or longterm cases are not retained in the infirmaries.

In May 1945 there were 72 workers of this type employed in the infirmaries. In June 1945 in the rapid treatment centers, 18 were em-

---

* This school was taking in 50 trainees a week during the war. The course is usually three months.

† On the day of the writer's visit to the infirmary in Vallejo, California, there were 27 patients, with five registered nurses and four practical nurses on duty. In the eighteen-bed infirmary at Marin City, there were two registered nurses and three practicals.

ployed to assist the registered nurses in clinic duties (15) (see pages 176–178 for typical duties).

Services to veterans in the field of vocational rehabilitation are already calling for both professional and practical nursing care. States have been asked by the United States Office of Vocational Rehabilitation of the Public Health Service to utilize practical nurses only under the supervision of graduate nurses employed by the official or voluntary health agency responsible for rendering service. In 1944 only about 55,000 handicapped persons had been rehabilitated but about 80,000 were expected to ask for help in 1945 (16).

OFFICE OF INDIAN AFFAIRS, HEALTH DIVISION

Under the Office of Indian Affairs (Department of the Interior) the Director of Nursing in the Health Division is responsible for the nursing service available to approximately 400,000 Indians representing 150 or more tribes. They are scattered over the states west of the Mississippi and in Alaska. More than 78 general hospitals, some quite small, serve the Indians, in addition to the public health services which reach even the most distant tribes.

Through the far-sighted plan of Elinor D. Gregg, former Director of Nursing, ably carried forward by the present Director, a school for nurses' aides was established in 1935 in Lawton, Oklahoma, for the purpose of training Indian girls to assist in the Indian hospitals at a level above a ward attendant but below that of a professional nurse. The school is the only one of its kind (17). The course is open to women of eighteen to thirty-five years who have completed high school and are in good health. Applicants must be one-quarter or more Indian blood. The length of the course is nine months (accelerated to six months during the war), but pupils who find the course difficult are retained for a longer period of supervision and practice—an outstandingly progressive plan in line with modern educational trends. Two classes are admitted each year. There are two full-time registered nurses in charge of the course and the girls are under supervision throughout the period. They live at the school and have their practice in the wards of Kiowa Indian Hospital in Lawton (150-bed capacity, 97 daily average). A three weeks' affiliation is given each aide at the Riverside Indian Vocational Boarding School at Anadarka, Oklahoma. Students receive $15 a month allowance during the course, as well as full maintenance and all supplies. The nurses' aides are definitely trained for service within the Indian reservations and not for employment as practical nurses in the general population.

More than 200 nurses' aides have graduated from the Kiowa School. Eight have gone on into professional nursing. Classes usually number 20 to 25.

The Indian nurses' aides are classified under Civil Service as SP-2, salary range $1,320 to $1,680 with overtime.*

In general their duties are assisting with records, bathing convalescent patients, taking temperatures of patients not acutely ill, feeding patients, giving evening care, passing bed pans, admitting and dismissing patients, assisting nurse with treatment; assisting in outpatient services; cleaning medicine cabinets, sterilizing and setting up trays; care of surgical supplies, linen, gloves; cleaning patients' rooms and units, nursery; putting babies to breast, giving bottles, changing diapers; assisting with nourishments and trays. They may give enemas to convalescent patients but have not been taught to give hypodermic injections or medications.

During the war they were called on to do more and more in the hospitals, as the registered nurse shortage grew. "It would be impossible," wrote Sallie Jeffries, Director of the Nursing Service, in a personal letter to the writer, "to carry on in some of our small hospitals were we not able to assign nurses' aides to supplement the nursing staff."

No estimate has been made of the number of nurses' aides which will be needed in the Indian Service in the future—Miss Jeffries believes a 50 to 75 per cent increase might be justified. Postwar plans include the possibility of developing a course to prepare nurses' aides to assist the public health nurses in the Service. Miss Jeffries writes that in her opinion there is "a definite place in the nursing picture for a well selected and well prepared nurses' aide."

THE ARMY AND THE NAVY

Prior to World War II the Army and Navy hospitals were not in the same position as the federal hospitals. Their attendant or practical nursing service was carried by corpsmen (enlisted men). This was especially true of the Navy hospitals where one of the major duties of

---

* There was a 15 per cent increase in base salaries in July 1945.

the registered nurses of the Navy Nurse Corps was to train and supervise corpsmen in nursing procedures. Many Navy corpsmen served on
battleships in place of registered nurses and as pharmacist's mates. The
ratio of corpsmen to registered nurses was often as high as 8 to one.
During the war, it was as high as 25 to one. The shortage of manpower
forced both the Army and the Navy to draw every available fighting
man into battle service, and with the shortage of registered nurses the
ratio of one nurse to every 8 patients changed to one to 15 and even
one to 22 (18).

The Navy was the first to train women as corpsmen. In April 1943 a
course was established at the Naval Hospital in Corpus Christi, Texas,
for WAVES who had completed their initial indoctrination period of
four to six weeks (19). This course began as one month and combined
theory (75 hours) and practice on the wards, and included anatomy
and physiology (8 hours), nursing (45 hours), hygiene and sanitation
(6 hours), first aid and minor surgery (10 hours), materia medica (4
hours), and metrology (2 hours).

By 1945, however, the course was increased to 16 weeks, and required 640 hours of theory and practice. Subject matter covered anatomy and physiology, 55 hours; elementary chemistry, 24; hygiene and
sanitation, 38; bacteriology and elementary laboratory technique, 18;
materia medica and toxicology, 46; minor surgery and first aid, 39;
nursing and dietetics, 48; pharmacy and metrology, 25. Practice in all
these subjects took 347 hours. Candidates for the course must have had
at least two years of high school.

The rating received by a WAVE on the completion of this course
could be up to and including that of pharmacist's mate, second class.
Approximately 150,000 corpsmen and corpswomen finished the
course.

The duties performed for patients by WAVES on the completion
of their course were far more advanced than those of trained attendants in most hospitals and, from report, exceeded those of the practical
nurse. Many of the WAVES had educational background superior to
that of the candidates for practical nursing. They were allowed to give
medications, do dressings, transfusions, injections, and other treatments not usually assigned to any but registered nurses.

The time allowed for teaching this group was about a third that advised for practical nurses. On the other hand, they were not taught

home management, nutrition, or care of mothers, babies, and children.

Questions are naturally arising as to how to utilize the returning veteran WAVE, trained and successful as a pharmacist's mate with one to three years' experience in nursing on busy medical and surgical wards (20). If she wishes to earn her living through nursing, what part of the curriculum in professional nursing should she be required to study and what credit can be given for her ward experience? If she is a suitable candidate for practical nursing, how are deficiencies in home management, preparation and cooking of food, care of mothers, babies, and children to be made up? It is not likely that these veterans will be asked to enroll for the complete training in either professional or practical nursing. They are desirable members of either group, however, and should be assisted to qualify for state registration or license, whichever proves appropriate, in as short a time as possible.

In 1943 members of the WAC were assigned to station hospitals of the Army for all sorts of non-nursing duties. By the end of 1944 the Army was forced to send medical hospital units overseas without registered nurses and asked to have WACs trained as corpsmen, medical and surgical technicians, and assistants. The Army's course for medical and surgical technicians was usually 12 weeks in length, and covered 468 hours of theory. Between Pearl Harbor and August 1, 1945, 36,428 men and women were trained (21).*

An abortive plan to employ Red Cross Nurses' Aides under Civil Service in Army hospitals on a pay basis† was announced in December 1944 (23). The duties of the Army Hospital Red Cross Nurses' Aides as described in the recruitment folder were to have been:

Under immediate supervision of a graduate nurse, to make beds, to give baths and to take and record temperature, pulse and respiration of other than seriously and critically ill patients; to carry food trays; to serve liquids and prescribed between-meal nourishment; to fill hot water bottles, ice bags and collars; and to perform such other related nonprofessional duties as will enable the graduate nurses to render greater professional service to sick and wounded soldiers in Army hospitals (24).

The last clause seems to be the redeeming feature about an otherwise

* By the summer of 1945, 60,000 professional nurses were serving in the Armed Forces (22).

† Red Cross Volunteer Nurses' Aides had been available to the Army since January 1943 and were on a pay basis in a few hospitals by June 1944.

drab job. The duties as described are considerably limited as compared to those performed by practical nurses.

It is possible that, if states had had fairly uniform standards for the preparation and licensing of practical nurses, and if a homogeneous body of these workers between the ages of twenty-one and forty-three had been ready for recruitment into the military services in 1941, the Army Nurse Corps might have called for licensed practical nurses to help out in the Army hospitals. As it was, in 1941, practical nurses were licensed in only a handful of states, inchoate, unorganized, inarticulate, and unprepared. Rounding up this scattered group and retraining them for military duty would have been too expensive in time, money, and registered nurse supervision to make their use feasible. Even a call for volunteers among the licensed practical nurses—the largest known number being about 31,510 in 1945 (25)—would have resulted in a very small group of military age who were free to leave home, in good physical health, and willing to go overseas. Many of the practical nurses are over forty, married, with dependents, and probably in no better physical condition than their sisters, the registered nurses, of whom about 20 per cent were rejected for military service on medical grounds. Many of the younger, well prepared licensed practical nurses regretted not receiving consideration for military duty and were particularly hurt when Uncle Sam called for paid Red Cross Nurses' Aides. The latter had had only 80 hours of theory as against the 200 to 300 hours of the practical nurses; they had had 150 hours of broken ward experience as against the practical nurses' six or more consecutive months of supervised student experience in general hospitals. "Of course," one bright young licensed practical nurse said to the writer (she had been on a surgical ward in a large general hospital for a year), "we can take the Red Cross Nurses' Aides course evenings and join under this paid aide plan, or we can enroll in the WAC or WAVES and ask to be put in a hospital, but either step would be a duplication of what we already know and would take time. I'm ready to go tonight."

When asked in 1943 regarding the responsibility for employing and training auxiliary hospital workers for civilian hospitals to relieve the nursing situation and release more young registered nurses for overseas military service, the subcommittees on Hospital and Nursing of the Health and Medical Committee, Office of Defense Health and

Welfare Services in Washington, replied that it was "neither desirable nor practicable for the federal government to foster a training program for hospital auxiliary workers. We feel this problem to be entirely local" (26).

So the licensed and unlicensed practical nurses lost out on recognition in the military nursing services of World War II.

War will probably always face the nursing profession with a mammoth emergency to supply skilled nurses at short notice in enormous quantities. It is too soon to say whether a different plan of recruiting and training for a "duration" type of practical auxiliary nurse would have been better than the plans we have followed in this war and the last. In the first world war, nurses' aides were used in army and civilian hospitals from the start (27). "Even," wrote Dr. Thompson in 1931, "conservative hospitals opened their doors temporarily and more or less reluctantly to the trained attendant" (28).

Canada has taken care of some of its army nursing problems through VAD service.

A VAD is a member of the nursing division of the St. John Ambulance Brigade or the Nursing Auxiliary Section of the Canadian Red Cross Corps, who has completed a period of probation and whose appointment has been confirmed. . . . Two VAD's replace one nursing sister in an establishment.

They are recruited by the Red Cross and St. John Ambulance Association and receive preliminary training in civilian hospital training schools. When required for duty in military hospitals, their appointment is approved by the Adjutant-General, through the Director General of Medical Services, on the recommendation of the Matron-in-Chief, RCAMC. The Matron-in-Chief makes her recommendation from the names submitted by the Director of Ambulance of the St. John Ambulance Commandery, and the National Commandant, Nursing Auxiliary Section, Canadian Red Cross Corps. They rank next and after members of the RCAMC Nursing Service, . . . VAD Nursing Members carry on simple nursing duties under the direction and supervision of a nursing sister, and are not employed where there are no nursing sisters (29).

Until the history of this war is written we shall probably not know how completely both Army and Navy nurses relied on the help of enlisted men and women, Red Cross aides, or any other workers they could find, to help nurse the wounded. An indication is given in a description of the work six enlisted men carried out in a shock ward in the E.T.O. (30). One man—a ward master—was carefully trained to supervise; the other five assisted the doctors and nurses. They were called on for emergencies, took blood pressures, gave hypodermic injections, and blood and plasma intravenously, and nursed the shock victims until they were able to return to the ward. It is not inconceivable that the lessons learned in the dire emergencies overseas will revolutionize our ideas of what practical nurses can learn to do, under supervision, in a short time.

REFERENCES

1 The classification pay scale (Form 2968, September 1942) may be obtained from the Civil Service Commission, Washington 25, D.C. An amended scale with increases of 15 per cent on basic pay rates went into effect July 1, 1945.

2 The fourth, first, and eighth Civil Service Regions have advertised this position, among others. In the main the positions were in veterans hospitals.

3 Quoted from an announcement of the Fourth United States Civil Service Region, Winston-Salem, N.C., November 27, 1944. Nursing Assistant.

4 "Classification of positions in Civil Service which assists in the differentiation in preparation, requirements and pay, is a tool to use in properly designating the duties of the practical nurse and trained attendant. . . . Back of every classification goes a complete job analysis. . . . It is essential that the jobs described, pay rates, and requirements be kept up to date." Ismar Baruch, "The classification of positions," Public Health Nursing 32:297–301, May 1940, at pp. 299, 300, 301.

5 Details of this shortage were discussed at the hearings on the Nurses Draft Bill, RH 2277, House Military Affairs Committee, Andrew J. May, Chairman, February 2–10, 1945.

6 See also news release in New York World Telegram, January 3, 1945, p. 16, or other newspapers of that date.

7 "Our veterans need more nurses; needs and opportunities for nursing service in the Veterans Administration," American Journal of Nursing 44:724–727, August 1944.

8 Instructions for hospital attendants in Veterans Administration facilities, revised, October 1941.

9 Courses of training, Veterans Administration; hospital attendants, mess attendants, maids and janitors, compiled by Mary A. Hickey,

Superintendent of Nurses, Veterans Administration, February 1935. A supplement to this outline for neuropsychiatric facilities (mimeographed, January 9, 1945) includes special material for newly recruited ward attendants (whether civilian or troops) to master before being permitted to care for patients.

The Veterans Administration was one of the first agencies to publish an outline of instruction for attendants. See Thyra Pedersen, "The ideal attendant," *U.S. Veterans Medical Bureau Bulletin* 4:475, May 1928; 5:305, April 1929; 5:997, December 1929.

10 Hickey (note 9), pp. 1–3.

11 Thyra Pedersen, "Training for attendants," *U.S. Veterans Medical Bureau Bulletin* 6:416–418, May 1930.

12 Katharine S. Read, *Nursing in Public Health Service*, Washington, Government Printing Office, 1944 (Supplement 176 to *Public Health Reports*), p. 6.

13 Dorothy Deming, "Some aspects of wartime nursing on the west coast," *American Journal of Nursing* 44:565–570, June 1944, at p. 568.

14 Jean C. McGregor, "Marin City saga," *American Journal of Nursing* 43:720–724, August 1943.

15 Information from the Public Health Service in correspondence with the writer, May and June 1945.

16 Dean A. Clark, "Nursing in vocational rehabilitation," *Public Health Nursing* 36:345–351, July 1944, at pp. 350–351.

17 Mary E. Gahagan, "Nurses' aides in the Indian Service," *American Journal of Nursing* 43:165–168, February 1943.

18 "Army nurse ratio is 1 to 22 patients," *Modern Hospital* 64:68, January 1945.

19 Esther L. Schmidt, "Training of WAVES for hospitals," *American Journal of Nursing* 43:717–718, August 1943.

20 See newspapers for current report of activities, especially *New York Herald Tribune*, February 9, 1945, p. 8. See also John S. Allen, "Service men's readjustment act," *New York State Nurse* 16:122–124, October 1944.

21 *Outline of courses for the training of auxiliary workers in the care of the sick by U.S. Army, U.S. Navy, U.S. Coast Guard, U.S. Maritime Service, American Red Cross*, New York, Joint Committee on Auxiliary Nursing Service, November 1945 [mimeographed].

22 United States Women's Bureau, *Outlook for women in occupations in the medical services; professional nurses*, Washington, Government Printing Office, 1945 (Bulletin 203, No. 3), pp. 8–9.

23 Ida M. MacDonald, "Nurses' aides for the Army," *American Journal of Nursing* 44:659–660, July 1944. See also report of paid nurses' aides in Army hospitals as early as June 1944, Mrs. Walter Lippmann, "Nurses' aides in Army hospitals," *Red Cross Courier* 23:11, 17, 22, June 1944.

24 See recruiting pamphlet issued by the Army Nurse Corps, November 11, 1944, *Nurses' aides in Army hospitals*.

25 "Licensed attendants and practical nurses," *American Journal of Nursing* 46:391, June 1946.

26 News item, *American Journal of Nursing* 43:302, March 1943. See also a quite complete plan for federal subsidy ($1,500,000) of a training program for 6,000 auxiliary nurses, described by Lucile Petry, "Increasing and using nursing auxiliaries," *Hospitals* 17:37–40, February 1943.

27 It is interesting to note that President William Howard Taft, calling for nurses' aides in 1917, wrote: "There is a limit to the number of our experienced nurses who can be spared for war service." *Ladies Home Journal,* September 1917. Quotation in *American Journal of Nursing,* November 1917, p. 81. See also editorial, "Training nurses' aides," *American Journal of Nursing* 16:681–682, May 1916.

28 W. Gilman Thompson, "The nursing situation," *New York State Journal of Medicine* 21:178, May 1921. See also New York State Medical Society, Committee to Study the Nursing Problem, Report submitted by Nathan B. Van Etten, *New York State Journal of Medicine* 30:668, June 1, 1930.

29 "Military nursing in Canada," *American Journal of Nursing* 43:729–730, August 1943.

30 Lorraine Setzler, "A shock ward in the ETO; shock ward setup and nursing personnel," *American Journal of Nursing* 44:935–937, October 1944.

CHAPTER TWELVE

Other Opportunities for the Practical Nurse

OFFICE NURSING

PRACTICAL nurses are finding the work in doctors' offices, when there are no highly specialized treatments or surgical procedures, suitable to their training and highly desirable as it pays well and frequently can be arranged on a part time schedule.

An office nurse should be able to type and take dictation and should know something about keeping accounts, billing, ordering supplies, and giving first aid in emergencies. It is especially important for her to secure complete directions from the doctor as to what he wishes done about telephone calls, visitors, and emergencies in his absence. The nurse will need to know how to assist the doctor in his examination of patients and how he wants his cabinets, files, and records kept, and she will learn his way of giving any special treatments.

She must at all times appear clean and carefully groomed, keep the office tidy, and learn to use the telephone as a friendly instrument of communication. In a sense, she is the hostess in the doctor's office, and his patients will be quick to sense her interest, learn to trust her, and feel welcome there. Some of the schools of practical nursing are making a special effort to see that students have information and preparation for this work.

Rates of pay range from 75 to 90 cents an hour.

SCHOOL AND COLLEGE INFIRMARIES

The work of practical nurses in school and college infirmaries is like that in any small hospital, except that age and sex groups are uniform. Their service is entirely under the supervision of registered nurses. Practical nurses may be permanent staff members or they may be called only in emergencies when the infirmary is overcrowded or the registered staff is ill.

As college infirmaries usually transfer seriously ill students to general hospitals, the average census shows mildly ill, slightly injured, or convalescent patients for whom practical nursing under supervision is appropriate. As these students are especially receptive to health education when it is imparted by a qualified professional nurse, practical nursing alone is not adequate.

Salaries are about the same as in small general hospitals (see pages 78 and 87) or they may be on a daily basis—$5 a day.

HOMES FOR THE HANDICAPPED AND CHILDREN'S INSTITUTIONS

There are many suitable and interesting positions for practical nurses in homes for the handicapped and for infants and children. Those in state or city institutions are usually under Civil Service and the practical nurse will be hired as an attendant or nurses' aide. Blind, deaf, crippled, mentally defective, and cardiac patients receive much of their routine care from nonprofessional personnel. Day nurseries, nursery schools, foundling homes, orphanages, and children's shelters can use practical nurses effectively. In many of these institutions trained practical nurses are very much needed.

The Child Welfare League of America recommends that a registered nurse be in residence in all children's institutions of 50 or more inmates, with assistance from house mothers, the latter being suitable positions for practical nurses. Modern child care policies recommend that small groups of eight to twelve children be housed together in the cottage system (1).

SUMMER CAMPS

Summer camping is a seasonal occupation for several hundred directors of camps and counsellors and for thousands of children of all ages each year. Recommended health standards call for the employment of a registered nurse when there are more than 50 campers. It is not advisable to employ a practical nurse alone, especially if the camp is far from doctors and hospitals. In a large camp, a practical nurse fits in well as an assistant to the registered nurse and can be of considerable help when the camp maintains a small infirmary or is taking convalescent children who need supervision. She relieves when the professional nurse is off duty, and assists her in any routine measures, such as weighing and examining on entrance to camp.

A thorough knowledge of first aid, of the early symptoms of communicable disease, and of simple bedside nursing procedures is necessary. The practical nurse works entirely under the supervision of the registered nurse.

Salaries vary greatly but are usually small, the camps believing that the staff benefits from the recreational character of the work—though as one weary camp nurse pointed out, in case of an epidemic, a siege of food or plant poisoning, or other disaster, this conception is farcical. Usually travel expenses to and from camp are paid and all maintenance is provided. Registered nurses receive from $50 to $150 a month, practical nurses less. It is usual, however, to offer a flat rate of $125 to $150 for the season of six to eight weeks.

Older practical nurses are advised not to take these positions.

OTHER POSSIBILITIES

A practical nurse who can qualify and who wishes to develop an additional skill will find it rewarding to study to be a physical therapist, an occupational therapist, an x-ray technician, a medical artist, a medical record librarian, or a medical secretary. The basic educational standards are fairly high; a course in practical nursing alone does not qualify one for entrance into these fields. However, evening courses in some of these subjects will enrich the nurse's experience and give her some welcome skills, even though she will not be able to secure a license in these special fields.

The writer interviewed practical nurses who had found classes in the following subjects useful to their patients as well as broadening to their own interests: typing, stenography, massage, arts and crafts, photography, kindergarten courses including story-telling for children, modeling, and dressmaking. Specializing in invalid cookery appeals to some. Many of the courses can be taken at the Y.W.C.A., at business schools, or in evening courses at local colleges.

Successful graduate practical nurses were found in allied fields of work where the physical strain was not so great as in bedside care, yet their nursing knowledge was of use. Some of these jobs were as matrons in industries and in girls' schools, running vacation homes, using their own homes as foster homes for children or selected mental cases, qualifying as masseuses, offering part time home nursing service for a small clientele, and assisting at blood donor centers.

REFERENCE

1 *Health program for children in foster care,* New York, Child Welfare League of America, 1939, pp. 11, 21. See also *Standards for children's organizations providing foster family care,* New York, Child Welfare League of America, 1941; *Standards and recommendations for hospital care of newborn infants, full-term and premature,* Washington, Government Printing Office, 1943 (Children's Bureau Publication No. 292), pp. 1–14.

CHAPTER THIRTEEN

The Schools of Practical Nursing

EXCEPT FOR "on-the-job" courses or classes to introduce hospital attendants to their work, no mention has been found in the records of organized schools for practical nurses prior to 1900 (1). This is not surprising because professional schools were not yet forty years old; only thirty-five of them existed in 1890. Canada had only four at this date (2).

Some of the early schools made a habit of sending student nurses into homes as part of their experience before graduation. The hospital benefited financially by such plans. Dr. Alfred Worcester, an ardent supporter of the idea known as the "Waltham Plan" (1888), reported that after three years the hospital accounts showed a clear surplus of $410.21 (3), and in 1878 a Hartford hospital earned $1,097.69 through pupil care of private cases outside the hospital. In 1910 Ysabella Waters reported that 39 hospitals were sending 73 pupil nurses into homes to nurse by the hour or day "irregularly" (4). The purpose of this arrangement, however, was not the training of nurses for practical work in the homes.

In 1900, 304 members of the Philadelphia Medical Society and College of Physicians lent their names to a project known as the Philadelphia Nurses Supply Association, which operated a ten-week "course" (5). Very little is known of its success.

The Thompson School for Training Attendants in Brattleboro, Vermont, was under the supervision of graduate nurses from the start in 1907, and set the pattern for other courses for some years afterward. It combined instruction in household duties and experience in both general hospital cases and maternity. So much has been written about the "Brattleboro Plan" that it is superfluous to repeat it here (6). Two unique features should be noted: the unusual plan of providing home nursing service by both professional and practical nurses for some 40,-000 people living within a radius of 30 to 40 miles from Brattleboro (7), and the later tie-up with the prepaid service plan of the Brattleboro Mutual Aid Association backed by the Thompson Trust Fund (8). This area is distinctly rural and we may thus say not only that

Vermont can claim to be the birthplace of formal practical nursing education, but also that it was the first state to offer rural practical nursing service under the supervision of graduate, later registered, nurses (9) and to promote an insurance plan which included nursing services in the home.

Mention must be made here of the much discussed and professionally condemned "course" organized in Chicago in 1921 by Dr. John Dill Robertson, Health Commissioner of the city (10). This course was eight weeks in length with 24 lectures on nursing subjects lasting one and a half to two hours each. The classes were free. It attracted thousands of girls and women who were then, according to the doctor, "ready to nurse the sick," frequently receiving the same pay as graduate nurses. Indeed, if interested, they could have an extension course of twelve lectures. There were 800 pupils at a time, and the "course" turned out 4,231 pupils in a year. "These women can be trained to do surgical nursing," wrote the doctor. As this "course" was not established for profit, it cannot be classed as commercial; the results, however, were probably as bad. It died in 1923.

As of July 1945, 46 schools for training practical nurses or licensed attendants had been approved by the state board of nurse examiners or other legally appointed authority in the state where each was located. There were six schools in California, three in Connecticut, nine in Maryland, ten in Massachusetts, twelve in New York, three in Pennsylvania, and three in Virginia. Not all these schools were admitting classes in 1945. (See Appendix, page 348.)

Six schools, one each in Ohio, Michigan, Minnesota, New Jersey, Vermont, and Washington, states in which there is licensure of practical nurses, had been approved by the National Association for Practical Nurse Education, and all were functioning in 1945. (See Appendix, page 349.)

There are estimated to be at least a hundred commercial schools or courses claiming to prepare practical nurses through classroom lectures, demonstrations, or correspondence. The graduates of these courses in states where the state board of nurse examiners or other legally authorized body approves schools of practical nursing are not admitted to state examinations for licensure to practice.

Of the 18 approved schools visited by the author in 1944 and 1945 and the three with which she had correspondence, none had capacity classes. Three had no classes because of a dearth of applicants and four had about a third of their usual prewar enrollment. In 1945 less than 500 students were graduated from the 52 approved schools. Many of the schools are accepting Negro students, some in large numbers.

Of the schools now in operation, the oldest are the Thompson School for Training Attendants, Brattleboro, Vermont (1907), the Ballard School of the Y.W.C.A., New York city (1912), and the Household Nursing Association, Boston (1912). Detroit organized a school (not the present one) in 1913. The first school for practical nursing for men was opened at Montefiore Hospital in New York city in 1940.*

TYPES OF SCHOOLS

No distinct classification as to type can be made of the half hundred approved schools now training practical nurses, for several combine the features of all. However, it is possible to pick out three general types, their differences relating mainly to sponsorship or support and educational plan.

Type I. The oldest type is the school that offers two or three basic elementary courses in theory, including home economics, during a period of residence in the home school, and then places the student in an approved hospital for a period of experience in which the rest of the theory and practice is taught. The major hours of theory and practice are given in the hospital, where the student usually lives, and are integrated with what the student has learned in her brief introduction in the home school. The student may or may not return to the home school for a final period of orientation to homes and community service. These schools ask a tuition fee. The hospitals pay a stipend during the students' experience. The Household Nursing Association of Boston is an example of this type of school.

Type II. A school of the second type is conducted wholly within the hospital. The students "live in" and have class work and demonstrations preceding and during ward service. The same instructors control

---

* Not to be confused with the Mills School—now closed—operated in connection with Bellevue Hospital which prepared professional registered men nurses, though in 1888 it was training attendants for wards of the hospital.

the educational program and ward teaching throughout the course. Many courses of this type are in special hospitals, and comparatively little attempt is made to prepare the practical nurse for duties in private homes or any other kind of outside service. Students may be paid a small allowance throughout the course. They are usually given full maintenance. Just about half the approved schools are of this type. The Central School for Practical Nurses, New York City Department of Hospitals (tax supported) is a large school of this pattern; the school in Caledonia Hospital in Brooklyn (120 beds) typifies a school in a small privately supported hospital.

Type III. The third and newest development is the so-called "vocational" course, which may or may not be connected with and conducted by a vocational school under a board of education. The school may or may not receive financial assistance from state and federal funds (the latter under the Smith-Hughes and George-Deen Acts). Theory and practice are given in a preliminary program of instruction (which may or may not be in a school building but usually is), lasting as a rule three months. The students live at home and attend as day pupils just as in any academic course. They do not care for patients at all during the classroom period. The three months of theory are followed by practice in a selected hospital; the students do not usually live in the hospital but they may. These schools do not customarily give supervised experience in homes, nor do they prepare for other specialized fields.

In a true vocational school, there is no tuition for residents of the state or county. Hospitals pay an allowance to the students during the practice period.

Students may take the course for credit as a part of a vocational training program in high school, in which case they are young—fifteen to seventeen—and may not practice their "skills" on a ward for a year or two or may not be licensed to practice until they are eighteen (the legal age in most states), leaving a period when they may attempt to nurse without a license.

The Essex County Vocational High School in Newark, New Jersey, is representative of this group in a state without a licensing law; the Rochester, New York, School for Practical Nursing typifies vocational training, on the level of adult education, in a state with a law.

The vocational-type schools conducted in rural areas by state extension services which assign their students to small but good rural hospitals for practice seem to the writer to offer a promising field for the future when under qualified professional supervision.

There are many variations in organization, support, and curriculum among these three general types of schools. Practice periods differ in length, place, and purpose. For example, one school prepares its students for service in homes and in nonacute institutions. The course is given in most attractive private home surroundings, practice is assigned in institutions caring for subacute conditions, and supervision of home service is offered from the school before the graduate receives her certificate. It can be seen that this is not a true vocational school as it is not receiving state or city funds and charges tuition; on the other hand, it does not belong to Type I or II because the graduates are not encouraged to nurse in general hospitals.

In another school, the educational plan is similar in that the acute hospital is not used for training and students are prepared for home service in a practice home, but this school does receive state and federal funds and is a part of the statewide plan of vocational training for practical nurses. This school arranges practice through the visiting nurse association for home cases and supervision of its students.

In still another vocational-type school, all theory and practice are given in a hospital for chronic patients. On the day of the writer's visit 90 per cent of the patients were over sixty years of age. The students live in a dim dormitory on the top floor of the hospital, their cots barely four feet apart; their classroom is in the basement. Students are on duty from 7 A.M. to 7 P.M. with two hours off. The students do much of the hospital's housekeeping. The course is nine months.

One of the newer type schools, under the auspices of the public school system, offers a unit (A) of 360 hours of theory (six hours a day for a five-day week) and then a unit (B) of seven weeks of supervised practice as students in a Marine Hospital (400 patients) without pay. The students work a thirty-hour week and live at home. They have no formal class work in the hospital. Unit C consists of 1,000 hours in a hospital or in home nursing under supervision but as employed workers. The director of the school tries to supervise the nurses working in homes. The state in which the school is located does not license practical nurses (11):

The reader's attention is called especially to the steps taken in organizing the School of Practical Nursing in Rochester, New York, and the present tie-up with the practice fields. While this school, which was organized in 1939, is vocational in character, it takes only girls and women over eighteen and gives practical experience in a maternity hospital and a county hospital for subacute illness. Tuition is free to Rochester residents, $60 for nonresidents (12).

Michigan has been most active through the State Board of Control of Vocational Education in promoting vocational courses for the preparation of practical nurses throughout the state, using in part funds available under the Smith-Hughes and George-Deen Acts. During 1942–1945, courses were organized in fifteen centers and some 500 practical nurses were graduated. While Michigan has not amended its nurse practice act to cover the licensure of practical nurses, there have been very definite control of these courses, supervision of the students, and high standards for entrance, faculty appointments, and placement, and no course is started without the active cooperation of the leaders in nursing and education. A full time consultant and adviser—a registered nurse—was employed in 1944 by the State Board of Control to organize these courses, assist in efforts to meet the state standards, and develop adequate practice fields. A few of these courses have given the students some hospital experience, others are patterned on the home-training plan (13).

There are also enormous variations among the schools in Types I and II. Policies in the schools in hospitals naturally reflect the pressures caused by number of patients and their condition on admission. In this respect the schools resemble the professional schools where, especially in small general hospitals, emergencies, shortage of personnel, and overcrowding always threaten the integrity of the educational program. In a tuberculosis hospital, on the other hand, the pressure is caused by the scarcity of professional nurses and the temptation to keep the practical student in the hospital's service as long as possible. The result is the extension of her course to eighteen months or even two years while she is learning just this one specialty.

The situation in a school connected with a state "infirmary" presents a different picture of Type II. Here the student may have theory and practice in a "practice home," with concurrent experience in wards admitting nearly every type and stage of disease: maternity, medical, surgical, pediatrics, tuberculosis, and mental disease. The care of chronic and convalescent patients can receive special attention in such an institution. Indeed, the only experience lacking is nursing in private homes.

On the other hand, some state institutions, such as mental hospitals of 1,000 to 2,000 beds, offer quantity (and quality in the specialty) but convey an undesirable impression of mass nursing service, and they seldom give experience in the behavior of normal people who are ill. For a young woman of eighteen or nineteen to have her introduction to nursing procedures and her first knowledge of what constitutes health —mental and physical—taught among mental patients in over-crowded wards seems to this writer little short of tragic, although she is warmly in favor of including the nursing of the mentally ill as a required experience for both practical and professional nurses before graduation or as a bona fide postgraduate specialty.

The content, length, and practice offered by the curricula in all these schools are described in Chapter XIV. It is well to note here, however, that the shortest courses, nine months from entrance to graduation, are given by the vocational schools (Type III), the longest courses, two years, by the hospitals training within their own gates (Type II), the intermediate, twelve to fourteen months, by the schools of Type I. This is again not a hard and fast differentiation but a generalization.

ADMINISTRATIVE POLICIES

Support

Support for the schools comes from almost every known source tapped by educational and charitable agencies: taxes (state, federal, city, county), gifts (direct or through community chests), tuition, earnings (such as rent of rooms), endowments, special benefits or projects (such as a coffee shop), and fees from registries. Schools supported by community funds in one form or another are organized under representative boards or committees, generally with medical advisory committees or councils. Alumnae associations of the schools also take a deep interest in their schools and assist in various practical ways, such as recruiting students and raising money.

The schools in Y.W.C.A.'s are supposed to more than support themselves. The schools in state institutions are probably profiting from the services of their students. Schools of Type I are always struggling to make ends meet, and their boards of management are familiar with the fatal red side of the ledger. Schools of Type III do not have to appeal to the public for voluntary support. All except "home hospital schools" (Type II) usually look to interested local committees and advisers in the community in planning to establish and conduct a school. The United States Office of Education recommends that a local committee sponsoring a vocational course consist of doctors, nurses from several fields of service, lay citizens, a school superintendent, and a hospital administrator—in all, possibly eight to twelve persons* (14).

School budgets are hard to compare since those of the vocational type use the space, telephones, equipment, etc., of school buildings, while those with nurses' homes have to include all household expenses. When all the student facilities are not used, they may be rented or shared with others.

Nor can detailed expenses (for equipment, for example) or salaries be satisfactorily compared. Sometimes the director of the school is also the superintendent of the hospital and does not know how to divide her time; usually it is all charged to the hospital. Instructors also may be serving in other capacities. Some are paid by the class or the hour; others receive part of their pay from the hospitals. Some give part time service to registries. Teachers of dietetics, home economics, or other non-nursing courses may be paid by the hour, for the course, or for each semester while they are holding jobs in a university. Some schools provide an excellent library, others depend on the hospital for this. Bookkeeping and cost allocations are chaotic.

The yearly expense budgets for schools of Type I would probably have a ceiling of $50,000 for an enrollment of 200 students; for those of Type II, perhaps $18,000 if salaries and other expenses just for the students could be computed; and a possible $5,000 for the vocational schools, largely in salaries, if use of school building and equipment is not included. However, the actual expenses of Type II and III schools are much less.†

Faculty

In all the schools visited there was a director and at least one assistant, but it is known that some schools employ only a director who is a

---

* In Rochester, New York, an even wider representation of interested groups sponsors the school for practical nurses.

† The cost of educating a professional student nurse was estimated in 1936 as $815 a year or $2,445 for the three-year course (15).

registered nurse and who is expected to carry administrative, supervisory, and teaching duties. The hospital used as a practice field is expected to pay the student instructor; the school may appoint her.

For teachers of nursing, qualifications were graduation from an accredited school of nursing, satisfactory experience, and acceptable personal appearance. A few nurse-instructors have advanced degrees, some have had previous teaching experience, and a handful have had experience in public health nursing. For subjects other than nursing, instructors must meet the qualifications of their own fields. For example, the home economics instructor should be a graduate from an approved course. Doctors are almost never asked to teach classes of practical nurses as they find it difficult to simplify the material. There was unanimous agreement on this point.

Size of Classes

During the war the classes in these schools varied in size from 5 to 36 students. In normal times, capacities were reported as from 12 to 60, but no director of nurses was ready to put a final ceiling on the size of the class which could be admitted provided instructors and space were available. Most of the instructors felt that classes of 20 were handled easily—fewer for demonstration and practice periods in care of patients and in cooking.

Most of the schools admit at least two, some four classes, a year. Three is usual.

The directors of schools pointed out that failure to fill classes during the war was not due solely to competing industrial wages in war jobs. Other reasons quoted to the writer were that the WAC and WAVES were attracting many young women; entrance requirements for cadet nurses in the professional schools of nursing had been lowered; family incomes were higher than formerly so there was no need for older women to earn a living; anyone with a smattering of nursing knowledge was getting good pay for poor work so women saw no reason for paying for a training course.

General Requirements for Admission

The following are the usual requirements for entrance: citizenship, eighteen years of age, good health (checked by entering medical examination), completion of grade school, acceptable appearance judged by picture and personal interview, genuine interest in nursing.*

Recruitment

In recent years the practical nursing schools have had to recruit strenuously for candidates. All the usual avenues of publicity are used —newpapers, radio, movies,† posters, leaflets, talks, and magazine articles. Schools have even run advertisements in country newspapers. The Central School in New York city launched a city-wide campaign on the opening of the school. Information, leaflets, and posters were sent to newspapers, schools, employment agencies of all types, the United States Employment Service, libraries, nurses' registries, social agencies, churches, and national agencies, and the New York city radio facilities were used (16).

Uniforms

Uniforms may or may not be required during class periods. They are required in hospitals and on duty with visiting nurse associations. They may be all white or colored, with or without cap; they may be specially designed by the school or the hospital. There is absolutely no uniformity about them except that they are all washable. Rules for wearing them differ, prices differ, the number required differs, as does the responsibility for buying and laundering them.‡

Tuition

Tuition in schools of Type I varies from $50 to $130 for the course. A few schools have scholarships. Most of them permit installment payments.

Tuition in schools of Type II is frequently free if the hospital is tax supported. In private hospitals the range is $50 to $100 for the course.

Residents seldom have to pay tuition for vocational school training (Type III). Nominal fees, seldom amounting to more than $5 to $15

* For the use of psychological tests before entrance, see page 21.

† An example is "A Real Career," a movie for school publicity prepared by the Household Nursing Association, Boston, in 1938.

‡ For discussion of uniforms for graduates in hospitals, see page 79.

per student, are asked for supplies, locker, luncheons, or use of certain recreation facilities.

Some of the vocational schools permit their students to take part time paying jobs weekends or evenings. Some "work out" their living where they board. If this work is in the form of caring for children or helping with the household, it would seem to be a desirable additional experience. It can even be made a supervised experience. A few instances were found where a student was working in a hospital weekends for pay to eke out her budget, in one case as a maid. This would appear to be not at all desirable unless the job were actually a learning experience approved by the director of the school.

Allowances During Field Practice

Most of the students receive allowances of $15 to $65 a month while having their practice in hospitals and other agencies. They usually "live in" and receive full maintenance, but this is not always the case.

Dropped Students from Schools of Professional Nursing

If a student has been dropped from a professional nursing school there is usually a good reason (17). Especially at a time when every pair of hands is needed, a school director thinks a long time and struggles hard with her shortcomings before dismissing a student. Reasons for dismissal, aside from a nurse's own decision to leave, are ineptitude, inability to keep up with classroom work, illness, and that subtle diagnosis "unfitted for nursing." Temperamentally, some girls just do not fit into nursing. A few take immediate dislike to the physical care of human beings. Others do not overcome a certain kind of clumsiness, others have definite personality problems and their approach to sick people is never successful. If such girls do not fit into a school of professional nursing, it is probable they will not be happy or successful in practical nursing. Yet all schools for practical nurses have some applicants from this group. This is not to say that all should be rejected. The undergraduate student nurse who dropped out because of a spell of ill health, because the pace was just a bit too swift for her, because of home responsibilities or other personal reasons may, if she cannot be persuaded to return to her professional course, be an ideal person for practical nursing.

A report, therefore, that a student has had some training in a professional school must be carefully investigated, the director's advice sought, and the candidate herself interviewed and tried before she is finally rejected for training as a practical nurse. Many of these girls say they do not want to be practical nurses if they cannot be professionals. It is unwise to try to change their minds, some directors pointed out, because they will probably be disappointed in the course and unhappy when they are thrown again with registered nurses. While this may be true in some instances, the director has a rare opportunity and a real obligation to present the service of practical nurses as one of dignity and satisfaction that fills a very necessary place in the care of the sick.

The reasons for withdrawal from a school of professional nursing are revealing and thought-provoking in the light of accepting "dropped students" in schools for practical nurses or of employing them without further training.

In 1943, the National League of Nursing Education analyzed the reasons for withdrawal of 6,207 professional students (18). In order of frequency the reasons given by the schools were:

1.	Failure in classwork	38.6 per cent
2.	Personal reasons	12.8 per cent
3.	Disappointment in nursing as a career	12.5 per cent
4.	Health	11.0 per cent
5.	Personality unsuited to nursing	6.6 per cent
6.	Failure to meet other standards of the school	4.0 per cent
7.	Immaturity	3.1 per cent
8.	Preference for other war work	2.7 per cent
9.	Failure in both class and practice	2.3 per cent
10.	Failure in clinical nursing practice	2.2 per cent
11.	Other reasons	4.2 per cent

If we combine reasons 1, 9, and 10, we find that 43.1 per cent withdrew for failure in classroom and practice. Some of these girls might succeed as practical nurses, others would fail again in nursing procedures. Time will take care of those in group 7, but it is doubtful if girls in groups 2, 3, 5, 6, and 8 would or should continue in any form of nursing, while health (No. 4) might keep a dropped student out temporarily or permanently from any work as demanding as nursing. If a student should disagree with her school's decision with regard to any of the reasons for her withdrawal, she may seek a shorter course, perhaps in a commercial school that claims to produce as good a nurse, able to command as high wages, as a professional. It is this hospital-connected but inadequately trained and unlicensed nurse of whom employers must beware.

From these reports it can be seen that a grave responsibility rests on the director of the school or on an employer, in accepting a "dropped student." Many school directors prefer to accept applicants less well qualified educationally than to take this chance. On the other hand, studies in 1931 showed that dropped students had low averages in high school, perhaps indicating that the school of professional nursing had made a mistake in the first place and should have guided these applicants into practical nursing (19).

WHERE SHOULD PRACTICAL NURSES PREPARE?

More than any other one subject related to practical nurses—with the possible exception of the number we need—the question of preparation, in theory and practice, demands thorough study and evaluation by those who are experts in the field of nursing and nursing education.

The following comments are offered with some reluctance. They are based on friendly visits to the schools, lasting seldom more than a day, not planned to "investigate" or evaluate educational methods or results. Probably several of the conclusions will meet with diametrically opposed opinion from experts and from the schools themselves. The writer hopes so, as that might be a spur to a thorough study of a very much neglected field.

Each type of school has its advantages and disadvantages as a training center. No school among the 18 visited can be singled out as a wholly desirable pattern for all to follow under all conditions. There are really very few good schools for practical nurses.

The writer presents three conclusions based on her observation of these schools:

In preparing this group of nonprofessional nurses, theory and nursing practice with sick people should go hand in hand—the closer in time and place the better.

A period of practice in a hospital is essential whether the nurse is being trained for home or institutional service.

Teaching and supervision of theory and practice must be much more constant than for the professional nurse and must be all of a piece—that is, carried through by the same instructor. To have a teacher teach and supervise practice in a classroom but never supervise her students' practice in those same procedures on a ward or in a home seems to this writer utterly unsound educationally—and futile. Some instructors do not even know the names of the head nurses under whom their practical students work or what special case experience the ward patients offer, and they do not plan progressive experience for their students with the head nurses. Notes made by the writer on visits to schools in an eastern state clarify this point:

A student in a vocational school classroom may be taught on October 1st to give a throat irrigation to a doll. On December 15th she is asked by the charge nurse on a ward in Memorial Hospital to give a throat irrigation to Mrs. Green. The student may not have reviewed the procedure taught her in class ten weeks ago, and she may not have seen a throat irrigation given with Memorial Hospital's equipment to a real person. The charge nurse is too rushed to take time to show her, the regular instructor of practical nurses in Memorial Hospital is engaged elsewhere. Is it any wonder that the student is nervous to the point of tears and that poor Mrs. Green gets a jet of tepid water over her face and hair? Is it any wonder that the charge nurse is irritated by the student's clumsiness, slowness, and lack of confidence?

The teaching and supervision of ward practice at the "home hospital" type of school, although centralized, may not be consecutive. Both can be bad because some hospitals are exploiting their students, not teaching them. The students provide a welcome form of cheap labor. In some hospitals a hasty introduction is given the student in class, she is shown the procedure by another nurse—any one on duty—at the patient's bedside; from then on supervision from anyone is sketchy. Conditions are much better in hospitals that employ qualified, full time instructors just for the practical students.

Those concerned with plans for the education of practical nurses would do well to review the discussion of the problem in the Goldmark report (20). The advantages and disadvantages of using hospitals for acute and for nonacute diseases and convalescent homes of various types as training centers for practical nurses are presented in this report, without mention, however, of any separation between theory and practice as occurs in some vocational schools. Miss Goldmark reminds us that care of the sick in hospitals has for many years given professional nurses the best preparation possible.

The drawbacks to training in hospitals are minor, though real enough. Administrators point out that

Girls and women of the type who apply for training cannot always arrange to leave home for six to twelve months

Some hospitals have a tendency to train students beyond their capacity, especially under pressure of the present shortages; others use them for housekeeping duties more suitable for maids

Some nurse administrators believe that if practical nurses are around cases of acute illness, observing treatments and medications, they receive a smattering of knowledge which they attempt to put to use later as "registered nurses"—the same complaint that used to be made by doctors who feared professional students would try medical procedures

The advantages in preparing practical nurses in large general hospitals are perhaps obvious, but are mentioned here nevertheless. The student has a variety of experience; a thorough grounding in routine procedure; a chance to understand hospital "ethics"; experience in working under pressure and in emergencies; the advantage of excellent facilities for teaching; usually plenty of professional supervision; access to a good library; and the advantage of observation and practice in specialized departments.

It would appear that the course of training could be given effectively in small hospitals if stipulations regarding the proportion of professional staff, supervision, teaching personnel, and equipment were complied with. While a small hospital offers less in quantity it can make up in quality of services and is a more homelike, friendly place and a better environment in many ways for girls and women to whom pressure and crowds are confusing. Conditions are more like those in private homes, and practical nurses are less "lost." They must learn to improvise equipment and frequently to get along without all the luxuries provided in a large hospital.

There is no doubt that the menace of exploited student service threatens all hospitals (21). Scores of substandard private and proprietary hospitals are ready to jump at any chance to get cheap nursing. Hospitals for training practical nurses must be chosen as carefully with relation to variety of clinical material, equipment, nurses' quarters, supervision, and faculty as for professional students.

In 1943 there were 200 professional schools of nursing in hospitals so small that their graduates were not eligible for military service. Should these schools be converted into schools for practical nurses? This has been suggested (22). There would be definite advantages in having faculty, equipment, and space at hand, although one decided disadvantage would be confusion between the previously graduated registered nurses and the practicals. The whole question needs study.

One hospital of 175 beds, on giving up its professional school in 1932, found it necessary to replace 21 students with 9 professional general duty nurses and 2 ward attendants (23). If a practical nursing school had replaced the professional, would 21 practical nursing students have done the work of 21 professional students? Certainly not. Yet the American Hospital Association reported after its study of nursing in 1916 that the training of nurses in small community hospitals to meet local needs is the only real solution of the problem of skilled nursing in such places (24). This conclusion was echoed as late as 1941, when *Hospital Management* commented editorially: "Our best bedside nurses came from these schools" in small hospitals (25).

We must not repeat the experience of professional nurses who are still fighting to make their schools educational institutions and not the labor supply of the hospital. To some extent both groups of students must and do meet the service demands of the hospital and we would not have it otherwise. Students must learn to be realistic and hospitals are always subject to pressures, but to employ young women and give them maintenance while promising to teach them nursing without meeting a standard of instruction usually results in more nursing care of patients than teaching of students.

Certainly, prerequisites to any acceptance of a hospital as a training center for practical nurses should be registration by the American Medical Association and American College of Surgeons and willingness and ability to provide adequate registered nurse supervision by a full time, qualified instructor for the practical student nurses. Training fields should be inspected regularly by the state board of nurse examiners or other authority legally vested with the responsibility of licensing all those who nurse for hire. The safeguard will, of course, be approval by the state board of nurse examiners of the school for practical nursing and the practice fields, with due publicity for those schools whose graduates may become licensed to practice in the state.

This is definitely the time to consider the elimination of substandard professional schools in small hospitals in the light of the need for preparing qualified practical nurses. It is quite likely that the preparation of professional students in the schools connected with small hospitals is only slightly above the level of the eighteen-month course offered practical nurses in one or two of the best schools. There should be a definite cleavage between the two groups. Professional nursing does not want poorly prepared nurses practicing under the title registered nurse, nor does it want licensed attendants expecting to perform —and performing—graduate nursing procedures. The wartime shortening in the period of training of the professional nurse from thirty-six to thirty months cut the margin between the preparation of the registered and practical nurse even more. Mrs. Public may well ask what vast difference in skill and knowledge six little months make, and will be inclined to accept the practical nurse's own assertion that she had had "just about the equivalent of a regular nursing course."

A word should probably be said here regarding the students who are graduating from two-year courses in specialized hospitals. Such a course may not be approved by the state board of nurse examiners, making it impossible for the graduate to be admitted to the state examination for professional nurse registration; or the graduate may, for some personal reason, have failed to apply for registration though she has completed an approved course. Many tuberculosis and mental hospitals give a two-year course within their own institutions, without affiliation in other services. These two-year graduates are often the "backbone" of the special institutions.* They know at least as much about the specialty as do registered nurses who have graduated from a general hospital not offering an affiliation in tuberculosis nursing, and in 1944 two-thirds of the schools of professional nursing offered no tuberculosis nursing (26).

The graduates of the two-year course within a special hospital may be licensed as practical nurses if the state has a law and if the "school"

---

* For example, in a tuberculosis sanatorium in Michigan there were, in 1945, 163 patients, 9 registered nurses, 18 attendant "graduate" nurses.

is approved by the state board of nurse examiners, or they may be licensed under a waiver. Affiliations in other outside services are recommended and may be compulsory. These "graduates" are not in a particularly happy position: they cannot qualify as registered nurses although they have worked for two years to learn to nurse; they spent fifteen more months than was necessary to become licensed practical nurses, yet they are not prepared after the two years in a single type of hospital to nurse in homes or to take care of mothers, babies, and children. The special hospitals, however, lean heavily on the "graduate" nurses for service. Graduates do just about everything registered nurses do in these hospitals.

The vocational school setting has certain advantages: superior educational facilities and equipment, health supervision (usually under the department of physical education), recreation, laboratory facilities, and qualified instructors in home economics and dietetics. The resources of related departments are at the disposal of the nursing director. The students have a chance to acquire credits. Most of the vocational schools can order any needed supplies, even expensive equipment, if they can also be used in other courses—for example, diathermy and metabolism sets, used also by those learning to be medical secretaries, office nurses, physical therapists, etc.

Of the disadvantages, the most serious has been mentioned: the divorcing of theory from practice with real patients. Some of the teaching staff in subjects other than nursing may be totally without experience in caring for the sick—the teacher of nutrition, for example. Or they may know only the institutional situation, not the home of a foreign-born family where there are a sick father, three children, and a limited income. One cannot teach the handling of sickness problems from books. The student's relationships to doctor, family, other nurses, and visitors are involved in everything the practical nurse learns and they should be instilled with each day's work and in each class—not saved for a massive dose on the ward three months later.

The supervisor who does not carry over her program of teaching into the hospital cannot use the knowledge she would gain of her student in helping her adjust to illness. Some students, she will know, must be pushed, some held back. The students themselves say, "I had to learn procedures all over again when I got to the hospital."

Girls in the high school credit courses are apt to be young, fifteen, sixteen, or seventeen. They take their class work casually. It's just another class, not a hospital. Youth may mean immaturity, undependable judgment, fear of life's crises. Learning self-discipline in the presence of patients, understanding how to organize the day's work, seeing the complete cycle of illness—these are not gained in a five-day week in a classroom. The young high school group is a difficult one to handle and the hospitals complain of their youth, undependability, and insufficient grounding in bedside procedures. They have to be retaught frequently. The girls appear overwhelmed when they are thrust into a ward full of real patients after three months of trying to imagine what it will be like.

It would seem from these impressions that the vocational school should be established in an approved general hospital where there is no school for professional nurses, that preference should be given to older girls and women, that free tuition should be provided and no allowance paid students if full maintenance is offered. If such a plan places too heavy a burden of theoretical instruction on the hospital, the central school idea should be tried.

Making a distinction between younger and older girls at once suggests the need in all our high schools (not vocational high schools alone, and not girls only) of required courses in homemaking, simple care of the sick, care of mothers and babies, and first aid, not as pretraining courses for nursing of any type but as basic, practical knowledge needed by every adult and especially every prospective parent. New Zealand has led the world in making such courses prerequisites for graduation from secondary schools. From among students informed in these elementary courses could well be drawn our candidates for practical and professional nursing.

The plan of a central school—joint, centralized theoretical instruction for all practical students in the area while living and practicing in their own hospitals—has not yet been tried, although it has been considered (see page 166). It is one of the many proposed experiments deserving attention. Nor have affiliations in the "specialties" been developed. Several schools attempt to give experience in more than one field, but no one school has a complete course of theory and practice in all the major services expected of the practical nurse. The school in the small general hospital comes close to a well rounded experience, as does the large state infirmary, but neither has all the services. Supervised practice in private homes is the most frequently neglected service.

THE SEPARATION OF PROFESSIONAL AND PRACTICAL SCHOOLS

There seems to be general agreement that it is preferable not to allow practical nurse students to be trained in a hospital with a professional school of nursing. The reasons are fairly obvious:

One can readily see that case experience, practice, and clinical facilities for students might run short, the pick in interest going to the future professional nurse.

A double teaching program on two levels puts a strain on the teaching staff. Actually, two faculties should be provided.

Professional nurse students need to do every simple procedure at least once to be good nurses and to be competent supervisors of students and families later. If a student practical nurse is always on hand to carry out the simple step, the professional student loses the experience.

In joint training, there is a temptation to turn over the unpleasant manual or "household" tasks to the student practical nurse, loading her down with these while the professional student takes over bedside nursing care. Each student needs some experience in both types of work and division in the first days of ward experience is practically impossible in a small hospital.

The practical nurse student should be trained in a hospital where her education is of first importance and receives major consideration from the doctors, superintendent of nurses, and all other personnel; otherwise, her position will always be that of a junior student.

If joint schooling is attempted, the hospital must be large enough so that student experience for the two groups need not be given in the same ward at the same time. Double student service is confusing to the patient.

There is some temptation for student professional nurses to supervise student practical nurses—a case of the blind leading the blind. Nor is it considered wise at present for the graduate practical staff nurse working on a ward to attempt to supervise the student practical nurse.

The gravest danger of joint training is the natural tendency of practical nurses to refer to their graduation from Blank Hospital, giving patients and doctors the impression that this graduation is from the school of professional nursing. This is the reason why it is undesirable to have a professional school change over directly to a practical nursing school. "A graduate of Blank Hospital" may then mean either a professional or a practical nurse. There can be no objection to licensed practical nurses working in a hospital where there are professional nursing students, but the mingling of two schools would seem to hold unsurmountable difficulties, except, as has been said, in carefully selected large hospitals.

COMMERCIAL AND CORRESPONDENCE SCHOOLS

Schools operating for profit and teaching by correspondence or by lectures in a classroom without contact with sick people have been the bane of the nursing profession for years. The claims made by these schools are extravagant, their charges high, and their graduates inadequately prepared to undertake the responsibility of nursing sick people. But so long as these schools do not claim to prepare professional registered nurses or licensed practical nurses and so long as their graduates do not take these titles, no present state law can touch them, and, in states with no control of the title practical nurse, they can claim to do anything short of preparing professional registered nurses. Many of the large schools have centers or branches in several cities and nearly all carry advertisements in newspapers all over the county, including small town and county weeklies. These ads list advantages of training, picture professional nursing staffs, and cite the highly paid jobs their graduates hold. Among the treatments taught are complete obstetrical care, surgical procedures, psychiatric nursing, and care of infectious diseases and cardiac conditions.

Most of these schools call themselves "schools for practical nursing," thus further confusing the public and interested applicants. The course may be anywhere from 60 hours to 6 months.

Undoubtedly the number of correspondence schools for nursing has decreased, thanks to the activities of the American Nurses' Association and to the publicity accompanying legislation for licensure. In 1912, Miss Goodrich reported one school which had produced 12,000 graduates in ten years. She wrote that 90 per cent of the women then practicing nursing in New York state had no preparation for it. She cited appalling samples of commercial school publicity (27).

Schools may prepare girls from one area of the country and send them to take state examinations in another. Schools change their names and move on to states without legislative control of practical nurses. They usually offer evening classes and urge the applicant to continue her regular job while she learns nursing. Promises of high wages, interesting work, and a continual demand for service after graduation usually accompany the school announcements.

In 1938, Miss Hasenjaeger reported that a school in the east was graduating 50 to 60 "practical" nurses every three months after 100 hours of class work. A pin and certificate were given on "graduation." Two registered nurses conducted the classes. Yearly profits were reported to be $12,000 (28).

Tuition for a few hours of class work, usually less than the instruction offered in Red Cross Home Nursing classes, ranges from $60 to $120. An applicant reported that when she explained she could not pay the $10 deposit required for enrollment, the director of the school offered her a job that night on a case at $25 a week (29).

In a New England state, two courses consisted of two hours, two nights a week for three months. In Toronto, until recently, persons could be taught various treatments at so much a treatment: an enema, $5, etc. (30).

In summary, the objections to many commercial schools are that they:

Exaggerate—without running foul of the law—the value of the instruction given
In many instances employ poorly qualified teachers
Frequently set up artificial and superficial situations for learning
Admit candidates indiscriminately—without education, without a health examination, at any age, with any personal qualifications
Claim to teach the care of the sick by correspondence, usually without having the pupil see sick people
Have limited equipment
Provide poor supervision
Charge the student high rates
Conduct the school for profit rather than for service
Make doubtful claims as to the students' capacities after the course
On completion of the course place students in jobs unsuited to their abilities
Present a certificate which the graduate may, if she wishes, show as her "registration" or "license"
Turn out men and women of such limited knowledge and training as to constitute a very grave danger to the public

There are, of course, schools for practical nurses that have not been approved by any agency and yet could not be classified as commercial. No one knows how many there are of these. Many of them are in states where there is no law to license practical nurses. In 1936, Katharine Shepard, superintendent of the Household Nursing Association in Boston, wrote to all the states to find out which had schools for attendants; ten states which had no legal control of graduates reported in the affirmative, including the District of Columbia. Between 1942 and 1944, a survey of Massachusetts disclosed about 40 schools of which only eight were approved by the state at the time.

For conclusions regarding the education of the practical nurse, see page 262.

INTEREST OF THE UNITED STATES OFFICE OF EDUCATION

For many years the Office of Education has been interested in the vocational opportunities for nurses and has been actively helpful in meeting the needs for special training courses of one type or another. Under the authority of the George-Deen and Smith-Hughes Acts (31), federal money is made available to states on the basis of certain population relationships (see page 1 of each Act), to supplement the salaries of teachers, supervisors, and directors engaged in vocational education. The states in turn may decide to which local projects they wish to allocate federal funds. Under this arrangement local vocational or trade schools wishing to develop courses for practical nurses may apply to the state board of education for a share of the federal funds. The states may also assist local boards of education from state funds, the local boards carrying the balance of the expenses.

Vocational schools for practical nurses have been in existence for some years, and vocational schools not strictly a part of local school systems have requested and received money from the federal funds available to the states. Certain conditions must be met locally in the use of such funds, the main ones being that these monies are definitely for the education of persons over fourteen years of age, that the local community must supply equipment, classrooms, practice centers or laboratories as appropriate, and that the course must meet certain standards as to length, size of class, quality of instruction, etc., set by the state.

In March 1944, with the evidence of a growing shortage of registered nurses and the need of bringing some order into a chaotic field, the Office of Education through its Vocational Division called a conference of national nursing organizations and others interested. As one result of the conference the Office of Education sent a bulletin (32) to the vocational division of each state department of education calling attention to the need for courses in practical nursing and the availability of federal funds for the purpose, urging that programs be set up on a long-term, not merely an emergency, basis.

Another outcome of the conference was the appointment of a committee, representing national and federal nursing agencies, home economists, practical nurse educators, employers, and practical nurses, to work out a job analysis of the practical nurses' duties. The committee has completed a breakdown of some 300 procedures believed to be wholly or in part within the ability of the practical nurse. When the analysis is complete a curriculum will be drawn up and recommended to the schools of practical nursing.*

With this material in hand, it will be possible to prepare criteria for the selection of practice fields, qualifications of instructors, minimum standards of housing, equipment, etc. It will be these standards which the vocational schools will be expected to meet for professional approval, for the receipt of state-federal funds, and for approval by state boards of nurse examiners. One may also expect, if the standards of the vocational schools are higher than those of existing private schools, that the latter will immediately take measures to meet the recommended level and new private schools will set such levels as their minimum.

It is the hope of those interested in the promotion of practical nursing education that the new schools established on a vocational training basis will be so good that graduates will be eligible for licensure in any state, even though they take their training in vocational schools in states without a licensing law.

For the moment, with the great scarcity of candidates and the dearth of qualified nurse instructors, it is unlikely that many new vocational schools will be started. Such periods of quiescence might well be utilized to develop adequate, supervised practice fields for the future students in vocational schools. The fact that residents of a state can secure free education at the vocational schools may discourage the opening of

* For latest information, write the U.S. Office of Education.

new private schools, especially as most private schools do not have many scholarships or large endowments, and so must charge rather high tuition.

REFERENCES

1 United States Women's Bureau, *The outlook for women in occupations in the medical services; practical nurses and hospital attendants,* Washington, Government Printing Office, 1945 (Bulletin 203, No. 5), p. 3.

2 Isabel M. Stewart, *The education of nurses; historical foundations and modern trends,* New York, Macmillan, 1943, pp. 128, 130.

3 Alfred Worcester, *A new way of training nurses,* Boston, Cupples and Hurd, 1888, p. 107.

4 Ysabella Waters, *Visiting nursing in the United States,* New York, Charities Publication Committee, 1909, tables, pp. 315–364.

5 Netta Ford, "Subsidiary worker and her place, if any, in nursing," *Hospitals* 11:91–94, November 1937.

6 Allon Peebles and Valeria D. McDermott, *Nursing services and insurance for medical care in Brattleboro, Vermont;* a study of the activities of the Thomas Thompson Trust, Chicago, University of Chicago Press, 1932 (Committee on the Costs of Medical Care, No. 17); Richards M. Bradley, "Attendant nurse solves puzzle of household nursing care," *Nation's Health* 7:735, November 15, 1925; Richards M. Bradley, "Household nursing in relation to similar work," *American Journal of Nursing* 15:968–975, August 1915; Richards M. Bradley, "Skilled nursing for all," *Survey* 70:9–11, January 1934.

7 Lillie Young, "The attendant nurse in the home," *Public Health Nursing* 31:166–168, March 1939.

8 See note 6.

9 Compare with the proposed plan for training practical nurses in Minnesota, "Minnesota plans for rural nursing service," *American Journal of Nursing* 44:147–150, February 1944.

10 John Dill Robertson, "Who shall nurse the sick," *Survey* 46:411–412, June 18, 1921.

11 Information from correspondence with the director of the course, January 1945.

12 Isabel H. Dill, "The Rochester School of Practical Nursing," *American Journal of Nursing* 45:373–378, May 1945.

13 Lottie Horn Waterman, "How Michigan produces a supply of carefully trained practical nurses," *Hospitals* 17:58–61, December 1943, at p. 59.

14 See suggested list on page 3, Bulletin VE-ND Misc. 3729, August 1944, Federal Security Agency, U.S. Office of Education, Vocational Division, Washington.

15 Basil C. MacLean, "Nurses—what next?" *Modern Hospital* 47:51–53, August 1936, at p. 53.

16 Information secured during visits to the school. See also Mary Ellen Manley, "The subsidiary worker in the nursing care of the sick," *Hospitals* 14:61–64, February 1940. For a description of New York state's practical nurse program, see Josephine F. Goldsmith, "New York's practical nurse program," *American Journal of Nursing* 42:1026–1031, September 1942.

17 In 1934, a frank statement of reasons for dismissing students included carelessness, immorality, untidiness, "not safe to be with patients." Elizabeth C. Burgess, "The subsidiary worker," *40th Annual Report of the National League of Nursing Education,* New York, 1934, p. 5. Dr. Worcester records sadly the dismissal of a student nurse "in disgrace after nearly two years of deception." Worcester (note 3), pp. 101, 107.

18 National League of Nursing Education, Department of Studies, "Student withdrawals," *American Journal of Nursing* 44:586–587, June 1944.

19 Helen F. Hansen, "Study of resignations and dismissals," *American Journal of Nursing* 31:739, June 1931.

20 Josephine Goldmark, *Nursing and nursing education in the United States;* report of the Committee for the Study of Nursing Education, New York, Macmillan, 1923, pp. 27–38.

21 Said in nearly the same words in an editorial, "Registration of attendants," *American Journal of Nursing* 12:277–280, January 1912.

22 Lucile Petry, "Increasing and using nursing auxiliaries," *Hospitals* 17:39, February 1943.

23 Comment, *American Journal of Nursing* 33:641, June 1933.

24 American Hospital Association, *Report of the Committee to Study the Nursing Problem,* Philadelphia, the Association, 1916, p. 7.

25 Editorial, "How can we meet the shortage of nurses?" *Hospital Management* 52:35, December 1941. This was also Dr. Alfred Worcester's opinion in 1888 (note 3).

26 National League of Nursing Education, Department of Studies, "Nursing specialties in the curriculum," *American Journal of Nursing* 44:680–682, July 1944.

27 Annie W. Goodrich, *The social and ethical significance of nursing; a series of addresses,* New York, Macmillan, 1932, p. 28.

28 Ella Hasenjaeger, "The subsidiary worker," *American Journal of Nursing* 38:772–776, July 1938, at p. 774.

29 See also description of schools in Pennsylvania reported by the State Nurses Association in *Study of the subsidiary worker in nursing service in Pennsylvania, 1939–1940*, pp. 34–36, and excerpts from their publicity material.

30 To counteract the effect of commercial school advertising in Maryland, the State Nurse Association authorized the release of a complete statement listing the approved schools in the state, emphasizing the wealth of clinical material, eligibility to state licensure, and that there is no tuition.

31 Smith-Hughes Act, passed by Congress, February 23, 1917. Public No. 347 (S. 703) to provide for the promotion of vocational education, and its mate known as George-Deen Act, Congress, June 8, 1936, Public No. 673 (H.R. 12120).

32 See note 14.

CHAPTER FOURTEEN

The Curriculum in Schools of Practical Nursing

THE TRAINING for practical nursing is not a short course in professional nursing. A pseudoprofessional course of inferior quality, which attempts to teach everything except advanced technical procedures in half the time necessary to produce a professional nurse, is plainly overdoing the preparation within the capacity and function of the practical nurse and underdoing that needed by the professional. Such a shortcut is definitely a threat to the desirable standards of both groups (1).

The curriculum most generally offered by the approved schools, including student practice, seldom exceeds twelve months in length. The shorter the course is, compatible with the subjects to be learned and their practice, the better, as this demonstrates to the public that the training is of different caliber from that of professional nursing, on a comparatively elementary level, and not under any condition to be confused with the two to three years' education of a professional nurse. The number of hours devoted to theory in class range from 164 to 540, but 200 is quite usual; two approved schools offer less than 110. The minimum hours of theory in the professional curriculum is 825 (2). Furthermore, the professional group has already advanced into the field of the specialties. Postgraduate courses are now usual in surgical, orthopedic, psychiatric, obstetric, pediatric, and industrial nursing, not to mention the academic year of study and practice necessary to prepare a public health nurse, nurse-midwife, hospital administrator, or nurse educator (3). The wartime "refresher" course in operating room technique, to take one specialty, offered to professional nurses by the U.S. Army was 75 hours.

Those with experience in planning these courses feel that nine months is the minimum and twelve to fourteen months the maximum time needed to teach practical nursing—more is unwise (4). During the study of the practical nursing situation in New York, Harlan H. Horner recommended that practical nursing be raised to a higher level of service by requiring a high school diploma, a year's training, self-maintenance, tuition, and a limitation of numbers. Candidates should be required to pass personality and fitness tests (5). So long as the majority of candidates offer less than high school graduation and make entirely satisfactory practical nurses, this recommendation for the present at least has not met with acceptance and no school for practical nursing requires a high school diploma for entrance (6).

The professional nurse has traveled far since the days at the turn of the century when the curriculum covered one to two years, based on a year of high school (7). Professional nursing is now as much advanced beyond practical nursing as is the practice of medicine beyond professional nursing. This distinction is important. It is ultimately most important to the patient, but the differentiation starts with the selection of the practical nurse student and what she is taught.

It cannot be said that the two programs of instruction are distinct at present (8). But the differences are emerging. There is general agreement that professional nurses need not carry on certain routine procedures for convalescent and subacute cases, while practical nurses should never attempt some of the expert treatments usually needed in acute illness. Confusion appears to rise, however, when it is realized that the "simple" nursing procedure—an enema, for example—must not be undertaken by the practical nurse if the patient is suffering from a condition which makes the enema difficult or dangerous, or if the situation is liable to change during the course of the treatment. On the other hand, the practical nurse may find herself called on to give an "advanced" treatment to a patient in an acute stage of illness where relief is essential to comfort, possibly to recovery. Catheterization is the classic example of this situation. It becomes plain that the condition of the patient and the doctor's orders determine which nurse should give the treatment. There are many patients with the same diagnosis, some of whom are completely safe in the hands of qualified practical nurses, some safe only in the care of professional nurses. The border-line or common-ground conditions and treatments need analysis, study, and trial under controlled observation in both hospitals and homes, for there is no doubt that a practical nurse may safely undertake a treatment under the constant supervision of a professional nurse in a hospital, with adequate equipment, which should never be attempted by her when working alone among the makeshifts of a private home. Curricula should not be "set" until such studies have satisfied a representative body of doctors and professional nurses qualified to judge where the lines should be drawn. It is not unthinkable that practical nurses should be given a list of treatments which they may perform alone in a home only under certain conditions. A public health nurse never, for example, gives an enema to a home patient without a doctor's order. Doctors and families appreciate these safeguards when the situation is explained to them.

The curriculum as generally set up at present for practical nurses as compared to that for professional nurses shows clearly and convincingly the difference between the qualifications and training of the registered professional and the licensed practical nurse. The comparison is presented here for the following purposes:

To show doctors, employers, and teachers the wide gap between the requirements for the two fields of service and the type of training now offered in each

To encourage practical nurses to see their field as a challenging, dignified, worth-while career in itself and to reassure those registered nurses who live in fear of competition from practical nurses that they have it in their power to place their profession on a plane of service so highly skilled that confusion between the two groups of nurses will be only a matter of history

To clarify for any nonprofessional reader what is meant by "professional registered nurse" and by "practical licensed nurse," and perhaps make it easier for him to choose the right type of nursing service the next time he is sick

Most of the differences in these lists are self-evident, but a few need further interpretation. The curriculum subjects compared were chosen at random. There would be greater significance in comparing what is taught each group in sociology, in trends in nursing history, and in professional adjustments. The professional student nurse received 20 to 40 hours in each of these subjects, with a list of some 50 reading references; the practical nurse receives barely three hours unless "behavior problems" are stretched to mean professional adjustments, then perhaps 15 hours.

The difference in the level of teaching all subjects should be stressed. We have only to skim through the approved professional nursing textbooks to see that we have a science in the making, built on a sound foundation of knowledge acquired preferably at college level by keen, trained minds accustomed to study, weigh, compare, and assimilate, and resulting in performance far above the "home nursing" level. We might draw a comparison from the field of industry: we

	PROFESSIONAL	PRACTICAL
	Admission Requirements	
Age	18 to 35	17 to 50
Educational qualifications	High school graduate, upper third of class; preferably science subjects	Completion of 8th grade
	Personal Qualifications	
	Many in common, including good health, poise, friendliness, neat appearance, integrity	
	Emphasis on evidences of leadership, versatility, breadth of interests, background, interest in people	Emphasis on common sense, maturity, eagerness to learn
	Length of Course	
Theory and practice	2½ to 3 years; 800 to 1,200 curriculum hours	9 to 18 months; 60 to 500 curriculum hours
Practice	In registered hospital, preferably 100 daily average census, all services (in affiliation if necessary), 2½ years, 44 hour week, 3,650 hours; or 3 years, 48 hour week, 5,000 hours	May be 6 weeks to 18 months in one hospital, in several hospitals, or in no hospital. May be in one specialized service only (mental or tuberculosis, for example). Hospital may be as small as 37 beds. May be 35 to 50 hour week
	Faculty	
	2 to 30 members, full time, 6 to 8 part time; usually college graduates, may have advanced degrees. Doctors give many courses. Laboratory periods under supervision. All specialties taught by specialists	1 to 3 members full and part time; college degrees unnecessary. Registered nurses and qualified home economics instructors. Specialties not usually taught by specialists. Doctors not found satisfactory as teachers of this group. No laboratory hours in accepted sense

Note. Average professional and average practical curricula and requirements are compared. The curricula in collegiate schools of nursing would show even greater differences.

	PROFESSIONAL	PRACTICAL
	Content of Course	
	Many textbooks on each subject but instruction not didactic. Students encouraged to do original work. Outside reading required. Freedom to specialize within curriculum framework. Experience sheets, case histories, etc., encouraged. Access to complete medical and nursing library	One textbook—at most two—used as basic reference, rest of material in pamphlet form of popular nature at high school level. Didactic teaching. No outside subjects encouraged, reading limited. Little record work required, no original research. Library very limited. All teaching at practical, "doing - with - the - hands" level
	Subject Matter	
Nursing procedures	In standard textbooks (9) tests and treatments cover 600 to 700 pages (one subject—diabetes—covers 20 pages)	About 100 taught. Text covers 40 to 100 pages in three standard textbooks (one subject—diabetes—covers 2 to 5 pages)
Total group of units	750 hours	90 hours
Materia medica	300 to 400 drugs and solutions; 200 to 300 pages in textbooks; 30 hours	Usually 40 to 50 remedies; 10 to 15 pages in textbook; 4 hours
Obstetrics	400 to 500 pages; usually 2 to 3 months' experience; unit of 60 hours	Delivery omitted. 10 to 20 pages; usually no experience, at most one month with babies; 10 hours of instruction
	Character of Instruction	
	In general, all treatments taught and practiced	Only simplest tests taught (sugar in urine, for example). About 20 common but skilled treatments never taught

have the unskilled but essential worker trained to use his hands as directed by his foreman and the more highly trained technician whose head dictates what his hands must do after careful analysis of the job to be done. Nothing illustrates this more vividly than the trained power of observation in the professional nurse. The position which a patient assumes in bed may look perfectly natural to the practical nurse but can spell trouble to the experienced eyes of the professional —as can the facial expression. The pulse may be described simply as strong or weak and its rate given. The professional nurse notes its rate, force, volume, or quality, rhythm, and tension (10). We could continue endlessly with these contrasts.

The faculty of observation is closely allied to an ability to rise to emergencies and to act swiftly and with good judgment. Manual dexterity can be acquired, but discrimination between significant and trivial symptoms, their implications, and the remedial steps to take calls for highly trained senses and the exercise of balanced judgment. The doctor takes it for granted that the nurse knows what to look for in a given condition. She may have his "s.o.s." (if necessary) or "p.r.n." (whenever necessary) order, but he relies on her to interpret the *if* and *when*.

Outside the hospital, in home contacts, public health nurses demonstrate the same trained ability to observe, size up, and interpret in a wider and slightly different area—that of social and economic conditions. It becomes almost automatic for the public health nurse to see the adequacies and inadequacies in a family, their characteristics, attitudes toward life, securities and insecurities, resources, and economic level.

The demand for trained minds in nursing is growing greater every year. Routine tests and treatments have increased enormously in the last ten years. It is nothing to find 15 or 20 of these currently in progress on an average ward (preoperative and postoperative routines; gastric, kidney, and heart functioning tests; transfusions and intravenous injections of various types) and to find patients who need expert professional nursing far beyond the capacities, knowledge, or skills of a practical nurse—for example, the diabetic in coma, the cardiac with an occlusion, the cardiac-nephritic, the patient with a brain tumor or an intestinal obstruction, the expectant mother in eclampsia.

Regular, frequent, accurate charting of blood pressure, exact measure of intake and output, use of suction apparatus such as the Wangensteen, apical and radial pulse readings, administration of insulin, urine analyses and "stabilizing" of the diabetic's diet, and special diet therapy are only a few of the skilled procedures professional nurses must carry out intelligently. It is necessary for the professional nurse not only to follow the doctor's order, but to keep abreast of his objectives in these treatments. Without a clear perception of the end in view, the hazards on the way, and the steps to take in an emergency, the nurse attendant on a critically ill person can hinder rather than help recovery (11).

The essence of professional nursing, then, as compared to practical nursing lies not in the mechanical details of execution, manual dexterity, speed, or accuracy in routine procedures, but in the possession and exercise of judgment, the training of a critical faculty, the development of a creative imagination, and ability to synthetize the symptoms observed or results obtained into a judgment upon which action will be based. To deduce, to build the new out of the old, to create, these capacities raise nursing above a trade or skill and transform it into an art—a profession.

On the other hand, let us once and for all cast aside the idea that practical nursing is unskilled or menial. Every procedure carried out for a patient should be skillfully done. The hands giving a back rub must be just as thoroughly trained in a practical nurse as in a professional nurse. The rendering of the humblest service to a human being, even the giving of a bedpan, should not be thought of as menial in the sense of a "servile" job. Anything that contributes directly to the cure of the sick person calls for skill, for sensitiveness and devotion. For their field of service, practical nurses need the highest type of instruction and the most careful drilling in techniques. In practice, instructors find practical nurses actually demand much effort and time, for the learning process is slower and the scientific foundation shallower than in the professional student. One of the salient differences in preparation observed by the writer on her visits with practical nurses is that a well prepared professional nurse knows several good ways to accomplish the same end and is guided by her past experience in choosing the one best fitted to each situation. Not so the practical nurse, who is usually taught one or two good, substantial, and reliable methods from which it is better for her not to deviate.

There is, however, one quality which all nurses of all ages have shared—the love of nursing. The same loyalty which makes a professional nurse stick to her task in the face of discouragement, fatigue, and danger can be developed in the practical nurse. The love of nurturing, of fostering the young, the sick, and the helpless is as elemental, as fervent, as glowing in "practicals" as in "professionals," say their teachers. Many older women and mothers have this enthusiasm even more strongly than the eighteen-year-olds. It is on this foundation that teaching is based and all good nursing practice rests.

VARIATIONS IN CURRICULA IN THE SCHOOLS OF PRACTICAL NURSING

Since 1907 all efforts to educate practical nurses have been experimental. There has never been a body of collective experience on which to draw in formulating a curriculum. A preliminary step in filling this lack is being taken as this book is being written by a committee of the Office of Education, which is making a job analysis of the practical nurse's service, based on the thinking and experience of a group of authorities in nursing and home economics (12). Their ultimate purpose is to draw up a curriculum based on this theoretical job analysis.

It will be possible to make an analysis from this list of the duties of the practical nurse, service by service, for use in hospitals. In 1937, Nell V. Beeby made a very complete study of the situations in obstetrics in which the professional nurse functions (13). More than 200 situations were reviewed. Some of these are now assignable to the trained and licensed practical nurse in the light of recent studies.

Even if a complete, theoretical job analysis is long in coming, there are simple, temporary expedients by which a school might arrive at a decision as to what to teach (14). In the meantime general statements of what approved curricula cover are obtainable from state boards of nurse examiners, from the National Association for Practical Nurse Education, and from the directors of the approved schools. During the last five years there has been more uniformity in hours and subjects taught as a result of sharing these lists, but the treatment actually taught, the place and hours of student practice, the amount and quality of supervision still show wide variations.

Subjects and Hours of Class and Practice

The general statement made by the National Association for Practical Nurse Education describing an acceptable curriculum suggests that the candidate have a minimum of 200 clock hours of classroom work, with six months' practice in the care of men, women, and children in institutions with a daily average of not less than 20 patients. The New York law states that six months of service in homes may be substituted for not more than two months in a hospital. In Michigan, 16 weeks (540 clock hours) of class work and six months (132 days) of practice under registered nurse supervision are recommended (15).

A nine-months course under Y.W.C.A. auspices offers 15 courses (380 hours) covering three months followed by practice, and additional classes in selected hospitals (six months). The courses are:

Bedside nursing	House management
Body structure	Methods of study
Child care	Mother and baby care
Chronic and convalescent	Nutrition
diseases	Personal and vocational
Community health	adjustments
Cookery	Personal health problems
First aid	Recreational therapy
Food buying	

The following curriculum, which is taught in a twelve-month course, is typical of those of the schools in Type II (see page 212).

	Class hours	Practice hours
Structure and functions of the body	25	
Personal health	12	
Diet in health and disease	16	20
Microorganisms	14	
Behavior and working relationships	7	
Nursing techniques	56	100
Administration of medicines	16	
Bandaging	6	
First aid	15	
Care of hospital and home environment	6	25
Care of mother and infant	9	
Care of children	6	
Care of the aged and chronics	5	
General medicine	14	
Total	207	145

One of the typical classroom curricula (13 weeks) in vocational schools of Type III (see page 213) includes:

Personal hygiene and development	20 hours
Behavior and working relations	5 hours
Nursing techniques	200 hours
Mother and child care	25 hours
First aid	20 hours
Occupational therapy	10 hours
Special cases	20 hours
Food and nutrition	75 hours
Care of home	25 hours
Total	**400 hours**

Variations in hours and terminology are evident in all the schools, and there are many additions to these basic lists. For example, a school connected with a large hospital for the chronically ill adds from two to six hours each in the care of heart disease, nephritis, cancer, paralysis, diabetes, orthopedics, urological disease, arthritis, tuberculosis, common cold, grippe, and old people.

A large state hospital offers in its course 12 hours of hydrotherapy and physiotherapy, three hours of massage, 12 hours of psychiatry, 12 hours "operating room, special."

A course in California for training licensed attendants divides the curriculum into:

Nursing procedures	26 hours class; 26 hours practice
Ethics	6 hours class
General housekeeping	2 hours class
Personal hygiene	12 hours class
Materia medica	8 hours class
Bacteriology	8 hours class
Medical nursing	12 hours class
Surgical nursing	10 subjects, time not stated
Anatomy and physiology	8 subjects, time not stated
Nutrition	10 hours; 20 hours laboratory
Tuberculosis nursing	6 hours
Total approximately	164 hours, plus review and examinations

A course of 585 hours includes:

Personal interviews	14 hours
Classes	
Personal problems	12 hours
Working relationships	18 hours
Nursing practices	120 hours
Recreation therapy	7 hours
Maternity and infant care	24 hours
Food and nutrition	64 hours
Home management	32 hours
Child care	24 hours
Supervised work experience	200 hours
Review and conferences	35 hours
Examinations	35 hours
Total	585 hours

First aid and care of the aged are included in nursing practice. It will be noted that there is no class period designated "materia medica."

The course offered student practical nurses in Ontario, Canada, which is approved by the Ontario Registered Nurse's Association, includes:

Professional, family, and community relationships	5 hours
Personal hygiene	15 to 20 hours
Basic instruction—anatomy and physiology	16 to 20 hours
Housekeeping	110 hours
Simple nursing care	8 to 12 hours
Feeding	
Rest—adult and juvenile patients	1 hour
Child psychology—rest and play, well children	3 to 4 hours
Elimination	12 hours
First aid procedures	10 hours
Simple massage	2 hours
Oral medicines	3½ to 6½ hours
Dressings, sterilization of dressings, simple dressing procedure	4 to 8 hours
Solutions	1½ to 3 or 4 hours
Sterilization, simple boiling method	½ hour
Isolation, colds—prevention and protection; care of kerchiefs, dishes, linen, etc.	2 hours

Practical cookery	48 hours
Simple treatments	50 to 60 hours
Care of infants and children	8 to 10 hours
Household economics and practical cookery	50 hours
Nutrition	5 to 6 hours
Charting	2 to 4 hours

Procedures

A check list of procedures taught and experienced by the practical student is kept by the instructor wherever the student is receiving her practice and a copy is usually returned to the school for the student's record. One such check list reads:

Nursing Techniques

Strip bed
Make open bed
Make closed bed
Make bed from one side
Make ether bed
Fan bed clothing
Use of bath blanket
Dress and undress patient
Move and turn patient
Make bed with patient
Remove patient's gown
Put gown on patient
Give bedpan
Give morning toilet
Give evening toilet
Prepare back rest
Put patient onto back rest
Get a convalescent patient onto chair
Care for patient's hair
Care for patient's teeth
Rub patient's back
Give simple body rub
Prepare and give s.s. enema
Prepare and give oil enema
Take temperature

Prepare and apply flaxseed poultice
Prepare and do irrigations
Prepare and do ear irrigation
Prepare and do eye irrigation
Prepare and apply hot application to eye
Measure drops
Measure medicines
Give medicine
Safety rules for giving medicines
Treat for poisoning (emergency)
Assist patient to void (10 ways)
Prepare and do turpentine stupe
Prepare and apply hot water bottle
Prepare and apply ice cap
Apply binder
Prepare and give pack
Prepare and give sponge
Prepare and give bed bath
Prepare and give perineal dressing
Collect specimens
Disinfect secretions

Take pulse	Do charting
Take respirations	Sterilize equipment
Prepare and give hypodermic	Supervise equipment
Prepare and pass rectal tube	Hemorrhage (first aid)
Prepare and apply mustard plaster	

Care of Young Child

Prepare for baby's bath	Prepare for feedings
Give oil bath	Feed baby
Give soft water bath	Give enemas, suppositories
Apply abdominal binder	Modify treatment for baby
Prepare solutions for tray	Arrange time and place for
Dress baby	sleeping
Buy clothing needed for baby	Prepare bed and carriage
Wash baby's clothing	Know normal development of
Care for diapers	baby
Prepare feedings, formulas	

The lists supplied by some schools show these additions: fracture bed, care of body after death, surgical dressings, catheterization, isolation technique, six types of hypodermics, restraints, charting doctors' orders, vaginal douche, tests of urine for sugar and albumen, bandaging, cleaning and care of oxygen tent, preparation of solutions, and assistance with special treatments and procedures such as pneumothorax.*

Not all lists included improvisation of equipment or use of electrical equipment (inhalators, bedpads, etc.). It is particularly important, if the practical nurse is having her student training in a hospital and has no home cases, to spend time explaining, demonstrating, and letting

---

* A sampling of typical treatments required of *professional* nurses in a general ward include (actual report): Blood pressure (usually at stated intervals); transfusions—blood, plasma (prepare for, assist doctor, watch); continuous intravenous fluids; clyses; suction (tracheotomies, chest cavities, throats, Wangensteen); bladder decompression; colostomy (cecostomy) irrigations; colonic irrigations; management of respirator; management of oxygen apparatus (tent, mask, catheter); lumbar punctures; approximately 230 dressings a day on 473 patients; catheterization; use of Danzer apparatus; some 1,500 medications daily (473 patients); care of patients with craniotomies, tracheotomies, amputations, lobectomies; thoracentesis, paracenteses; phlebotomies. Among the tests for which they were responsible were basal metabolisms, phenosulfonphthalein tests, gastro-intestinal series, blood tests, gastric analyses, cystoscopies, and assistance with electrocardiograms (16).

her use the homemade appliances and electrical equipment she will inevitably have to handle in homes.

When practice is given in a maternity hospital or ward, a school may require the student to have experience in the following procedures:

Care of Mother

Antepartum care—general routine
Observation of normal delivery (pupil not to assist)
Postpartum care—general routine for convalescent mother
    Breast care for nursing mother and for non-nursing mother
    Diet
    Bed bath
    Morning care
    Evening care
    Perineal care
    Rest and exercise
    Elimination
    Temperature, pulse, and respiration
Care in case of threatened abortion
Care after abortion or miscarriage
Instructions given mother upon discharge from hospital
Vaginal douche

Care of Baby

Preparation for birth: layette, basket, identification
Observation of normal delivery
Immediate care after birth: tying of cord, cord dressing, drops in eyes, oil bath, etc.
Daily routine after fifth day
    Bath—table or lap (oil)
    Care of cord and navel
    Care of skin—irritations, impetigo, etc.
    Handling baby—dressing and undressing
    Care of bassinet
    Feeding: breast, artificial, formula making
    Daily rest and exercise
    Elimination: meconium, normal stool
    Weight and temperature—charting
Observation of circumcision—daily care
Signs of illness
Demonstration tub bath before discharge

Homemaking

As has been said, the amount of instruction and practice in home-making varies to an even greater degree than the hours devoted to nursing practice. Much depends on the preparation and interest of the instructor and the facilities of the school. A completely hospitalized environment neither looks nor acts like a home. In schools where experience is in a practice home, the instruction is far more complete, more realistic, and prepares the student for almost any situation she is likely to meet in private duty. To indicate the fundamental nature of the activities taught students, the writer has taken a list of typical duties from the procedures taught in three well established schools, all of which have home "laboratories."

Plan meals in relation to budget, balance, ration points, family size, and condition of patient; go to market; order by telephone; prepare all types of simple meals for well people, growing children, the sick; use of leftovers; clean kitchen; care of range (coal, gas, electric), refrigerator (ice, mechanical), laundry tubs; dusting; cleaning furniture, floors, drapes; simple washing including baby's garments and silk lingerie; mending; darning; scheduling activities for day; care of linen, blankets and beds, silver; dish washing; answering telephone and door; welcoming visitors; care of bathroom; cleaning agents and removal of spots; prevention of fire, home accident; care of plants, flowers, pets, books, first aid cabinet; reading meters; fuel and heating; ventilation; use of disinfectants; sterilization of dishes; ironing; care of woolens and furs; use of washing machine.

At the school for practical nurses at a state hospital, these subjects are described as "Hospital housekeeping, 30 hours, to be assigned on wards."

WHERE SHOULD PRACTICE BE GIVEN?

Practice of varying lengths (one month to 18 months) is now offered in hospitals, large and small, general and special, with and without professional schools of nursing; in institutions for the aged, for the convalescent, for the handicapped, and for infants; in nursery schools and child care agencies. Some approved schools offer no home service under supervision; some approved schools offer no general (acute) hospital experience of any kind. Many approved schools offer practice in only one institution which may be highly specialized. Instruction in homemaking may be confined to a diet kitchen, care of student's bedroom and school living room, with purely theoretical planning of family meals, or it may be a realistic living together in a "practice house" where meals are planned, bought, prepared, and eaten by the students and the routine of housekeeping, cleaning, scheduling of duties and recreation are experienced week after week.

Of uniformity there is none; standardization awaits study and the establishment of an authoritative, accrediting body outside the school directors which can stand in the same relation to the schools of practical nursing that the National League of Nursing Education stands to schools of professional nursing.

Twenty-five years ago, Miss Goldmark wrote:

If the leaders in nursing education will apply to the evolution of adequate training for the subsidiary group, the same courage and determination which have won their way in nursing education against the heaviest odds, they will have provided for a no less imperative public service which should rightly be under the direction and support of the nursing profession (17).

In Hospitals

As has been said the problem of supplying less expensive nursing service to hospitals should not be allowed to dominate the problem of training practical nurses. Institutions should rely for service on salaried graduate practical and professional nurses and not on student practical nurses. On the other hand, to have small hospitals with ideal clinical material for practical student nurses go unused seems unfortunate, especially as there are many approved schools looking for practice fields in hospitals and, if vocational aid for instructors' salaries could be secured, many hospitals without professional schools could guarantee a highly satisfactory educational experience to students.

The tie-up with the hospital is vital, the writer believes, for two reasons: it must precede hospital employment of the licensed practical nurse if the hospital is to have any confidence at all in its employee and feel her salary is justified; hospital experience under supervision yields a breadth and frequency of experience in repeated procedures and develops a sense of responsibility which private duty in a home or visiting on an hourly basis can never accomplish. Students see and care for more patients in a day in a hospital than they meet in a week of private duty service in homes. There is a chance to see that each listed treatment is satisfactorily performed and the techniques taught in class are fixed in a routine of habit; this can seldom happen in a series of homes all differently equipped and confusingly varied. There is an indefinable discipline acquired in nursing in a hospital which is valuable in any type of position chosen later. Supervised hospital experience would seem to have the same importance for the practical nurse as it does for the professional. Here is where sick people are assembled, here is where the doctors decide what needs to be done, here is where nurses carry out their orders. Adaptations of hospital methods may be made in the homes—and should be taught. Practical nurses learning only in homes will be seriously handicapped when they go into a complicated hospital setup and try to translate the informalities of the home. However, as late as 1930 the Committee on the Costs of Medical Care concluded that less than half of the practical nurses serving in homes had had institutional or formal training, yet they were willing to accept any type of case and in many rural communities were the only nurses available (18).

The hours of practice under supervision in hospitals required by the approved schools have so wide a divergence in arrangement that it has been difficult to figure totals. Hospitals require eight, ten, and twelve hours of duty a day, sometimes including classwork. Length of practice may be one month on a forty-hour week or two years on a fifty-hour week. Students may attend five days a week, day duty only, or may form the nursing staff of the hospital. A few of the situations found by the writer in her visits are cited.

In the Baltimore City Hospitals clinical experience was divided as follows:

Chronic medical	
Chronic surgical	25–30 weeks
Maternity	10 weeks
Children	6 weeks
Tuberculosis	8–10 weeks
Diet kitchen	2 weeks

The Massachusetts State Board of Nurse Examiners has suggested the following division over a period of 10 to 12 months:

Female medical	2 months
Male medical	1 month

Female surgical	1 month
Male surgical	1 month
Postnatal care	2 months; care of mother 5 days postpartum
Infant care	2 months; including formula room for 2 weeks
Child care	1 month; nursery school experience may be substituted for hospital experience

The description of the course in Ontario, Canada, states: "Students should obtain practical experience in hospitals for non-acutely ill, institutions caring for well children and homes under direction of registered nurses."

The Rochester, N.Y., school stipulates 1,150 hours of ward practice and assigns students for six months of service in the Monroe County Hospital and the Batavia City Hospital (maternity). Observation of well children in a nursery school is included.

In Massachusetts, Katharine Shepard has found that 12 months in a hospital of 65 beds and 25 bassinets, with a staff of 14 registered nurses for 18 practical students, is a safe arrangement. A full time instructor is a prerequisite (19). Small hospitals have been used for student practice in Massachusetts since 1917.

"The writer," wrote Florence Nightingale in 1860, "honestly believes that it is impossible to learn it (practical manual nursing) from any book and that it can only be thoroughly learnt in the wards of a hospital" (20).

In Homes

It is one of the fundamental principles of the project method of education that the student shall be taught to solve problems in the circumstance in which they arise. Translated . . ., this means that nurses who are to serve in homes should have training in homes, under supervision (21).

At present, experience in home care of the sick under supervision is given in only eight schools. To the writer's knowledge, two of these give the practice period through an affiliation with the staff of the local visiting nurse association, one gives it from the hospital outpatient staff, and the others supervise from their own teaching staff. From the point of view of good community relationships and the presence of a highly skilled type of supervision, the visiting nurse association would appear to be the logical agency with which to arrange the practice period if the case load is large enough to permit a selection suitable for the student care and if adequate supervision can be provided. The connection with the visiting nurse association has five decided advantages:

It accustoms the visiting nurse association staff and the families under care to the presence and service of supervised practical nurses

A pattern of "student affiliation" is already at hand in these agencies for professional students which makes adaptation to the needs of the practical nurse easy

The variety of cases under care in the average visiting nurse service is ideally suited to a graded experience for the student, starting with simple bedside care of a chronic case and advancing to more and more demanding cases

Patients are never "exploited" or assigned care unwisely, because the professional staff makes all first visits and supervises at least once a week

Practical nurses thus learn as students to like and seek professional supervision of their home cases

Some of the schools require that the experience in home care under supervision be completed before the school certificate is granted. This experience may last from six weeks to six months, and may be on a visit basis or full time. Supervision may be on a routine schedule or as needed. The student on full time may be paid by the family, but if she is the rate is less than for the licensed practical nurse. It is usual to have the home experience follow the hospital training, but this is not always so. Many of the directors of schools spoke hopefully of the day when home practice would be a requirement of their course. All agreed it was highly desirable.

The visiting nurse associations themselves are enthusiastic about this service. It is a relief, said two public health nurses in different services, to the writer, to place the care of chronic patients in such capable hands. Past experience—in Detroit especially—bears out this conclusion (22).

The report of the American Hospital Association in 1916 in regard to the practice field for this group is significant. The Committee to Study the Nursing Problem concluded that the class of worker undertaking care of both home and patient should be prepared in homes, under fully qualified nursing supervision, thus building up a reliable corps of household nurses for every community. No certificate or period of "graduation" was recommended. This "community center for household nursing" was at all times to be under the direction of a trained graduate nurse and the practical nurses would be supervised in all their work.* In a small community, the practical nurses from a community bureau would serve in the hospitals as needed. The committee was emphatic in saying that a "broad statesmanlike view" must be taken in planning to fill all types of nursing needs in a community and that business organization on an efficiently run plan should be back of both home and hospital service. "The chief difficulties in regard to hospital training for this class of workers are that most of those who have had even a few months of experience in a hospital object to doing housework." Many of the younger women who have had short courses in hospitals "do not carry the double responsibility of the home and patient well" (23). This, too, is a present-day complaint.

In Tuberculosis Hospitals

In tuberculosis hospitals offering affiliations to professional or practical nursing students, as much supervision as possible is given. Health is checked before, during, and at the close of employment. Follow-up x-ray of chest is advised three, six, and nine months after leaving the tuberculosis hospital. It must be remembered that the incidence of tuberculosis among young nurses is higher than in like age groups of other women (24).

There appear to be two points of view regarding the safety of allowing practical nurses as students in tuberculosis hospitals. One holds that the practical nurse is more liable to infection because she does not understand her danger. She has had a very shallow grounding in bacteriology, communicable disease, and aseptic techniques. At best, she has not had more than six months in her school of practical nursing and general hospital. She needs closer supervision, repeated lessons, and drills over a longer period than her professional sister.

The other point of view is that the pupil practical nurse is far more afraid of tuberculosis than her better informed sister, that she obeys instructions to the letter, is not bored by routine, and takes no chances. She may be an older and more mature person.

---

* Bureaus of this type were then in existence in Brattleboro, Detroit, and Boston.

Further discussion of this specialized field for practical nurses appears in Chapter 7.

Other Practice Fields

It has been suggested that practical nurses should receive their training only in institutions where nonacute cases are cared for, such as convalescent homes, old people's homes, homes for chronics, and the various institutions for the handicapped.. Apart from the one-sided experience this plan offers, it is a little hard to see how young women would be attracted to a training course solely in, say, a home for the aged.

In 1919, Anne H. Strong suggested the use of children's homes and homes for crippled, feebleminded, and epileptics as suitable institutions in which to train practical nurses (we would rule out the last two) and added that the visiting nurse association should provide instruction in home visiting (25).

The advantages and disadvantages of this type of training have never been evaluated. Indeed, the writer could find no comparative studies of time, content, supervision, or appraisal of student experience. No one has determined through study of present practices whether a period of four, six, or twelve months of practice is desirable, or how much experience in one type of agency is equivalent to practice in another.

It would appear desirable to consider these institutions as experience fields in affiliation with the basic hospital practice work, and for the most part this is the use to which they are being put at present. Training received only in these institutions should not be accepted as preparation for licensure as a practical nurse.

PROBLEMS IN TEACHING

A certain number of students withdraw from schools of practical nursing, and for much the same reasons as do professional students (26). In the 18 schools visited, approximately 10 per cent of the students withdrew before graduation. Reasons included health, dislike of the work, unfitness for nursing, and failure in class work. Home situations accounted for several resignations.

The examinations at the end of the practical nursing course, the reports of supervisors, and the candidate's own adjustment form control points in the supply. The state examination for licensure may also weed out the incompetent. Occasionally a student may have to be dropped on the completion of her course, but dismissal should take place within the first weeks. Rarely, also, a nurse fails to make happy personal contacts or conducts herself unethically during her hospital or home nursing practice and has to be dismissed before the completion of the course.

That incompetent practical nurses will be reported to the proper authorities by the public, by doctors, and by professional nurses and will be automatically dropped seems to be largely a theory. In actual practice, practical nurses are so much needed that even the poor ones continue to find work and no one bothers to report any but criminal action. Most private individuals are discouraged by the red tape involved in bearing witness, collecting testimony, and appearing in court to testify. Therefore, the responsibility for producing safe nursing service rests primarily on the schools (27).

It may sound simple to plan the rather elementary courses of instruction to be offered the practical nursing students and to set up the program, gather applicants, teach and graduate classes. Actual experience proves otherwise. The first factor which complicates instruction is the "ungraded" nature of the student body. Women from eighteen to fifty, native and foreign born, fast and slow, with and without experience in nursing the sick; women who read fairly constantly and widely, girls who glance at the headlines and occasionally pick up a story in a movie magazine; women who have been homemakers, girls who have never boiled an egg; students with poise, calm, and common sense and excitable, nervous, shrill-voiced, shy students; women who have had families and know how to meet life's crises firmly, jittery girls in the throes of their first love affairs. All types, ages, degrees of maturity and intelligence appear in class. The teacher's first task is frequently to take time to size up the class and weld it into a teachable whole. Here is a woman who must be taught elementary English so that she can take notes, speak acceptably, and gain self-confidence. She will be given extra lessons in English after hours. Another is woefully lacking in a knowledge of how to dress, how to keep clean and dainty, how to meet people. Individual conferences are scheduled for her.

Is it worth while? Yes, because all these women have the fundamental thing that makes good practical nurses: they want to take care of sick people. In the end, after nine to twelve months of rigorous personal, class, and hospital supervision, they emerge neat, quiet, self-assured, reliable, and trained practical nurses. The change is very nearly miraculous.

So one of the first essentials in planning a curriculum for this group is to anticipate time for extra tutoring, to keep the teaching speed at an average rate which will be right for the majority, not too boring for the best students, not too speedy for the slower readers.

Nearly all the schools visited by the writer discouraged the use of just one textbook. A standard text was on hand for reference, occasional chapters were assigned for reading, the illustrations and tables were used, but the class did not take chapter after chapter in lesson form. All sorts of elementary reading and visual aids form the course. These may be reprints from authoritative popular magazines, health education booklets from such government sources as the Children's Bureau, charts from the National Dairy Council and similar organizations, and movies. In one school all textbooks were out of sight and files of leaflets, posters, charts, and pictures took their place. In another school four textbooks were used for various subjects. "No one book gives just what we need," directors remarked again and again. The lesson material was of the type suitable for junior high school age.

Assistance of all sorts is given to make learning easy. All the devices used in teaching pupils twelve to sixteen years old are employed in these classes—visual aids of every kind, summaries of yesterday's class, lessons repeated if difficult, outlines, quizzes, preexamination reviews, supervision of class notes, demonstrations of various activities with the pupils themselves taking part. The material is easy, calls for little reasoning power, does not depend on a basic knowledge of the sciences, and in every respect is training for the practice of a limited number of manual skills.

Another point was evident to the visitor listening to the teachers of practical nurses: instead of recalling to the students by a brief review the basic facts of, say, biology and then proceeding to the application of those facts to asepsis, sterilization, etc., as in a class of professional students, the teacher of practical nurses states one or two characteristics of bacteria (called germs) and at once outlines the duties of the practical nurse in preventing their spread and proceeds to demonstrate how to kill them. The fact and the act are tied together. Theory is simplified and every piece of information leads to something the practical nurse must do about it. It is teaching at the doing, manual level, if one may express it that way.

In the same way, when a system of the body—the respiratory system, for example—is under discussion, diseases of that system are studied at the same time: pneumonia, bronchitis, and the common cold—but only in relation to prevention, symptoms, and care in convalescence. Diseases such as scarlet fever, poliomyelitis, typhoid, which call for a differentiation in nursing dependent on a detailed knowledge of each, are not studied in detail (28).

Vocabulary is another point of departure. Every effort is made to keep away from any but the most common scientific terms. A glossary of perhaps 200 words used in the everyday care of the sick appears in nearly all textbooks. Definitions are in terms of description, not the underlying cause of a reaction. Just enough information is given to help the practical nurse understand what the doctor means when he speaks of symptoms and orders treatment.

One of the most difficult subjects to teach this group, instructors agree, is personal relationships or what the professional nurse thinks of as professional adjustments—formerly called "ethics." The practical nurse's responsibility, loyalty, attitude, and obligation to her patient, the family, the doctor, and other nurses are discussed at length. Such problems as emergencies, standing orders, reports to the doctor, family disagreements, and cooperation with professional nurses are all aired and sensible, workable advice is given. The students hark back to their own experiences. The writer heard the following questions asked by young nurses having their first practical experience in homes: "The family wants to get rid of Dr. S. and try Dr. M. What shall I advise them to do?" "My patient wants me to go to a hotel with her at the seashore and does not want me to wear my uniform. Will that be all right?" "Please tell me what to do: Mr. Y. has asked me to take twenty-four-hour duty so that I can be with the baby while his wife is in the hospital. He will sleep in the living room. Shall I take the case?"

Even more difficult to inculcate in this group is the spirit of personal helpfulness and thoughtfulness. "Put yourself in the patient's place," "Remember what it was like the last time you were sick," "If this were your mother, what would you do?" The time is very short—200 hours —in which to teach all the theory, techniques, the point of view, the "ethics," and the spirit of nursing to the practical student. Nearly everything rests with the instructor's own attitude and personality. If she always treats her demonstration "patient" as she would her own mother, her students will, too.

Problems of personal adjustments frequently include talks by experts in the field. Typical subjects are poise, use of cosmetics, keeping one's temper, attitude toward disagreeable situations, what to do in the presence of death, spiritual growth, proper recreation, books to read. Even mature students blossom under the skilled guidance of the instructors and to the younger women the course is, as one twenty-year-old girl told the writer, "the making of me."

Overtraining can be a serious danger. The practical nurse who has a course of more than fifteen months (theory and practice) gets a false impression of her abilities and builds up the unwarranted belief that she can practice as a professional nurse. If her qualifications are as good as those of a professional nurse she should have taken up professional nursing in the first place, which would have involved only a few more months of training. Some of the successful two-year graduate practical nurses at the top of their classes probably should have been guided into professional nursing, and there is no doubt that a few of them are better nurses than the ill prepared students now graduating at the bottom of their classes from small, poorly staffed professional schools. Doctors are prone to give these superior practical nurses a false impression of their competence by praising them and urging them to do nursing procedures they are not prepared to carry out.

What really disturbs professional nurses in these situations is the knowledge that when practical nurses are taught to carry out professional nursing procedures they are given skills to use anywhere and everywhere. Said a supervisor in a visiting nurse association, "We warn them never to catheterize a patient unless the doctor will take the responsibility for teaching them but we know they do." A director of nurses in a hospital of 135 beds reported, "We teach practical nurses to catheterize because we know they will be asked by doctors to catheterize patients in their homes. They should know how to do it correctly." And if, asks the realist, they can be taught to catheterize correctly—which means safely—why are they not taught in their schools? Furthermore, if catheterization is safe, why not bladder irrigation, colon and colostomy irrigations, or other treatments calling for an equivalent amount of skill, knowledge, and judgment? It is hoped that the job analysis of the practical nurse's duties being prepared by the United States Office of Education (12) will throw light on this vexatious problem. To the writer, the crux of the matter seems to be, not what the practical nurse can be taught to do, but when she should be allowed to do it. The judgment of doctors and professional nurses should govern these decisions, based on the condition of the patient under care.

The courage and daring of the overconfident or poorly trained practical nurse are boundless and cause deep apprehension among professional nurses who realize the risks to the patient in treatments that are incorrectly administered. The mistakes made by untrained women calling themselves practical nurses would be ludicrous if not so fraught with danger for the patient; for example, the woman who stood on a chair holding the douche bag up near the ceiling to give her patient a "high" enema; the untrained practical nurse who irrigated both ears on the general principle that what was good for an infected ear was good for a well one, and did not sterilize the catheter between irrigations; the unlicensed practical nurse who served all yellow and white foods because the doctor ordered a "blonde" (bland) diet. Other "crimes" of the ignorant on record include the application of heat to inflamed appendices, massage of painful legs of obstetrical patients causing emboli, application of salves to "lumps," and the release of traction on a fractured limb. One practical nurse is said to have reported to the doctor over the telephone that her patient was sleeping peacefully. The patient never woke up. Nothing the self-trained nurse had learned taught her the difference between coma and natural sleep (29). There was the "practical nurse" who urged the patient with pneumonia to keep coughing to get rid of the poison, the attendant who figured that if a saline douche was effective one of bichloride of mercury would be more so.

The writer found such stories all too prevalent. They should serve as a warning against the untrained nurse, for in every instance when the occurrence was recent and known to the narrator, the writer found the nurse was neither trained nor licensed.

CONCLUSIONS

It would seem shortsighted, in the light of our experience in the last few years and the probable future need for practical nurses (see page

34), to confine the preparation and practice of the practical nurse to any one type of service or patient—home or hospital, young or old, acute or subacute. "The nurse," wrote Miss Nutting, "should not be prepared to serve a single person or a single purpose; she should be trained to meet the need of the entire community" (30). We do not know what proportion of her service a practical nurse will give in home or hospital after graduation, but the hospital is the source of techniques, treatments, equipment, methods, and safeguards (31). It should serve as a base or take-off for home nursing, and it is the home where we have and will always have hundreds of sick people needing practical nurses.

A study of community needs, resources, qualified faculty, and practice fields should always precede the establishment of a new school. Upon organization, the school should have community sponsorship and consultant service of a representative and expert character.

Educational entrance standards should not be set so high or the course made so long that they approach the requirements for professional nursing. This means a definite limitation of the field of recruitment to high school students, not necessarily graduates, who are not eligible for training as professional nurses.

Theory and practice must go hand in hand during the student period, in two major fields: the general hospital (preferably one without a school of professional nursing) and supervised home experience. For how many weeks, in what size hospital, and under whose auspices in homes must be determined after evaluation of the best present practice. To offer less to the student in practical nursing is to have her unprepared for the future demands of her chosen occupation.

Supervision must be continuous and closely coordinated with classroom instruction.

The possibilities of the small hospital (less than 100 daily average) should be studied as a training ground for hospital experience and those of the visiting nurse association for home nursing experience.

A prerequisite to effective planning for a practice field is the sponsorship of representative professional and lay groups. A hospital or other agency which offers to receive students, "educate" them, and use them to care for patients should be preparing future community workers—practical nurses capable of serving anywhere in any suitable type of illness. Many of the schools in hospitals are now training practical nurses to be staff members within their own walls only. "We get a lot of employees from among our graduates." This narrow viewpoint limits unfairly the training of the practical nurse. The curriculum committee deciding on practice opportunities for the students must be as representative as possible of all future fields of usefulness in the community, the state, and the nation.

Evaluation of curricula, practice fields, and results of training should be undertaken, leading to accreditation of schools by an authoritative national body that is not made up of the school representatives themselves.

Wide publicity to accredited schools and vigorous promotion of state licensure for practical nurses will go far toward inhibiting the activities of substandard schools as will the development of local community nursing bureaus for the distribution of qualified nursing service of all types to employers.

It cannot be emphasized too strongly that the training of practical nurses is an educational undertaking requiring an adequately prepared teaching staff, standard equipment, a wealth of case experience, and close supervision. A school for practical nurses in a hospital has as its primary purpose the preparation of practical nurses for state licensure to practice anywhere, not the provision of cheap labor for this hospital and this hospital only. If the situation is not recognized we will have a tide of poorly prepared subsidiary workers flooding the market. Professional nursing fell over this stumbling block in its early years and spent most of the time between 1920 and 1935 picking itself up and dusting off its uniform. The same pitfall awaits the practical school which places the needs of the hospital first.

REFERENCES

1 In 1919 Anne H. Strong discussed the use of attendant nurses and their training at some length, expressing many of the viewpoints of today. "On the training of attendants," *Public Health Nurse* 11:245–246, May 1919.

2 Effie J. Taylor, "Yesterday, today and tomorrow," *American Journal of Nursing* 33:689, July 1933.

3 Editorial, "Few experts in nursing," *American Journal of Nursing* 44:526–527, June 1944. See also Charles T. Stone, "Levels of nursing; practical nurse, trained nurse, specialized nurse, and their rela-

tions to economics of illness," *Southern Medical Journal* 24:902–906, October 1931, at p. 903; John Winslow Hirshfield and Matthew Ashton Pilling, "Injuries of the hand," *American Journal of Nursing* 44:967–973, October 1945, at p. 971; Margaret G. Reilly, "Teaching dermatologic nursing; a suggested outline of minimum requirements for nurses in dermatology," *American Journal of Nursing* 44: 1169–1172, December 1942; Raidie Poole, "Army course in operating room technic," *American Journal of Nursing* 44:270–271, April 1945.

4 Katharine Shepard, "Massachusetts pattern for training attendant nurses; course aimed at home and small hospital duty," *Hospitals* 17: 29–30, November 1943.

5 Harlan H. Horner, *Nursing education and practice in New York State*, Albany, University of the State of New York Press, 1934, p. 12.

6 See also *Minimum standards for practical nursing schools approved by the National Association for Practical Nurse Education*, 250 West 57th Street, New York 19, N.Y. Curriculum hours should not be less than 200 clock hours.

7 Taylor (note 2), p. 689. In 1896 the maximum hours of theory for preparing trained nurses was 105. See also Anna Fillmore, "Scene—U.S.A., 1900," *American Journal of Nursing* 41:913–915, August 1941, at p. 914.

8 Nor were they in 1925–1935. See Harlan H. Horner, "Looking facts in the face," *American Journal of Nursing* 33:15, January 1933: "Will the new concept of professional nursing emphasize skills or knowledge or both?" Father Schwitalla points out that until we know what constitutes professional nursing we will not know how long it takes to teach it; A. M. Schwitalla, "Changing concepts of nursing seen as one result of war program," *Hospital Management* 57:60, 62, 64, June 1944. See also James A. Hamilton, "The lady upstairs," *American Journal of Nursing* 43:746–749, August 1943: "If a student concentrates solely on such a basic nursing course, it should not require 36 months to receive adequate theory and experience."

9 Margaret A. Tracy and others, *Nursing, an art and a science*, 2d ed., St. Louis, Mosby, 1942; Bertha Harmer and Virginia Henderson, *Textbook of the principles and practice of nursing*, 4th ed., New York, Macmillan, 1944; and Katharine Shepard and C. H. Lawrence, *Textbook of attendant nursing*, New York, Macmillan, 1935; Kathryn O. Brownell, *Textbook of practical nursing*, 2d ed. rev., Philadelphia, Saunders, 1944; Florence Dakin and E. M. Thompson, *Simplified nursing*, 4th ed., Philadelphia, Lippincott, 1941.

10 Tracy et al. (note 9), p. 165.

11 Josephine Goldmark, *Nursing and nursing education in the United States;* report of the Committee for the Study of Nursing Education, New York, Macmillan, 1923, p. 477.

12 Scheduled for publication in 1947 by the Government Printing Office, Washington, D.C.

13 Nell V. Beeby, "Where and what shall we teach? an analysis of the situations in which the nurse functions in obstetrical nursing," *American Journal of Nursing* 37:64–79, January 1937.

14 See, for example, Ruth Ingram, "How much is necessary for the education of the nurse," *American Journal of Nursing* 31:1431, December 1931; Florence K. Willson, "Ward study units," IN *Medical nursing,* Philadelphia, Lippincott, 1935.

15 Lottie Horn Waterman, "How Michigan produces a supply of carefully trained practical nurses," *Hospitals* 17:58–61, December, 1943.

16 Clare Dennison, "Maintaining the quality of nursing service in the emergency," *American Journal of Nursing* 42:774–784, July 1942, at pp. 776–777.

17 Goldmark (note 11), p. 481.

18 Allon Peebles and Valeria D. McDermott, *Nursing services and insurance for medical care in Brattleboro, Vermont;* a study of the activities of the Thomas Thompson Trust, Chicago, University of Chicago Press, 1932 (Committee on the Costs of Medical Care No. 17), p. 39.

19 Shepard (note 4), p. 30.

20 Florence Nightingale, *Notes on nursing, what it is and what it is not,* Boston, William Carter, 1860.

21 Stephen Rushmore, "Community nursing needs," *New England Journal of Medicine* 217:861–864, November 25, 1937, at p. 863.

22 Leona B. Stroup, "Preparation of nursing aides for the home," *Public Health Nursing* 31:223–227, April 1939, at pp. 225–226.

23 American Hospital Association, *Report of the Committee to Study the Nursing Problem,* Philadelphia, the Association, 1916, pp. 15–19. See also Edith M. Ambrose, "How and where should attendants be trained?" *American Journal of Nursing* 17:993–1002, October 1917, at pp. 998–1001. She urges both urban and rural experience.

24 Fannie Eshleman and A. W. Hetherington, *Nursing in prevention and control of tuberculosis,* rev. ed., New York, Putnam, 1945, p. 59.

25 Strong (note 1), p. 248.

26 Out of 12,569 students admitted to professional schools in 1943 in a three-month period, 16.5 per cent had withdrawn at the end of nine

months. Blanche Pfeffercorn, "Student nurse survey determines why they quit," *Hospitals* 18:58, June 1944.

27 Stella M. Hawkins, "Disciplinary actions under nurse practice act," *New York State Nurse* 17:65, April Quarter 1945. The report cites 15 cases in which action had been taken since 1938, only one of which involved a practical nurse.

28 Dakin and Thompson (note 9), Preface, p. iii, describing purpose of course, and p. 48. Compare with case studies expected of the professional nurse: Muriel E. Burgess, "A plan for nursing care," *American Journal of Nursing* 41:215–218, February 1941.

29 Edith M. Stern, "Impractical nurses or how practical can practical nursing be?" *Survey Graphic* 29:27–28, January 1940.

30 Adelaide Nutting, *History of nursing*, New York, Putnam, 1907.

31 Netta Ford, "Subsidiary worker and her place, if any, in nursing," *Hospitals* 11:91–94, November 1937, at p. 92. Miss Ford makes the point that nursing habits must be inculcated under continuous, expert supervision which is possible only in the hospital wards.

CHAPTER FIFTEEN

Supervision

THROUGHOUT this book the importance of supplying supervision of practical nursing service has been mentioned with purposeful frequency because it is one of the five essential steps in improving the nursing care of sick people.* From the day the student enters the school for practical nurses until she retires, her service to the sick should be thought of as complementary to that of the professional nurse. A logical corollary is that the professional nurse is primarily responsible for the care of the patient under the direction of the doctor and with his approval delegates as many tasks as possible to the practical nurse. This is virtually what happens in general hospitals. When the service is extended to homes, however, in the form of private duty, the relationship breaks down. Only occasionally are practical nurses on private duty supervised by professional nurses. The vast majority of practical nurses serving in homes receive no professional nursing supervision and the official professional registries have made little effort to provide supervision for either their registered or their practical registrants, (1) with the one exception of District 14 in Brooklyn. The weakest link in the chain of training various types of workers as assistants in hospitals and homes during the era of W.P.A. and N.Y.A. projects was, according to the reports, the lack of professional supervision (2). As long ago as 1916 the American Hospital Association was urging close and continuous supervision of the practical nursing group working in the community, and had suggested a plan of supervision similar to that provided for midwives by local boards of health (3).

Over the years, there have been sporadic attempts to improve the home supervision of private duty. In District 14 (Brooklyn) in 1940, the Nursing Committee of the Kings County Medical Society called physicians' attention to the fact that practical nurses were not prepared to nurse acute illness. The Nurses' Bureau, a professional registry, offered to send an experienced registered nurse, without charge, to any

---

* The other four being selection and training of candidates, licensure, placement, and the education of the public in the use of this type of nurse.

home where there was a nursing problem to assist the family and physician to decide on the type of nursing care needed. Very little use was made of the service, however (4). An effort to supervise home care of professional nurses from this registry likewise was not particularly successful. The professional nurses were not prepared to accept the idea, and the supervision was not organized along the lines found effective in public health nursing. It was felt that if the registry had been paying the registrants there would have been some "control"; without such an arrangement the nurses were independent.

Private-duty professional nurses would undoubtedly like to see more home supervision of practical nurses, primarily for the safety of patients but also because they feel that practical nurses working alone undermine the field of private duty, discourage young girls from going into professional nursing ("Why spend two and a half years learning to be a nurse when you can earn as much money after a nine-month course?"), and give an exaggerated impression of experience and training to doctors who fail to inquire into the background of the worker. The fact, however, that they have not developed home supervisory service for themselves weakens their position in the eyes of the practical nurses. Private-duty nurses especially have always been free lance workers and this reluctance to develop a desirable source of help has been due partly, administrators believe, to the fact that the function of the supervisor has been so poorly interpreted and demonstrated in many hospitals that staff nurses long for the day when they can get as far away as possible from anyone vested with that kind of power. This condition of affairs is changing rapidly for the better, however, and in most large institutions it is now a far cry to the days when supervision meant checking, spying on, and following up a worker. The function of supervision of nursing service is like that of the foreman in industry: to improve service (the product), to schedule production efficiently without waste of time or skill, to train new workers or to teach workers new processes, to relate the work to other departments (use of community resources), and to develop workers' skill to maximum capacity. Beyond all these well known objectives there is in nursing supervision a function we generally call interpretation, which includes explaining the service to families, patients, the medical profession, and the public, and promoting harmony through understanding among staff members, administrators, and the people served. "There must be an imaginative appreciation and manipulation of both human and social factors" (5) to produce a good supervisor. "Supervision," runs one definition, "may be defined as a cooperative educational process which has as its objective the improvement of nursing service . . . facilitated through the fullest possible development of each staff member; by the achievement of integration between service and community; and by the development and constructive use of scientific procedures" (6). Inherent in this function and paramount in importance is the obligation of protecting the patient from poor care.

This failure to provide experienced help to the home nurse is the more surprising because the principle of supervision has been accepted in schools for both professional and practical nurses, in public health (7), in most hospitals, in the Army and Navy, in education, and, of course, in nearly all business and industrial firms. When the supervisor is prepared and qualified for her position, students and graduates not only welcome but seek her aid and counsel. Public health nurses new to a job even demand supervision as their right and have been known to refuse a position not providing it. They know their experience will be richer, their chances of promotion greater where there is dynamic, intelligent, and understanding leadership from a well qualified supervisor. Practical nurses receiving supervision on the staffs of visiting nurse associations frequently expressed their appreciation to the writer for the careful introduction to their work and the continued supervision offered them by the professional staff. Many of the colleges, the Civil Service positions, and the administrative jobs in nursing admit only those candidates who can show a record of "experience under supervision."

WHERE ARE PRACTICAL NURSES SUPERVISED?

At the present time, practical nurses are routinely supervised by registered nurses in the following situations:

During study and practice in the schools for practical nurses
In all general and special hospitals of more than 30 beds*
In a handful of industries
In all visiting nurse associations, public health clinics, and outpatient services

---

* It is necessary to make the statement in this form because small hospitals, infirmaries in homes for the aged, etc., may have practical nursing staffs only. They consider themselves under the supervision of the doctor.

By a very few registries in an opportunistic way
In all federal institutions caring for the sick

It goes without saying that the amount and quality of supervision in these situations vary greatly. In many hospitals it may be purely nominal, intermittent, or in the best militaristic style of forty years ago. In agencies where the doctor is the "supervisor" of both professional and practical nurses, he may be only a part time worker or on call. He gives orders, checks to see they are carried out, and leaves the nursing staff to do its own planning. There are still many situations in which the nurses proceed without standing orders.

During the Student Period

During the practice period arranged by schools for practical nurses, supervision is routinely provided—indeed required by the better schools in both institutional and home service. Every effort is made in the good schools to integrate theory and practice, and to the field supervisor or educational director or both—whatever they may be called—falls the heavy job of teaching and supervising. Practice in the homes of patients may be under the supervision of the local visiting nurse association (as in Detroit), may be supplied by the school's placement service (as in Cleveland and Boston), or may be provided more or less jointly by registry and visiting nurse service (as in Ontario). All methods call for careful records and reports of experience (experience sheets), and the setup is not very different from the introduction of professional student nurses through public health agencies. The opinions of patients who have had their practical nurses some time are usually sought, as an aid in supervision, either by a visit from the supervisor or in writing.

The following letter is sent by the Hamilton Branch of the Victorian Order of Nurses for Canada to families who have had practical nursing students working in their homes.

Would you be so kind as to write a few words in the space below regarding the practical nurse student who had experience in your home? Did you find her helpful with the patient? with the children? with the meals?
Student's name:
[Space for report]

Unfortunately, while the principle is accepted in theory by all schools, in practice supervision of the student's experience, both in homes and in the hospital, is frequently the weakest spot in the school program. A full time supervisor is needed to coordinate the program adequately but she often has a heavy teaching schedule at the school. Supervision of practice on the wards may be irregular and institutional pressures and changes may confuse the student who does not have them interpreted to her. Many schools provide no home practice whatsoever. The whole picture is spotty and unsatisfactory in the extreme, except in three or four schools.

Several schools with placement services connected with the institution offer no home supervision to their graduates although they are in an ideal position to do so (Y.W.C.A.'s, for instance).

In Institutions

Hospitals are beginning to recognize the value of assigning to a full time nurse the responsibility for the auxiliary workers and, where enough practical nurses or aides are employed, of having their orientation and service supervised by an educational director who may in turn arrange in-service programs or delegate supervisory responsibility to ward or department heads (8). More than a year before Pearl Harbor, editorials in the *American Journal of Nursing* urged hospital supervisors to be ready to provide adequate supervision for the nonprofessional workers joining hospital staffs, otherwise such service "will be disastrous to good standards of nursing care and so to the profession itself" (9). "Every effort must be made to prevent an unregulated flow of such [untrained subsidiary] workers into our hospitals" (10).

The principle of professional nursing supervision in industrial medical departments has only recently been promoted, although its need was noted in 1919. Of 435 establishments, only 48 per cent reported that they were providing nursing supervision in 1942. "Plants employing large numbers of nurses did not always employ nursing supervisors" (11). In two plants, professional supervision was from the local visiting nurse association under contract to supply nursing service.

In industries where a number of practical nurses are employed, the oldest one in service is usually in charge of the work but not necessarily as a supervisor in the modern sense. Of 753 nonprofessional attendants employed in 22 per cent of the plants surveyed by the Committee to Study the Duties of Nurses in Industry, only one-third were reported to have nursing supervision (12). Supervision of practical nurses by registered nurses in industry should be as natural an arrangement as it is in the ward of a hospital where the registered nurse is responsible for assignment of duties.

In Community Services

In a small way, the experiments in community nursing service in Brattleboro, Vermont, and Rhinebeck, New York, assisted by the Thompson Trust Fund of Boston, attempted to provide professional nursing supervision of all practical nursing care in homes. Both projects were connected with schools for practical nurses and were therefore in a sense merely extensions to graduates of the required student supervision. Yet in both instances, voluntary requests came from the practical nurses to the registered nurses to visit with them in the homes. In Brattleboro, the terms of the insurance policies providing nursing care sometimes made visits obligatory to determine the type of service needed by the insured family. In Rhinebeck, the hospital* which conducted the school for practical nurses maintained a placement service, and the graduate practical nurses were supervised by the public health nurses of the community nursing staff (13).

In Ontario, Canada, a professional nurse (the registrar) in each registry where practical nurses are enrolled is available day and night to respond to questions from practical nurses, and some of the registries have an agreement with the public health nursing staff of the Victorian Order of Nurses to make a supervisory visit to a home where a practical nurse is working if need arises. This service is offered to the practical nurses as one of the advantages in belonging to the professional registry. The graduates of the approved practical nursing courses agree to serve two years through the professional registry (14). The plan for their supervision is described as follows.

For the information of persons concerned with the supervision of practical nurses, working through Nursing Registries, an outline of policy for supervision of these workers, and frequency of reports of supervision as approved by the Registered Nurses Association of Ontario is set forth as follows:

---

* The hospital at this time had 35 beds, eight bassinets, six registered nurses including the supervisor, and five practical nurses.

1. (a) Practical nurses to be supervised once monthly during the first three months, if the cases are suitable
    (b) Twice yearly following this three month period unless contraindicated
    (c) Group conferences as a means of supervision be arranged at the discretion of the supervisor. (Note: It is suggested these conferences be held at the registry office where possible in order to strengthen their tie with the registry)

2. *Reports of Supervision.* It is recommended:
    (a) That a report of each student be filed with the registry at the end of the first three months following initial registration and once yearly thereafter
    (b) That the report form for reporting the work of practical nurses be a narrative type of report
    (c) It is recommended that a general report of the work done by the supervisor be sent to the registry once yearly and that this report include data, criticism and suggestions for improving the service and any related point of interest

Public health nursing agencies established the principle of supervision in their earliest organization and it is so much a part of their service today as to be inseparable from other features of the work, including the employment of practical nurses as decribed on pages 164–173. Administrators find that a home visit made by a practical nurse under the supervision of the professional public health nurse accomplishes four desirable purposes:

It brings more thorough and appropriate service to the individual patient
It interprets to family and doctor alike the distinctions between the grades of service
It develops the skills and stimulates the interest of the practical nurse
It frees the professional nurses' time for the preventive and educational work which they are prepared to give

The ultimate result is a more far-reaching program of service to the community, with safeguards in quality and character of care for the individual patient.

THE NEED FOR SUPERVISION

Even a brief description of a few typical cases, chosen at random, which were visited by the professional supervisor of one of the approved schools during the nurse's practice period reveals the need of help from such a source. These reports are from the Household Nursing Association in Boston which has provided home supervision from the day of its founding.

Patient: a middle-aged woman with pleurisy, living in a four-room tenement in a poor section of town. Husband, a retired sailor, kept the kitchen very clean and did the cooking.

Work of practical nurse: the physician ordered brandy for stimulation and morphine by hypodermic for pleurisy pains, fluids to be forced. A practical nurse was on twelve-hour day duty and followed physician's orders, keeping a written record. The family lived in such a small, crowded apartment that the nurse went home to sleep and the husband took care of the patient at night.

Work of the supervisor: to watch one demonstration of giving hypodermic, suggest variations in fluids, assist in rearranging household equipment for convenience in use, be assured husband was giving safe care.

Patient: a very nervous, high strung young woman in the fifth month of pregnancy whose physician advised complete rest in bed to avoid miscarriage. She lived in a modern three-room apartment. No servant.

Work of practical nurse: attendant gave patient cleansing bath every morning, cooked all the meals for patient, husband, and herself, serving attractive trays to patient. She kept the three rooms orderly and well dusted and was otherwise kept constantly busy doing errands and waiting on patient. On twelve-hour duty and went to her own home at night.

Work of supervisor: mostly suggestions to maintain patient's peace of mind and an adequate diet. Supervisor also protected practical nurse from overfatigue in waiting on an exceedingly difficult patient.

Patient: a young married woman, totally blind; husband and housekeeper ill with grippe. Modern five-room apartment.

Work of practical nurse: the nurse waited on husband and housekeeper who were both in bed for one week. She planned and cooked meals and kept the rooms neat and orderly. After the housekeeper recovered she went home for a week's rest, and the young couple kept the nurse to run the house.

Work of supervisor: to assist in planning, arranging schedule, and caring for the helpless people.

Patient: a middle-aged woman, crippled by arthritis, ill fifteen years. Absolutely helpless, had registered nurse in charge of case and practical nurse on night duty. Well-to-do home with several servants.

Work of supervisor: to promote good relationships between nurses and interpret work of each.

Patient: the mother of three children, tried to do too much after returning from hospital with third baby. Developed phlebitis. Lived in a cottage house, six rooms and bath. Could not afford servant. Her mother came to help with housework.

Work of practical nurse: physician ordered patient to rest in bed with ice bag applied to left thigh. Nurse took entire care of the month-old baby. She gave a cleansing bath to the patient daily, kept the ice bags filled with ice as needed, and served attractive trays. She made all the beds every day, kept the bathroom clean, and helped the grandmother with the cooking whenever possible.

Work of supervisor: to keep general oversight of situation as the nurse actually had two patients.

WHAT THE SUPERVISOR DOES

When visiting patients cared for by graduate and student practical nurses, the writer was accompanied on several occasions by a professional supervisor. The following notes made at the time indicate clearly the definite ways in which the supervisor was helping and guiding the nurse for the benefit of the patients' families and the nurse's own improvement.

Case A. Elderly woman with cardiac condition

Supervisor spoke to practical nurse in private about the completeness of her record for the doctor, pointing out that she had omitted to chart patient's refusal of her midnight s.o.s. sleeping pill; called attention to patient's habit of scratching her scalp, suggesting dry shampoo; suggested change in location of bed to shield eyes from glare on snow outside; reminded practical nurse of her promise to have her own eyes examined as she had been having headaches.

In presence of patient, talked over diet that would be more welcome for next few days than cereals which patient was tired of, discussed increasing fluid intake (ordered by doctor). Supervisor asked patient, in absence of practical nurse, how she liked her nurse, whether she was making her comfortable, whether her meals were hot and nicely served. Patient asked if she could have practical nurse for her daughter who was expecting a baby, asked charge; only thing she could complain about was practical nurse's inability to play bridge! Supervisor made note of this.

Case B. Cancer of breast

Very difficult patient in last stages of cancer. Supervisor watched entire nursing procedure in giving enema, doing dressing, giving bath, and making bed. Assisted several times at difficult points; unobtrusively showed practical nurse better arrangement for dressing tray, and by her own example emphasized washing hands before and after the dressing; discussed fluid diet; with husband of patient, planned time schedule for nurse so that nurse was given time off duty for a walk in open air each day. Out of earshot of both patient and husband, discussed possibility of hemorrhage and what must be done when patient's condition grew critical.

Practical nurse asked whether she should increase frequency of morphine (doctor had left order to do so if nurse felt it necessary); when she should call patient's minister; how she could tempt patient's extremely poor appetite; how she could keep relatives out of patient's room as they tired her and she begged not to see them. Besides these questions the supervisor and nurse talked over question of more rest for nurse; desirability of persuading distraught husband to visit his son's house (around the corner) once a day for a change; fee to be charged family for what was almost constant twenty-four hour duty; frequency of doctor's visits, as he depended on nurse; nurse's uniform (she wished to wear an apron and old dress to save new uniforms and avoid problem of laundry).

Case C. Young man, discharged from hospital, convalescing from pneumonia

Graduate practical nurse had just replaced a "nurse" family had employed through a newspaper ad, who had disregarded doctor's orders and misinterpreted them. Fortunately, wife had known enough about illness to report to doctor and "nurse" was discharged at once. Supervisor took name and address to report to Health Department, calmed down excited family, helped practical nurse set up plan of care that involved changing bedrooms for convenience to bathroom, talked over diet with wife and at her urgent request supervisor promised to telephone next day to "find out how things were going."

Nurse asked supervisor in private what she ought to guard against with this highly nervous young man, who had been very sick and received sulfa drugs in quantities; whether she should call the doctor if patient's pulse remained over 100. She requested supervisor to talk with her when she called patient's wife the next day.

On returning to the office, the writer received a cumulative report of the student practical nurse on Case A from her supervisor, a report covering the following points: appearance, poise, tact, judgment, nursing care (technique, gentleness, thoroughness), records (completeness, neatness, accuracy), homemaking (time schedule, planning meals, serving patient's meals), relation to rest of family, resourcefulness in use of materials, in entertaining patient, in care of children, ability to plan work, character of reports to doctor, adjustment to family situation and handling problems presented by this special case, improvement since last visit. Notes made by the supervisor regarding this nurse on earlier cases included three significant items which perhaps epitomize the outstanding values of professional supervision.

The nurse had been invited to attend a group meeting at which the home care of a patient in a cast was to be presented by a prominent professional orthopedic nurse

The nurse had been shown how to prepare for the return from an Army hospital of a patient who was being allowed home between stages of surgery on an injured back

The supervisor had visited a family to explain that their little girl, ill with flu, who had been cared for by this practical nurse, must now have professional nursing care as the chest condition had developed into pleurisy, with probable congestion of the lungs—pneumonia. The doctor on the case had been consulted by the supervisor when she read the practical nurse's report, and he had been greatly relieved to learn that a professional nurse would continue care. He at once requested to have the practical nurse take one of his less acutely ill cases. The change had been made the same day

A supervisor's own report summarizing work in supervising practical nurses gives a vivid picture of the responsibility she assumes and also the need for her counsel. In two months, a supervisor visited 45 students on cases, saw 95 different patients, and made in all 135 calls. The types of problems encountered in the homes were roughly classified as:

Adjustments in household routines, arranging schedules, etc.	50 per cent
Personality problems (nurse, patient, family attitudes and dispositions)	33 per cent
Nursing techniques and procedures	17 per cent

She reported that nine of the nurses showed marked progress since her last visit. The work of three of the group receiving supervision was described as follows for their final record.

Miss A. B., a nice-appearing, wholesome woman, particularly well suited to practical nursing. Creates a pleasant atmosphere and takes excellent nursing care of patients. Can take over management of the house easily and cook appetizing meals. A capable, dependable nurse who can be sent on any type of case. Would suit a fastidious patient very well.

Miss C. D., a stocky, heavily built young woman, very impressed with her own importance. At first she was immature and wanted attention and praise for her work, while she needed guidance and was inclined to be untidy about her uniform. By the end of the eighth week under supervision she had picked up noticeably; made remarkable improvement and showed more common sense. Supervisors received excellent reports of her work at end of the six-month period; one noted: "I think this nurse should be sent on cases where patients require routine nursing care. Miss D. will need occasional visits as she may slip back into careless ways."

Mrs. E. F., a youngish woman. Mrs. F. did good work on field duty under supervision. She appeared to be interested in her patients and they usually liked her. It was frequently necessary for supervisors to criticize her carelessness in appearance and untidy hair. She seemed grateful for advice and immediately improved, but she was inclined to slip back into careless personal hygiene. She was advised to work in an institution and is now employed in a hospital.

It is evident from these brief summaries that a guidance job is under way, for not only do these suggestions bear on the nurse's immediate improvement but they serve as a guide to the registry in placing the nurse on future cases. Above all, from the community standpoint, Mr. and Mrs. Public will not be subjected to "grab bag" chances in hiring a nurse.

Helen Z. Gill, assistant superintendent of the Household Nursing Association, Boston, Mass., to whom I am indebted for the foregoing material, believes in supervision of home practice because the practical nurse faces at least two difficult adjustments in every home: the nursing of the patient and the care of the home. Miss Gill stated in a personal communication: "It seems unfair to throw her on her own resources before she has learned to correlate what she has been taught during her course. Therefore, the school helps her to assume her new responsibilities by sending a registered nurse to visit once a week on each case until the practical nurse has worked for six months and earned her diploma."

Here is an example of how an inexperienced practical nurse was helped to adjust as reported by Miss Gill:

Miss G.'s first case was with a woman artist of uncertain age and demanding nature who was suffering with arthritis. On the first visit, the supervisor saw that Miss G. was quite equal to keeping the four-room apartment neat and orderly, besides preparing appetizing meals for the patient and a hot dinner for the husband at night. The patient was comfortably fixed up and no medicine bottles were in evidence to remind her of illness. But the nurse was at a loss to know how to fit in the ordinary household details with the various treatments for the patient and do errands at odd intervals. Nor did she know how to be tactful when the demands were unreasonable.

The supervisor suggested that a part time worker be engaged to clean the apartment each week. The patient agreed readily to this arrangement. It had not occurred to the practical nurse to ask for this help. Then the supervisor helped to plan the treatments so that the patient could have longer periods of rest. This made it possible for the nurse to be off duty in the afternoon for three hours.

When the professional supervisor functions through a registry, an employment agency, or a community nursing bureau, she adds to the duties of selecting cases, supervising nurses, and guiding policies the sizable task of keeping on the alert for new avenues of service to the community. An example of this was the offer to supply a practical nurse who had a special aptitude in caring for children to a day nursery for very young children, while a registered nurse called daily to supervise her work and care for any special problems.

It is evident from these descriptions of supervised service that many direct benefits accrue to patients, nurses, and employers. Some of these are:

Better service to patient, family, and doctor
More efficient distribution of nursing time, thereby saving the employer money
Smoother relationships between employer and employee, resulting in an atmosphere conducive to recovery
Protection of the nurse from overfatigue, thereby assuring the patient of better care
Prompt investigation of complaints
Extension or adaptation of service as recognized by the supervisor, thereby reaching more patients

Prevention of overlapping into field of professional nursing (15)
Better placement through sizing up the practical nurse's ability and spe-
cial aptitudes
Opportunities to fill community needs

OPPORTUNITIES TO DEVELOP SUPERVISION

What can be done to provide and improve the home supervision of
practical nurses by registered nurses? Here is a group which needs
continuing guidance and help even more than public health nurses
who have accepted the principle of supervision and seek it no matter
how long their experience in the field or how complete their professional education. Will professional nurses accept the concept that they
are responsible for the care offered by practical nurses to home patients
and develop supervisory services from their registries, visiting nurse
associations, and community nursing bureaus? Will practical nurses
resent the implication that they cannot handle home cases without
help, although they accept close supervision and strict limitation of
their duties in hospitals? Both groups should remember that until the
time arrives when practical nurses have a recognized standard of training and have met a legally established minimum requirement for
licensure, Mr. and Mrs. Public are exposed to all kinds of unregulated
service; the public will continue to employ any grade of nursing it can
afford—which is bad business for professionals and practicals alike—
and will continue to think a practical nurse is just as good as a registered nurse, thereby continuing to encourage correspondence and commercial schools in turning out keen rivals for their jobs.

A prerequisite to developing any plan of supervision of practical
nurses in homes or hospitals is their acceptance by professional nurses
as partners in the care of the sick. Encouragement of a spirit of mutual
helpfulness wherever the two groups meet—in hospitals, registries,
and homes—a genuine concern to help qualified practical nurses attain
legal recognition, and friendliness in the informal give and take of
every-day contacts will go far toward laying a foundation upon which
to build such a program. Registries that do not offer supervision to
professional nurses will hardly be in a position to thrust it upon practical nurses, but visiting nurse associations are already in line and indeed might go a step further and offer home supervision to student
practical nurses and all registrants of community nursing bureaus (as

in Detroit). The most effectual and natural way to establish such a service in homes would be through the placement bureau of a true community nursing service where all types of nursing under qualified supervision are available. As hospitals, industries, visiting nurse associations, and other organized health agencies add practical nurses to their staffs, the supervisory problem will take care of itself, but the homes being served on a private-duty basis by anyone calling himself or herself a nurse remain a no-man's-land of chance and possible danger. Professional supervision should be extended to them, not just as a tool in teaching students, but as an essential to good nursing care of patients.

REFERENCES

1 Alma H. Scott, "Economic security for private duty nurses," *American Journal of Nursing* 33:1031–1038, November 1933. See also Leona B. Stroup, "Home nursing aides; a community project in Detroit, Michigan, for the training, placing and supervision of subsidiary workers in homes," *American Journal of Nursing* 40:255–260, March 1940, at p. 260.

2 Mary C. Jarrett, Housekeeping service for home care of chronic patients, W.P.A. Project 165–97–7002, December 31, 1938.

3 American Hospital Association, *Report of the Committee to Study the Nursing Problem,* Philadelphia, the Association, 1916, p. 20.

4 "Registry and medical society cooperate," *American Journal of Nursing* 40:217, February 1940.

5 Ruth B. Freeman, *Techniques in supervision in public health nursing,* Philadelphia, Saunders, 1944, p. 15. See also Mary M. Wayland and others, *Hospital head nurse; junior executive and clinical instructor,* edited by Isabel M. Stewart, 2d ed., New York, Macmillan, 1944, chapters I and II.

6 Freeman (note 5), p. 16.

7 For general policy regarding supervision of practical nurses, see National Organization for Public Health Nursing, *Board members' manual,* 2d ed. rev., New York, the Organization, 1937, pp. 27–28.

8 "Supervisors of subsidiary workers at Charity Hospital [New Orleans]," *American Journal of Nursing* 40:1411, December 1940.

9 Editorial, "One nation indivisible," *American Journal of Nursing* 40:1017–1018, September 1940.

10 Editorial, "To the colors—or?" *American Journal of Nursing* 40:1134, October 1940.

11 Olive M. Whitlock, Victoria N. Trasko, and F. Ruth Kahl, *Nursing practice in industry,* Washington, Government Printing Office, 1944 (Public Health Bulletin No. 283), p. 35. See also Anna M. Fillmore, "Part-time nursing service to the small plant," *Public Health Nursing* 37:130–137, March 1945.

12 Whitlock et al. (note 11), p. 44.

13 Marion Wetzel and Beatrice Tremper, "Community nursing service; an interesting experiment in northern Dutchess County, New York," *American Journal of Nursing* 40:40–46, January 1940, pp. 40, 42, 46. See also Richards M. Bradley, "Household nursing in relation to other similar work," *American Journal of Nursing* 15:968–970, August 1915.

14 Information gathered during visits to registries, registrars, and practical nursing courses in Toronto and Hamilton, Ontario, November 1944. See *Rules and regulations,* Community Nursing Registry, Ontario Registered Nurses Association, 1942 (revised).

15 "The activities of subsidiary workers should be reviewed to see whether they are safely done by a non-professional person, well selected, really useful to the service and well supervised." Freeman (note 5), p. 70.

CHAPTER SIXTEEN

Protection through Legislation

VIRGINIA had the first law providing for the training and licensing of practical or attendant nurses under the title "licensed attendant." The governor signed the bill in April 1918 (1). The Act gives the reason for such a bill as the war shortage of nurses and it was passed as a war emergency (2). Administration was placed under the State Board of Examiners of Graduate Nurses, and rules, regulations, and supervision were assigned to the Board. The law was to be in effect only until July 1922, but is still in effect. It is separate from that governing the practice of registered nurses (3).

Legislation in the other states followed slowly, with constant setbacks, amendments, and lapses. The American Nurses' Association has complete information about the dates of introduction of bills and the ever-changing status of the laws in all the states. The Association also has prepared valuable aids for those considering the introduction or revision of legislation, and the reader is referred to this source for details (4).

In point of fact, however, with all the discussion of this question over a period of 45 years and its acceptance (on paper) ten years ago by the national professional bodies, the results in state legislative action make a poor showing. It is a satisfaction to record a greatly increased expression of interest in the problem within the last few years. Maine, Tennessee, Alabama, Arkansas, and the Territory of Hawaii passed legislation in the spring of 1945. Discussing at present the problem of amending their nurse practice acts are West Virginia, Pennsylvania, Washington, Colorado, Montana, Mississippi, and Iowa (5). By the time this book is off the press it is probable that several other states will have legislation.

Anyone who wishes to do so may nurse for hire in the United States; there is no law in any state at the present time against such practice so long as the title registered (professional) nurse (R.N.) is not used, or, in 19 states, the title licensed practical or attendant nurse. The 19 states are Alabama, Arkansas, California, Connecticut, Florida, Georgia, Indiana, Maine, Maryland, Massachusetts, Michigan, Mississippi, Missouri, New York, Oklahoma, Pennsylvania, Tennessee, Virginia, and Wisconsin (6). Laws which make it illegal for anyone to nurse for hire who is not either a registered (professional) nurse or a licensed practical or attendant nurse have been passed in only two localities, New York state and the Territory of Hawaii. The latter passed its mandatory law in 1945.

The mandatory clause in the New York law prohibits anyone from nursing for hire who has not qualified as either a registered professional nurse or a licensed practical nurse. The enforcement of this clause was postponed until one year following cessation of hostilities to permit the civilian public to get nursing service of some sort in the face of the military demands on registered nurses.

When the New York law goes into effect, it may cut down somewhat the general supply of practical nurses in the state as it will prohibit certain classes of workers to give nursing care under other titles. Orderlies, for example, if serving as nurses, must be licensed. There will probably be an increase in licensed men practical nurses qualifying from the orderly and attendant levels.* Hospitals and employers everywhere will be asked to scan the credentials of those hired to give nursing care on any level, to urge proper preparation, and to abide by the law by insisting on state license or registration. There will follow, presumably, a clearer line of demarkation between duties of the orderly or attendant and the male practical nurse.

At the present time, only persons who have completed a prescribed course or period of training can secure a license to practice as a trained attendant in California, Connecticut, Indiana, Michigan; as an undergraduate nurse in Georgia; as a licensed attendant in Massachusetts, Oklahoma, Pennsylvania, Virginia, and Wisconsin; as an obstetrical nurse in Missouri; as a licensed practical or practical nurse in New York, Maryland, Alabama, Tennessee, Arkansas, and Hawaii. However, except in New York and Hawaii, so long as these titles are not used, anyone may don the uniform, imitate the methods, language, and procedures of practical nursing without so much as a bowing acquaintance with illness—and at any rate of pay. A manicurist may walk out of a beauty "shoppe" today and appear at your bedside tomorrow,

* At the annual conference of the State Hospital Association in Buffalo in May 1938, hospital administrators recognized this clause in the law as a means of raising the standards of nursing care rendered by male attendants to male patients (7).

decked out in white cap and uniform. A barber, seeing an advertisement in the newspaper for a male attendant for a chronic invalid at $50 a week plus maintenance, may appear in the old gentleman's home looking the part in white suit and rubber-soled shoes but with only the skill of a barber. Yet the condition of the invalid with a decompensating heart calls for highly skilled nursing.*

A distracted mother, searching desperately for help in time of illness, may place the care of a child in hands far less skilled than those ministering to a sick dog, for a veterinary must hold a license to practice and must give evidence of training to secure that license. A person must secure a permit to hunt deer or fish for trout, and he may hunt and fish only at stated seasons. But it is always open hunting for the "practical" nurse. She may shoot drugs into the human body without knowing how to sterilize the hypodermic syringe, measure medicine, prepare the skin, or inject the solution. She probably will not know the purpose for which the drug is given let alone its effects or the contraindications for its use. From birth to death we are surrounded by operators— doctors, midwives, pharmacists, chiropodists, beauticians, taxi drivers, barbers, and undertakers, to name a few—licensed to serve us under a law, ordinance, or departmental regulation, who must present evidence of previous training and fitness in their chosen fields, except in the case of practical nurses who deal with the intimate problems of life and death. Moreover, as practical nurses do not come under the health regulations affecting food handlers, these persons may carry an infectious disease.

The present situation of uncontrolled, unregulated, and unpunishable "hiring out" to nurse is fraught with great danger in the transitional period when registered nurses are scarce and the best practical nurses are either snatched by hospitals to relieve the professional staff or have qualified for highly paid jobs in industry. What is left on the market is likely to be the least skilled, elderly, least desirable would-be "nurses," ready to charge exorbitant fees for poor work. Furthermore, most families, knowing the pressure on doctors and nurses, call for a nurse only under dire necessity. To produce the poorest type of practical nurse at the moment when the most skilled care is needed is hazardous to the patient and disillusioning to the family—a bad reflection on the good practical nurses. Economists know that when a commodity

* These are actual examples from the reports of nurse registrars in New York and Cleveland.

is scarce, then is the time to beware of counterfeits, adulterations, and shoddy substitutes. Nursing is no exception, and in the case of nurses such a substitution may be fatal.

Any person who nurses for hire, who enters a home or institution to assume responsibility for the health and life of individuals, is in truth a public servant. His or her employment should be safeguarded by compliance with minimum standards of training, with permission to use that training granted under authority of the law, with penalties for violation of its practice.

The public will be safeguarded only when there is state control, in all states, of all those who nurse for hire. A "permissive" law which allows anyone to charge for nursing the sick so long as certain titles are not used leaves wide loopholes for unscrupulous and untrained individuals and makes the prosecution of violations practically impossible (8). A "mandatory" law virtually making nursing for hire a closed calling to anyone who cannot qualify as either a registered professional or a licensed practical nurse may seem a drastic measure to the states without any legislation relating to practical nurses, but in the interests of public safety such control is long overdue. For those states with nurse practice acts which already protect the titles of registered and practical nurses, it should not be too difficult to secure public and professional approval to back a mandatory amendment.

Protection through restrictive legislation is due the practical nurse. She, like the professional nurse, has put time and money into preparing for her occupation. Practical nurses who have qualified under a state law and are practicing their calling are eager to put an end to the competition from inadequately trained graduates of commercial and correspondence schools or those who have learned only in the school of experience (more correctly described as inexperience), yet who practice under such high sounding titles as "certified nurse." The well qualified women also recognize the danger of the one-sided training offered in special hospitals, especially tuberculosis sanatoria, mental hospitals, and proprietary hospitals, and are striving to keep practical nursing education out of the field of cheap labor for these specialized institutions. When the New York state law was in its early stages as a bill, practical nurses who were graduates of recognized, well established schools fought for its enactment; the opposition came from the untrained groups.

It is confidently hoped that when the practical nurses have secured nation-wide state licensure, they will do much to protect their title and report violations. Their status will become precious to them, something to be proud of and to defend. This is the way the registered nurses feel about their position under the law.

The purposes of state licensure for practical nurses are:

To raise the standard of practical nursing care given to the public wherever they may be sick, in home or hospital

To provide the public with a clear-cut distinction between the registered professional nurse and the practical nurse

To furnish the physician with evidence that the practical nurse employed by his patients has met state qualifications for the practice of her trade

To protect the practical nurse herself who has qualified for licensure from competition of untrained workers nursing for hire

To protect young women wishing to enter practical nursing from exploitation by commercial and correspondence schools

To weed out those individuals who, qualifying under a waiver, prove in practice to be unsafe to give nursing care, and to offer a legal means to prosecute all those guilty of misdemeanor

THE ESSENTIAL POINTS IN A GOOD NURSE PRACTICE ACT

A satisfactory nurse practice act should protect the public from unsafe nursing service in these ways:

By stating the minimum educational qualifications of a candidate desiring to enter this field of work

By stating the age limits for candidates eligible to take the state examinations for licensure. This controls to some extent the age of acceptability in the schools of professional and practical nursing

By limiting candidates for state examination to those graduating from approved schools or presenting satisfactory evidence of equivalent training and experience

By defining the practice of nursing as clearly as possible so that violations of the act will be obvious and easily understood

By creating a board of qualified individuals (usually the state board of nurse examiners) to set up rules and regulations for administering the act, such a board being especially concerned with minimum standards of preparation (curriculum content, hours of theory, practice, length of course, etc.), approval of schools, examination of candidates, and violations of the act. The board should be authorized to employ executive and secretarial personnel and should have authority to recommend the endorsement of applicants (with evaluation and acceptance of "equivalents")

"The right of the state to prescribe reasonable standards for, and to control the practice of, medicine, osteopathy, dentistry, and other branches of the healing arts including nursing, has been upheld as constitutional by the U.S. Supreme Court in a number of decisions" (9). "A license," James A. Tobey states, "is not a contract, but permits the enjoyment of a privilege granted by the State." Its refusal or revocation for proper cause may be contested in the courts, but it is not a deprivation of liberty or property (10).

It is important, of course, that a good law "seek to maintain the highest standards consistent with good practice and consistent with other professional laws designed to protect the public health" (11). The law should define the practice of nursing for each class, and the board of nurse examiners (or whatever may be the name given the authorities vested with the administration of the law) should enunciate the rules and regulations governing such practice.

Every state should know its own nursing situation, especially the need for practical nurses, before "legislating." This is important not only to plan wisely with relation to representation from the practical nurses' group or their formal associations, but also because no state legislature will accept data from another state. Facts and figures must be recent and pertinent and compiled specifically for that state so that they speak for themselves (12). Legislators must have the problem presented to them personally so that it hits home, and nothing is as convincing as actual examples of malpractice within the borders of their own state (13). The consumer must be shown that legislation for the control of this group is vital to the public safety.

A waiver or clause postponing the full application of the act permits time for those with limited training or experience to qualify and recognizes up to a specified date the right of individuals to register who can present length and recency of experience in lieu of formal training. Most states license only persons who have completed a prescribed course or period of training, but there are still many persons practicing who hold only waiver licenses. Some are acceptable in certain situations, but employers need to be discriminating on this point.

The handling of a waiver is a ticklish though necessary business. In justice to those with acceptable experience and qualifications but no formal training, a certain amount of publicity must be given to the regulations. At the same time, all those with any experience whatsoever will wish to register to avoid the later restrictions of formal training and a state examination. A few undesirable candidates will be licensed, inevitably, and they can only be weeded out through natural causes or the conviction of malpractice. Many states have offered refresher courses of one type or another to assist these practical nurses to do better work.

The waiver is admittedly a weak spot in the law, but it is a constitutional right and must be included to allow time for those to qualify who wish to do so and for out-of-state applications, and for the setting up of a workable file and the issuance of license cards after all references have been checked.

Practical nurses claiming all kinds of abilities will seek registration under the waiver of a new law. New York state reports a would-be licensee who claims to have expert knowledge of the care of mother and baby during delivery. Should the baby, she asserts, come feet first, she would "push real hard and rotate the baby." Another has a panacea for tuberculosis—corn whiskey and honey, one full glass every three hours; another speaks of cow dung as a cure—and this in the Empire State, in the year 1938 (14).

In the existing laws, penalties for violation range from a fine of $10 to $1,000 with revocation of license of a licensee, to imprisonment for not more than six months or a fine, or both, for a second offense. Many people feel that these penalties are not sufficiently severe to be effective in preventing malpractice. Hearings before the state board are usually granted before court action is taken.

Many violations of the law hinge upon definitions. While the definition of professional and practical nursing is most difficult, experience and expert advice both urge a broad but specific and understandable description or definition of each (15). (For definitions, see page 291.)

Another ticklish point in the law, liable to controversial opinion but essential to the clarity of the act, is the definition of duties or typical service of the practical nurses. A recent typical law states:

Such duties as are required for the physical care of chronically and mildly ill patients and in carrying out the medical orders as prescribed by licensed physicians, requiring the understanding of nursing but not requiring the professional services of a registered professional nurse (16).

The same law defines the difference between the duties to be performed by the registered professional nurse and the practical nurse. The practice of nursing is defined as follows:

A person practices nursing within the meaning of this article who for compensation or personal profit (a) performs any professional service requiring the application of principles of nursing based on biological, physical and social sciences, such as responsible supervision of a patient requiring skill in observation of symptoms and reactions and the accurate recording of facts, and carrying out of treatments and medications as prescribed by a licensed physician, and the application of such nursing procedures as involve understanding of cause and effect in order to safeguard life and health of a patient and others; or (b) performs such duties as are required in the physical care of a patient and in carrying out of medical orders as prescribed by a licensed physician, requiring an understanding of nursing but not requiring the professional services as outlined in (a).

The proposed Michigan bill, which was withdrawn in 1945, reads as follows:

The term practical nurse is defined as one who has been authorized by the state to care for semi-acute, convalescent, and chronic patients requiring service under public health nursing agencies, or in institutions, or in homes, working under the direction of a licensed physician or the supervision of a registered nurse, and is prepared to give household assistance when necessary.

When a satisfactory bill has been prepared by a legislative committee, it is important to have the wording reviewed, not only by the committee's lawyer hired for the purpose, but by the state's legislative reviewer or reader of bills, if there is one. It should be cleared by the state's attorney as to conformity with existing laws covering attendant, aide, or orderly service and as to the terminology used by governmental departments (for example, attendants under Civil Service in state institutions, prisons, etc.). A member or members of the legislative committee, preferably nurses experienced in lobbying, should be on hand to watch the progress of the bill. This may also be a duty assigned to the lawyer representing the backers of the bill.

Obviously, any state legislation which would admit to examination only graduates from approved schools of practical nursing and prohibit anyone to nurse for hire who could not qualify as either a registered professional or a licensed practical nurse would be unpopular with correspondence and commercial schools (17). With ample funds for subtle publicity, wide experience in lobbying, and ability to arouse organized opposition, these groups frequently become strong and crafty opponents of nurse practice acts. They can be more than a match for the casual, disorganized, and inexperienced supporters of a bill. When, as occasionally happens, the opposition is strengthened by the tacit support of members within the registered nurses' ranks who do not approve of practical nurses, it can be seen how easy is the way to defeat.

Registered nurses know now that the successful passage of a well worded mandatory nurse practice act takes endless hard work, financial means, much preliminary publicity among all groups, lay and professional, and the best legal advice money can buy.*

ADMINISTRATION OF THE LAW

The state board of nurse examiners is responsible for administering the law relating to licensed practical nurses in all but two of the 19 states with laws. In California the State Department of Public Health administers the Act. In Georgia, responsibility is shared, as the Act covers dental hygienists or dental nurses as well as licensed undergraduate nurses. The former section is administered by the Board of Dental Examiners.

The state board of nurse examiners may be appointed by the governor on recommendation from the state nurses' association. In the majority of states the board is composed of registered nurses only. Representatives from nursing, the medical profession, teaching, and the lay public may serve in others. At least five members are recommended.† In Michigan's proposed bill (withdrawn) it was suggested that a licensed practical nurse serve on the advisory committee to the state board.

Within the rules and regulations for licensing practical nurses

---

* Direct help and consultant service in all problems relating to legislation for nursing may be secured from the American Nurses' Association.

† For further details, see material published by the American Nurses' Association.

passed by the state boards of nurse examiners or other body vested with this authority are many variations in details, although the boards are assigned oversight for the same general problems. The standards to be met by schools of practical nursing for approval by the board is one example of these variations.

Maryland gives approval to schools offering from nine months to two years of training, Missouri requires eighteen months (18), while several states make no stipulations. The California law states that the course of not less than twelve months (for trained attendants) shall be given in a reputable hospital or sanatorium connected with a school for trained attendants. The Massachusetts approving authority describes the minimum curriculum, equipment, and teaching staff in detail, including the supervision and housing of students, and sets a minimum of twelve months for the basic course.

There are also some variations in the statement of qualifications for candidates asking to take state examinations for licensure. However, the present state laws with closed waivers usually require the applicant for a license to be eighteen years or over, a citizen, of good moral character, to have completed eighth grade of grammar school, and to have passed a state examination after the completion of a training course of nine months or more in an approved school. The state examination covers such subjects as elementary anatomy and physiology, personal hygiene and behavior, elementary nursing procedures, home management, simple nutrition and training in child care, care of chronic and convalescent patients.

NEW YORK STATE'S EXPERIENCE

In New York, the committee charged by the State Nurses' Association with the job of getting the bill passed had a five-year task. The bill was killed in 1937 and reintroduced in 1938. Legal assistance was retained by the Association; a state-wide educational campaign enlisted the interest of lay and professional groups; a speakers' bureau and vigorous press and radio publicity contributed to the final victory. It was public support, however, more than any other one thing that resulted in the passage of the bill (19). The outstanding lesson learned from this experience, according to the state executive secretary, was that it is necessary to reach the public with information before the introduction of the bill. The wholehearted backing and understanding of medical and professional nursing groups precede even the approach to the public.

Experience in setting up the New York bill revealed certain weak points in procedure. These have been summarized by Stella M. Hawkins, executive secretary of the State Board of Nurse Examiners, and are cited here for the benefit of others (20):

The law should carry financial provision for putting it into effect.

"Residence" should be clearly defined. Time should be allowed to clear citizenship status of applicants.

Ample time should be allowed between the filing of applications and the issuance of licenses; also for surveying schools of practical nursing from which graduates are to be accepted for licensure. The department responsible for handling applications must expect and prepare for increased secretarial service in handling waivers.

It is highly important to check all educational and employment records directly with their source and to accept only original or photostatic copies. Enough instances of inaccurate and false records came to the attention of the department to justify these extra steps.

A suggested course (curriculum and minimum standards) should be ready to recommend to substandard schools.

Funds should be generous enough to permit visitation and consultant service to the schools. A survey of need for a school in a given area should precede its establishment whenever possible.

Ease in handling two classes of nurses is promoted by assigning and maintaining two colors throughout all forms, records, filing cards, and correspondence.

Finally, it must be remembered that the law once passed must be guarded against amendments or conflicting, competing new legislation which will weaken or confuse the original act. This means eternal vigilance on the part of state nurses associations and their legislative committees, and reserve funds.*

DETROIT'S CITY ORDINANCE

Because so many states will have to mark time until another session of the legislature rolls around, a temporary expedient for the control of practical nursing is described here.

---

* This was pointed out as long ago as 1901 at the Congress of the International Council of Nurses, Buffalo, New York.

In the absence of a state nurse practice act which covered practical nurses, the city of Detroit, wishing to have some control over the heterogeneous group of women representing themselves as "practical nurses," revived and adapted an old city ordinance which now stipulates that a person practicing for hire as practical nurse or home nursing aide must obtain an annual permit from the Department of Health (21). Power to make rules and regulations governing the issue of this permit is vested in the Department of Health (Division of Special Investigation), as is authority to withhold the permit if upon satisfactory proof the applicant "is not qualified to perform the duties of a practical nurse or is not a proper or suitable person to engage in such occupation." To receive a permit, an applicant must be twenty years of age, a grammar school graduate, a citizen, and of good moral character. Fitness is investigated on the basis of the information contained in the application blank; a personal interview; a physical examination recorded on forms supplied by the Department, including chest x-ray; four letters of recommendation (two of these preferably from doctors); satisfactory completion of a written examination or completion of the course at the Detroit Council of Community Nursing; and formal visits by a public health nurse to the homes of three recent employers. The applicant must supply two passport pictures.

There is no charge for these permits or renewal of permits. Some 300 practical nurses now hold permits, renewed annually or withheld for just cause. The best possible relationships are fostered by the members of the Department who try to convey to the practical nurses that they want to help them give satisfactory service. The practical nurses frequently drop in with problems or seek advice on such matters as rooming accommodations. Every effort is made to help them understand the reason for the regulations of the Department.

If an applicant fails to qualify because of lack of experience or evidence of insufficient knowledge of nursing, the head of the Department, working in cooperation with the local Council on Community Nursing, urges her to take one of two refresher courses offered at the School for Practical Nursing. One, of 100 hours, is a review of home nursing principles; the other of 24 hours, emphasizes relationships, behavior, and the practical problems arising out of the nurse's experience. These courses have been popular with the practical nurses, more than 70 enrolling to February 1945. The permit is issued to an applicant who promises to take such a course. It can be withheld the following year if the nurse has not completed the work satisfactorily.

The applicant agrees to abide by certain rules of the Department, such as keeping it informed as to change of address and giving the Department the name of the physician and address of patient while on probation. She promises to carry out the orders of the physician in charge of the patient in her care and be loyal to him, to accept supervision from the Department of Health, to be neat and clean about her person, to wear uniforms that can be boiled, to refrain from giving nursing care or treatments to a patient who is not under the care of a physician, from prescribing, advising, or administering drugs, diets, or treatments on her own responsibility, and from posing as a graduate nurse or a trained attendant or demanding fees equal to either.

The procedures to follow in the case of certain conditions are also stipulated, such as notification of the physician and Department of Health in case of suspected communicable disease.

Violation of this ordinance carries with it an unusually heavy penalty. Upon conviction, a fine of not more than $500 or imprisonment for not more than 90 days, or both, may be imposed by the court. So far, there have been no court cases. A warning or threat to withhold the permit has sufficed to remedy conditions.

The personal references given by the applicants are investigated by letter, the individual being asked to comment especially upon the practical nurse's ability in housekeeping, care of children, and nursing service. Has she been willing, cheerful, patient, efficient, painstaking, and neat?

A much more detailed letter goes to doctors, including such points as type of care given, reaction of patients, ability to plan, to carry out orders, etc. Further comments are solicited. On visiting the homes where practical nurses have been employed, the public health nurse fills out the most complete report of all, covering some nine main headings and 40 subheads.

By the time all this information is secured, backed by personal contact, a very good "profile" of the applicant has been secured.

Both the professional and practical nurses of Detroit approve this temporary expedient to regulate practice, pending the state law to license the group.

ATTITUDES OF THE PROFESSIONS TOWARD LEGISLATIVE CONTROL OF PRACTICAL NURSES

The medical profession is on record through some of its state organizations as being in agreement with the effort to control practical nursing through legislation (22), and previous studies of the situation by physicians have stressed the step as preliminary to a campaign of recruitment and training. Other professional bodies have expressed some uncertainty as to the wisdom of legislative control.*

Conscientious private physicians naturally prefer the service of the *licensed* practical nurse upon whose training and minimum qualifications a state board representing professional nurses and doctors has passed, but in the absence of legal recognition they will accept anyone at hand, sometimes going to considerable pains to teach a promising worker. Less cautious medical men will go so far as to train their own "practical" nurses and are irked by limitation of state licensure (24). Opposition to the idea of controlling nurse practice by law is the exception among doctors, however, although some may object to the phraseology and penalties stated in the present laws.

A few hospital administrators have not been wholehearted in their support of legislation for practical nurses (25). They see in it a threat to the service of many employees now giving nursing care in their hospitals who have had no preparation for the work other than that given on the spot. More preparation usually means higher wages and some administrators are interested in keeping costs at a minimum. This is especially true in proprietary hospitals.

The three national nursing organizations—the American Nurses' Association, the National League of Nursing Education, and the National Organization for Public Health Nursing—have officially recognized for more than 25 years that state control of all those who nurse for hire is fundamental to public safety (26). They have re-

---

* For example, in the fall of 1944, the Catholic Hospital Association adopted the following resolution:

"Be it further resolved that . . .

"The Practical Nurse may, under conditions existing today and under conditions likely to exist for some time to come, find an important place of usefulness in the hospital as well as in the home. The Association believes, however, that the legislative recognition of the position of the practical nurse may entail implications of the utmost seriousness for the profession of nursing and for the nursing care of the nation" (23).

The implications were not described.

peatedly urged their constituencies to initiate and support legislation controlling the practice of *all* those who nurse for hire, not registered nurses alone, and have advocated an all-inclusive nurse practice act rather than two separate acts, one for registered, one for practical nurses (27).

They have gone further. They have insistently emphasized that state legislative control is a *first* step, an essential preliminary, to establishing schools for the preparation of practical nurses, to adopting a curriculum, and to recruiting students (28).

Nevertheless, in 1944 in five states* without laws controlling practical nurses there were ten schools "approved" by a national association, and, on the other hand, in seven states† that had laws protecting the title there were no approved schools (29). In some of these states the law does not contain provisions for approving schools.

The far-thinking registered nurses as individuals—administrators and staff workers alike—have harped consistently on the need for state control of practical nurses. The place of the registered nurse whose preparation and practice are controlled under the law is threatened when there is no control of any kind of those with less than graduate nurse education who are free to nurse for hire. In the past (and unfortunately) a few professional nursing leaders and state nurses' associations have opposed legislation. This opposition was epitomized in 1912 by Lavinia L. Dock, for years the able spokesman for the profession, in a letter to the editor of the *Journal*.

The suggestion that nurses should amend their own registration acts so as to provide for a class of legally recognized trained attendants seems to me a most destructive and despairing proposal, opening the way to a complete confusion as to nursing standards. . . .

Let their own leaders come forth and state their aims. We have no more right to create and control the training of a class of attendants than physicians have to create and control nurses. . . .

The nursing movement was to lift women up, but an attendant movement is to press them down (30). . . .

Undoubtedly, the confusion in all the thinking of those years was not helped by our entrance into the First World War and the demand for nurses—any nurses—and the effort to shorten courses.

* New Jersey, Ohio, Minnesota, Washington, and Vermont.
† Florida, Georgia, Indiana, Mississippi, Missouri, Oklahoma, and Wisconsin.

The tide of opinion ebbed and flowed, but by 1920 most members of the medical and nursing professions were strongly urging mandatory legislation to license two groups of nurses (31). As professional nurses had started their own fight for state registration in the late nineties and the first state law was enacted in North Carolina in 1903, they were beginning to feel sufficient security to consider licensing a secondary group. Alice Shepard Gilman, touring the state of New York in 1920 in behalf of a nurse practice act which would include attendants, pointed out the menace of the untrained horde of "nurses," and the *Journal* stated: "It is the desire of the nursing body to give the trained attendant a dignified status in a field which will be peculiarly her own" (32).

The now famous report of the committee that studied nursing and nursing education in the United States in 1923 stated:

Before training or seeking to enlist additional numbers of girls and women, the first imperative need, the crux, the sole safeguard of a subsidiary group, is to include in state licensing laws subsidiary nursing attendants as well as graduate registered nurses. In no other way can the sick be protected so that they may know by the title of the sickroom attendant what grade of service they are receiving (33).

Between 1930 and 1940 it is more difficult to find expressed opposition to legislation among the professional nursing groups, and by 1940 its only evidence was the failure to discuss the matter in state meetings, to propose and to secure legislation. Certain states have had so negative an attitude toward practical nurses that only the most courageous have promoted their service. Others have gone on record as favoring legislation but have taken no action. For example, in 1938 the New Jersey State Nurses Association sponsored a study of the subsidiary worker (34) and was on record as approving the licensure of all those who nurse for hire (35), but the state is still without legislative control of the group.

Reasons for delayed professional sponsorship of legislation as revealed in professional opinion expressed in reports and published articles over a period of thirty-five years are cited on page 354. These statements represent for the most part past opinion and are no longer relevant or held by the majority of professional nurses today.

In summary, it may be said that previous to Pearl Harbor, those of the nursing profession in favor of state control felt that unless the profession stepped in and assumed leadership, undesirable outside interests might control the group, low standards of preparation would continue, and the numbers of untrained practicals would increase to the menace of professional nursing.

Those opposed to a move of this nature contended that to assist this group by giving them legal status implied approval of their service, much of which was bad, that to open the door through state recognition meant a general lowering of all nursing, that the public would be confused by two groups on different levels, and that such a step would merely serve to encourage practical nurses to charge more for their services, already overlapping the fees for professional nursing. Any legal recognition of a group using the word "nurse" seemed dangerous to the opposition (36).

PUBLIC EDUCATION

Whenever the public has had the need of legislation presented and the chaotic—nay, dangerous—existing situation explained, its support of a valid and adequate nurse practice act has been wholehearted and vigorous. Experience in all the states that have recently enacted laws indicates that it is worth spending time and money—even delaying the introduction of a bill if necessary—to win public support through careful interpretation of the purposes in the proposed bill (37). A widespread, carefully timed publicity program, reaching especially the women's groups, not only will aid in the passage of the bill, but will also create a genuine understanding of the provisions of the act, thus enabling the public to select the type of nursing service needed with greater discrimination and intelligence.

It would seem logical to infer that those who require the services of a nurse—lay people as well as the medical profession—will cooperate when they are convinced that something more than merely the status of the professional group is at stake, and I am of the opinion that the convincing is our [the professional nurses'] responsibility (38).

The safety of the public in using the practical nurse also lies in the *education* of the public in her use, and in this the doctors are of primary importance. They must be reached first and the law explained to them. The success of the law depends on the recognition of the difference between the two classes of nurses, recognition in relation to their preliminary education and background, training, procedures, skills, judgment, and, least important, charges for service. The outward symbol of this difference is the nurse's registration card or license which she is expected to carry with her and to renew at stated intervals in many states. Asking to see a nurse's legal permit to practice should become as automatic as looking for the word "pasteurized" on the milk bottle or expecting to show a driver's license on demand. At present the routine is seldom followed. An excuse not to show the card should be regarded with suspicion. Qualified nurses are proud to show their state authorization to practice. The card should bear the official state seal. If there is any doubt about the card, the state board of nurse examiners in the state capital will verify the nurse's license or registration.

As no law however strict can guarantee protection from misrepresentation, fraud, or malpractice without the fullest cooperation of all concerned, every use of nursing service carries with it a civic obligation in assisting to prevent persons not registered or licensed from practicing, remembering that the safety of all the public is at stake. It is always possible to find out from the state nurses' association what fees are being asked by registered and licensed nurses. An exorbitant charge is an indication that one is dealing with an unlicensed nurse. Others are disregard for the doctor's orders, neglect of nursing duties, and untidiness.

A safeguard is to employ nurses only from reputable sources. The professional "official" registry (which may be listed as nurses official or professional registry), a registered hospital, the visiting nurse association, the department of health, or your own licensed physician are more reliable sources than newspaper ads, telephone directories, drug stores, or commercial registries.

CONCLUSIONS

State licensure is no guarantee of safe nursing or of good work, especially during the period when those licensed under the waiver are still functioning, but at least such a law demands a minimum of preparation and attainment, which is preferable to nothing and to the dangerous gamble of hiring the first person in sight to nurse for pay.

In view of the leniency of the law, the ignorance of the public as to what constitutes practical and professional nursing, and the great difficulty in securing public testimony to violations, it is predicted that rigid control of practical nurses will be exceedingly difficult. In addition to an adequate nurse practice act, the remedy would seem to lie in widespread, pertinent, and continual public education in the difference between registered professional and licensed practical nurses; insistence that every employer demand to see evidence of a nurse's state registration or state licensure; consistent differentiation between the two classes of nurses by title, color of uniform, insignia or initials, and salary; wholehearted, sincere support of the law by doctors and hospital administrators; stiffening of the penalties for violation of the law as it becomes understood and effective.

It is disheartening to see new legislation for practical nurses perpetuating some of the mistakes made by professional nurses. One of these is the barrier set up by differing state regulations—length of training being an outstanding instance—with individual state examinations and standards, making it impossible for a licensed nurse to move freely from one state to another without considering the law controlling her practice. The variety of titles, of which there are no less than six recognized by law in 19 states, does not help matters and is vastly confusing to the public.

Just as the American Nurses' Association through the state nurses' associations fought an uphill fight to secure state registration for all professional nurses, so now the practical nurses of America are in the throes of securing this recognition, protection, and title. They need help from every reader of this book (39). Its most urgent message is to urge support of nationwide mandatory state legislative control of all those who nurse for hire under protected titles with suitable penalties for misdemeanors.

Professional nurses know what is good nursing. They are vehement and quite articulate when control by labor unions or commercial interests threatens their professional status. They feel strongly that practical nurses themselves, because their service is part and parcel of nursing as a whole, should not proceed as a separate group to educate, legislate, or establish placement services not under the control of professional nurses. Is it not contradictory, however, for a professional nurse to say, "You are not able to walk alone, but we will not help you"? This is a clarion call to action to state nurses' associations to help practical nurses to serve safely and well, protected by an adequate nurse practice act—and the time is now.

REFERENCES

1 The bill was printed in full in *American Journal of Nursing* 18:929–930, July 1918.
2 *Ibid.*, Article 8.
3 American Nurses' Association and National League of Nursing Education, *Nurse practice acts and board rules; a digest,* 1940, p. 62.
4 See especially ANA Committee on Legislation, "Organizing a legislative program," *American Journal of Nursing* 42:275–280, March 1942.
5 Information from 1943–1945 issues of *The American Journal of Nursing* and correspondence between the writer and the various state boards of nurse examiners.
6 "Trained attendants and practical nurses; the ANA report on licensed attendants and schools for training attendants," *American Journal of Nursing* 44:7–8, January 1944.
7 Ethel G. Prince, "New nurse practice act for New York," *Hospitals* 12:89–91, July 1938, at p. 91.
8 "Permissive legislation is useless. The value of the law lies in the compulsion to register, to qualify, to practice under the provisions of the Act with penalties for malpractice." Elizabeth C. Burgess, "A good nurse practice act," *American Journal of Nursing* 34:655, July 1934.
9 George V. Fleckenstein, "Nurse practice acts," *American Journal of Nursing* 36:230–234, March 1936, at p. 233. For examples, see James A. Tobey, *Public health law,* New York, Commonwealth Fund, 1939, p. 49.
10 Tobey (note 9), p. 50.
11 Fleckenstein (note 9), p. 230.
12 Compare preparation for passing New York legislation. Harlan H. Horner, "Looking facts in the face," *American Journal of Nursing* 33:13, January 1933; also Emily J. Hicks, "A crusade for safer nursing; how New York's new nurse practice law was won," *American Journal of Nursing* 38:563–566, May 1938. Information about studies carried on in New York, Pennsylvania, and New Jersey may be obtained from the executive secretaries of the state nurses' associations whose names and addresses are listed currently in the advertising section of *The American Journal of Nursing.* See also Program of

Pennsylvania State Nurses Association, accepted by House of Delegates, October 24–25, 1944, p. 1, revision of nurse practice act. Recommendations from the study of subsidiary workers in New Jersey are in part as follows: All who nurse for hire should be licensed; nurses' registries throughout the state should enroll licensed nursing attendants; and appropriate publicity should be given these steps. See Ella Hasenjaeger, "The subsidiary worker," *American Journal of Nursing* 38:772–776, July 1938, at p. 774; also News note, "San Francisco district to study use of practical nurses," *American Journal of Nursing* 40:329–330, March 1940.

13 See comments by Stella M. Hawkins, *Law and legislation;* report of conference of members of state boards of nurse examiners in Philadelphia, 1940, New York, American Nurses' Association (mimeographed), pp. 4–5, 7.

14 Ellen G. Creamer, "Practical nurses; their preparation and sphere," *Hospitals* 13:64–67, August 1939, at p. 65. There was also the woman who wished to obtain a license as a practical nurse and sent her photograph. She was recognized as a maid discharged from a mental institution; Edith M. Stern, "Impractical nurses or how practical can practical nursing be?" *Survey Graphic* 29:27–28, January 1940, at p. 28.

15 For definitions of "registered nurse," see "Professional nursing defined," *American Journal of Nursing* 37:518, May 1937; "Industry and the professional," *American Journal of Nursing* 44:420, May 1944; Editorial, "The National Nurse Planning Committee," *American Journal of Nursing* 44:1109–1110, December 1944; Ester L. Brown, *Nursing as a profession,* 2d ed., New York, Russell Sage Foundation, 1940, pp. 9–10.

16 New York Education Law, Article 52, Para. 1374, University of the State of New York, State Education Department, Albany, N.Y.

17 See the stand taken by correspondence schools in lobbying against legislation to control this group. "Nursing legislation, 1939," *American Journal of Nursing* 39:974–978, September 1939, at p. 977, and comments by Jessie W. Gardner, Chairman of the Legislative Committee, California State Nurses Association, at p. 978.

18 American Nurses' Association (note 3), pp. 61–62.

19 A vivid description of how this interest was roused and the points to be safeguarded may be found in Hicks (note 12), p. 566.

20 Hawkins (note 13), p. 7.

21 Ordinance of the City of Detroit, Michigan, Chapter III, p. 1936, Section 4, Practical Nurse. With regard to local situations, practical

nurses welcomed a question regarding numbers and licensure of their group suggested by Miss Colcord which should be investigated when lay people (or others) are making community surveys. See Joanna C. Colcord, *Your community; its provision for health, safety, and welfare*, 2d ed., New York, Russell Sage Foundation, 1941, p. 95, No. 59.

22 See "Need of trained attendants," *American Journal of Nursing* 3: 884, August 1903; "Recommendations of the Committee on the Costs of Medical Care," *American Journal of Nursing* 32:1291, December 1932. In 1937, Dr. A. Charles Zehnder, chairman of the Committee on Nursing and Nursing Education of the New Jersey Medical Society, urged the licensing of practical nurses; for discussion, see "New Jersey Hospital Association," *American Journal of Nursing* 37:321, March 1937. Nurses were in apparent agreement.

23 "Resolutions pertaining to nursing education and service, Catholic Hospital Association of the United States and Canada, 29th annual convention, 1944," *Hospital Progress* 25:277, October 1944. See also *Twenty-eighth annual report*, 1922, of the National League of Nursing Education, "Resolutions," p. 16.

24 Compare Dr. W. A. Newman Dorland, in an address before the Philadelphia School of Nurses, *The sphere of the trained nurse* [1908], pp. 29–30. He feared that registration for all would mean the same fee for all—good and bad alike—"a nurses' trust."

25 Nellie Gorgas, "What is the future role of hospitals in nursing education?" *Hospitals* 20:35–38, February 1946, at p. 38. This is a report of the Educational Conference of the American College of Hospital Administrators at Purdue, November 1945.

26 The Committee on Nursing of the General Medical Board of the Council of National Defense (Chicago, December 1918) recommended that the three national nursing organizations take over the training of attendants and regulate their practice. *American Journal of Nursing* 19:331, February 1919. "We must license all those who nurse for hire" (p. 333). The American Nurses' Association approved the training of attendants, Cleveland, May 1918; *American Journal of Nursing* 19:415, May 1919.

27 State associations were urged by the American Nurses' Association and the National League of Nursing Education to work for mandatory legislation, January 1919; see report, *American Journal of Nursing* 19:474, March 1919.

28 See "Progress report of the Joint Committee to Outline the Principles and Policies for the Control of Subsidiary Workers," *American Jour-*

nal of Nursing 39:917–918, August 1939; also Editorial, "The subsidiary worker," *American Journal of Nursing* 37:283–285, March 1937.

29 American Nurses' Association (note 3), p. 80.

30 Lavinia L. Dock, letter to the editor, *American Journal of Nursing* 12:500, March 1912.

31 The New York City League of Nursing Education went on record in 1920 as endorsing trained attendants and their licensure. See *American Journal of Nursing* 20:95–96, October 1920.

32 Editorial, *American Journal of Nursing* 20:280, January 1920.

33 Josephine Goldmark, *Nursing and nursing education in the United States;* report of Committee for the Study of Nursing Education, New York, Macmillan, 1923, pp. 4, 15, 28. See also Effie J. Taylor, "Present trends in nursing as affecting nursing education and nursing service in hospitals," *Hospital Management* 46:31–34, 57, November 1938, at p. 57.

34 Hasenjaeger (note 12), p. 773.

35 Editorial, "The subsidiary worker" (note 28).

36 It is of interest to note here that this problem of the untrained nurse was agitating the world of nursing. See comments in the *International Nursing Review,* January 1932, p. 3, and England's radical step in 1942 making nursing virtually a "closed profession." None but state registered and state enrolled assistant nurses may nurse for hire. "Nursing to be a closed profession," *Journal of the American Medical Association* 120:779, November 7, 1942.

37 Hicks (note 12), p. 565.

38 Effie J. Taylor, "The auxiliary worker in the care of the sick," *I.C.N. International Nursing Review* 13:314–321, December 1939, p. 321.

39 "General education of the public in relation to the practice of nursing and care of the sick in any form should be the function of the organized profession." Taylor (note 38), p. 321.

CHAPTER SEVENTEEN

Hiring a Reliable Practical Nurse

To the average person in any large city seeking a reliable practical nurse, the situation is utterly confusing and discouraging. He is confronted with a dozen sources of supply and no assurance that he is hiring a competent nurse. It is not unusual to find that nurses of several kinds are available through commercial employment agencies, hospital registries, doctors who have names of nurses they customarily call for their cases, visiting nurse associations on a visit basis, and occasionally from Y.W.C.A.'s and welfare agencies; there may be lists in the classified telephone directory (1) and in drug stores.

In 157 cities there are professional (official) registries organized by, affiliated with, or approved by state or city registered nurses' associations (2). This is a lamentably meager coverage to serve 140,000,000 people, 2 per cent of whom are said to be currently incapacitated through illness or accident, especially as 76 of these registries are in only seven states.* Illinois, for example (population 8,000,000), has only one professional registry. Nearly all the registries are in large cities, and it is in the small cities where practical nurses are most in demand (3).

In addition to the confusion in types of distributing agencies, there are differing policies in effect among them. Not all registries supply practical nurses; hospital registries do not as a rule. Hospital and school registries usually restrict placement to their own graduates. In cities where practical nursing schools are located (either commercial or nonprofit) there may be employment bureaus run in connection with the schools in order to give graduates employment (4). If other local professional registries are not placing practical nurses (only 36 out of 106 were doing so in 1943; see page 317), the nonprofit school may operate a registry in order to provide safe service to the public through registrants supervised from its office (5).

The professional nurses' registry does not take the place of other types of employment agency or of hospital registries. In New York

---

* California, Michigan, New York, Ohio, North Carolina, Texas, Iowa. Compare with the 20 professional registries serving the Province of Ontario with a population of 3,000,000.

city where all forms of registries function, including a professional registry,* hospital registries are very active. So far as is known, there is no employment agency organized and administered solely by and for practical nurses. Many commercial agencies are conducted by registered nurses.

In spite of the multitude and variety of sources from which to secure nursing service, typical of the average city, the agencies are not coordinated in any way in a clearing house and are not organized to meet known needs in a community or to prevent duplications and gaps in service. A nurse may be listed on several registries if she wishes to pay the fees; she may "register against" special types of cases or refuse calls when she wants to. Except in small towns, there is no one central bureau where Mr. and Mrs. Public, a doctor, a hospital, or an industry may call and be assured of obtaining reliable nursing service. A registry may be unable to fill a call for a nurse and make no effort to relay the request to another agency. It may limit the number of registrants to suit its budget or staff. In no registry visited by the writer was there a waiting list of practical nurses, yet no registry was referring calls for practical nurses to any other source of help, although two professional registrars said they usually suggested that the family "try a commercial agency."

In most of these registries, calls for professional nurses were also going unfilled—as high as 60 per cent of the calls. Practical nurses or visiting nurses might have taken care of these patients, but no attempt was made to find out whether they could. No routine referral to any other source of help was in order; the patient, doctor, or hospital simply received a courteous refusal of service. Nor was there any uniformity among them in practice, fees, standards, or coverage.

In 1938, Grace Reid, studying the problem of calling a nurse in Rochester, New York, reported, as chairman of a subcommittee to study nursing needs in the community, such situations as these: Patients without nursing care, cost of service prohibitive, uneven distribution of nursing service over the area, lack of integration of services, confusion in the names of agencies supplying nurses to the public, too complicated procedures in obtaining a nurse, no uniformity in policies and regulations of service (6).

* In January 1945, the Manhattan professional registry was not placing practical nurses. There were 55 commercial registries in Manhattan, 88 in all the metropolitan area.

In several cities, hospital administrators were asked by the writer where they had secured the practical nurses they were employing. All but two had been unable to secure practical nurses through the professional registry, either because the registry did not list practical nurses or because they were all on cases. Some had used commercial registries, one had advertised in the newspaper, six had telephoned or written the director of an approved school for practical nurses, but the majority had found their staffs through other nurses, registered or practical—friends telling friends of the job. A doctor had referred to a hospital a candidate who had served as practical nurse in his office, and in two instances the practical nurse had just walked in and asked for a job. A director of a visiting nurse association, formerly affiliated with a nurses' registry, knew of four excellent practical nurses on whom she could call for emergency service or replacement of present staff. "But I am lucky!"

This chaotic situation is not peculiar to wartime conditions. It has existed for years (7). The result not only is confusing to the public but fails to bring patients needed care and nurses needed jobs when jobs are scarce. Also, the lack of a central bureau which will investigate fully and stand back of the service offered puts an extra strain on institutions employing practical nurses (8). In states where practical nurses need not be licensed and may apply for positions without formal training, administrators report that they or their staff spend the first months of employment in training applicants for their jobs. There is always a long probationary period during which teaching and close supervision must be given. References from previous employers and doctors are secured by many hospitals, but are admittedly unreliable. The evaluation of references is a specialized job; even the registry which sends practical nurses into home situations is often not able to obtain valid credentials for them (9). Without the service of a well organized, disinterested vocational bureau, each administrator becomes his or her own employment agency, using considerable office time for the investigation of each practical nurse.

Furthermore, while institutions employing an adequate supervisory staff of registered nurses can weed out unsatisfactory practical nurses fairly promptly, or assist the promising ones to improve so that patients do not suffer, the smaller hospitals are not so equipped.

In homes the situation is even worse. If the placement agency sends a wholly unqualified, unlicensed, and unsupervised practical nurse to care for a patient, anything may happen and the family has no redress. A dismissal is usual in the case of obvious inefficiency, untidiness, laziness, rough handling, or gross misdemeanor, but few families know enough about illness to detect the type of carelessness which is potentially dangerous to the patient, such as failure to carry out the doctor's orders as he intended them. Few families take time to observe the thoroughness of the nurse's work. They usually turn over all responsibility for the patient to the nurse the moment she enters the door. A complaint to the commercial registry only serves to pass the unsatisfactory worker on to another family. A professional, hospital, or school registry usually investigates the difficulty. In times of shortage, however, only serious dereliction would remove a nurse's name from a registry and, in the case of a commercial registry, it would probably be necessary for the family to testify in writing against the nurse to secure her removal.

The commercial schools for practical nurses operating in states where no law controls the title "practical nurse" find it to their advantage to maintain placement bureaus, not only as an additional source of income but in order to recruit candidates for the school by advertising immediate employment in well paid positions, steady work, and an opportunity to earn money while learning a new trade.*

We can be sympathetic with a "Dr. Jones" who exclaimed, "Nurses, nurses! . . . Fourteen agencies distributing nursing service in this town and still one can never find the kind of nurse a patient needs, when he needs her, at a price he can pay. . . . Where can I get a reliable woman who will see that Grandma doesn't get bedsores and who won't give the baby soothing syrup when he cries!" (10).

THE UNITED STATES EMPLOYMENT SERVICE

Since 1930, a new employment agency has been in the field of nurse placement: the United States Employment Service, with local offices in every good sized city and regional offices in other areas and with facilities to study supply and demand, survey opportunities, and advertise needs—the daily radio announcements describing openings

* A commercial school advertised in 1939 that its graduates had become hospital superintendents, directors of private hospitals, and assistants to well known physicians.

for war workers were an example. The U.S.E.S. seems to many the logical distributing center for every type of nurse. Whether the U.S.E.S. would be willing to handle private-duty demands for nursing personnel as well as institutional positions, or whether Mr. and Mrs. Public would turn to a public employment agency for this type of private service, seems at present doubtful. The rate of turnover among registered and practical nurses assigned to private homes may prove too expensive for a public agency to handle, since such service seldom lasts more than three weeks, often only a day or two. The transfer of employment to the U.S.E.S. would certainly be unpopular with the commercial agencies and it would take time to accustom physicians to use this type of agency. Professional nurses would wish to be assured that the quality of vocational guidance was superior to that now offered in their own professional registries before turning over the placement job, because long experience has shown that placement, vocational guidance, and counseling are inseparable (11). On the other hand, the war emergency definitely revealed ways in which the U.S.E.S. and professional nursing placement services can be mutually helpful (12) and it is quite conceivable that the placement of registered and practical nurses in long-term salaried positions in public and private institutions could be undertaken to the advantage of all by the vocationally skilled placement staff of the U.S.E.S. in consultation with professional nurses, leaving the private home calls to be filled by professional registries or a voluntary agency such as a community nursing bureau.

THE POSITION OF THE REGISTRY

It is impossible to say whether, if all the practical nurses available in a given area were registered at a central bureau, there would be a supply sufficient to answer all calls as there is no city where a test of this kind has been made. Estimates would have to take into account the supply of registered nurses and the total need for both types of nursing care in homes, hospitals, and other institutions in normal times. Where commercial agencies enter the field of placement, the situation is complicated by the fact that these agencies are in business for profit, and most of them will send a practical nurse to anyone who will pay for service, without more than an oral inquiry as to the type of care really needed. If registered nurses are not available, a practical nurse may be sent regardless of the request from or the condition of the patient (13). It is assumed that this would not happen in a professional registry where a registered nurse registrar discriminates between the patient needing a professional nurse and the one for whom a practical nurse can serve safely (14). A professional registry will not knowingly send a practical nurse to an acutely ill patient requiring highly skilled treatments. If it does in an emergency, the doctor must take the responsibility and the family must be made to understand the nature of the placement.

Several professional registries visited by the writer reported that owing to the present demand, unlicensed practical nurses and "temporary registrants" were being sent to homes in answer to urgent calls. However, in each instance the registrar explained to the family that the nurse was unlicensed and that the registry could not vouch for the character of her work. The fact that registries in some localities have been sending practical nurses to cases where they would normally send registered nurses while registries in other localities have refused to enroll practical nurses for any cases distorts the picture of the demand for practical nurses, and any survey of community need would have to take these factors into account.

Doctors and nurses themselves do not always support the effort of the registry to serve the public. "There is a black market in practical nurses in our city," a registrar stated to the writer, "but why not? A doctor finds two or three well qualified, acceptable practical nurses. He has enough cases to keep them busy every day of the year. Why should they pay the registry fee and stick to the charges our board sets? They can get all the work they want at higher wages. You can't blame them."

"I don't blame the practical nurse," another experienced registrar commented, "I blame the public for being willing to pay an exorbitant price for mediocre service." But must not the profession shoulder much of the blame for being aware of the critical situation and recognizing the poor service, yet doing nothing to protect and warn the public? This is not a case of exonerating the practical or the professional nurse on the grounds that the buyer should beware (*caveat emptor*). "A well-recognized principle of economics has it that *freedom of choice should be limited where the consumer is not a proper judge of the quality of the ware*" (15). (The italics are mine.)

We, as professional nurses, have done little to protect the public's choice of nurses. They are not in a position to judge the quality of the ware; we are.

"Gradually, our practical nurses are leaving the registry to nurse 'on their own' or go into war work," another registrar complained. "They go where there is more money. That is the difference between a professional worker and one in a trade" (16). Yet professional nurses also left the registries during 1944–45. Similar experiences were reported by registrars in three other cities. It was generally agreed that these nurses would return to the registries after the war when industrial jobs will be less abundant.

The Committee to Study Nursing Education in the United States in 1923 pointed out that someone must be responsible for deciding whether a patient needs a practical or graduate nurse (17). Ordinarily, the report states, this would be the physician. It is frequently the registrar who never sees the patient or family. The public using this source can be safeguarded only by state legislation providing for the licensing of nurses' registries (this is usual now) and the approval of professional registries by some authoritative body, possibly the state board of nurse examiners or the American Nurses' Association. Also, unless the registry has command of most of the nurse power in a community, it cannot do much to meet the needs of the public, distribute service equably, and in times of shortage stretch nursing service by a judicious adjustment or spreading of each type to suit the patient's changing condition. For example, professional nursing service may be needed during the acute stage of illness, relieved gradually by practical nursing part or full time, with visiting (registered) nurses coming in to give special treatments. The combinations of service are many. Is it too much to hope that the day is not far off when the judgment as to type of home care needed will be based on a visit to the patient, made by a professional nurse from the visiting nurse association or registry, who, in consultation with the doctor, decides on the type and amount of nursing care needed for that particular case?

So long as a professional registry receives official approval from the registered nurses of the state or district, the impression is given to the public that its registrants and personnel practices meet the standards set by the authoritative national nursing organization—the American Nurses' Association (18). This is true in general, but the American

Nurses' Association does not attempt to visit, accredit, or approve each registry in the sense that the American Hospital Association approves ("registers") hospitals or the National League of Nursing Education accredits schools of nursing. The official list of professional registries is composed of registries which have been approved locally. They are expected to conform to the standards recommended by the American Nurses' Association (19). Many registries do not meet all the standards, many exceed the minimum requirements. Without doubt, a nonprofit professional registry is the safest place to secure a registered nurse at the present time, but there are far too few of them to meet the need and they are too weak in organization to serve the whole community effectively.

The American Nurses' Association has urged that nonprofessional registrants be listed with the professional registries, to give bedside care in the hospital or home where skilled nursing service is not needed and to assume nonprofessional and household duties (20). The registration of such personnel is not a requirement for recognized status as a professional registry, but the national nursing bodies are decidedly in favor of it.

The professional registries which do not list practical nurses give the very understandable excuse that the variations in training and ability and the difficulty in securing reliable evaluations of past performance of nurses without formal preparation make the handling of such enrollment impossible for a small office staff. The placements take longer than do those of professional nurses. Some registrars have never seen the very excellent work of well prepared licensed practical nurses and they are skeptical of the advantages in adding the group to their lists (21).

An argument which appeals to the registries for accepting the responsibility of placing practical nurses is that of increased income. With the falling off of professional nurse registrants through enlistment in the military services, more salaried jobs in institutions, and the ability to find continuous employment in one home after another without the aid of a registry, income from fees has been steadily declining and some registries are "in serious straits" (22). Practical nurses' fees offer a new source of revenue.

The professional registries which do not enroll practical nurses may not have qualified applicants or the district may have voted against their admission. Many registries are set up under all-professional boards or committees without a governing body representative of the community as a whole, although this also is one of the recommendations of the American Nurses' Association (23). There is therefore no way in many registries for the employer and consumer of service to have a voice in registry policies.

In June 1944, on the recommendation of the Subcommittee on Registries, the Board of the American Nurses' Association voted that practical nurses be invited to act in advisory capacity only to nurses' professional registries which were placing nonprofessional registrants (24).

PRACTICAL NURSES ARE NEEDED, WANTED, AND LIKED

When the registrars were asked how families and doctors liked the practical nurses, the response was nearly always the same—favorable if experience with their service had been satisfactory. "They like to use them if we will recommend them," was a frequent comment made to the writer. Families, especially, frequently prefer the practical nurse. "She's easy to get on with," the daughter of a bedridden lady of eighty told the visitor. "She doesn't make trouble for us."

The attitude of the registered nurse toward the practical nurse on the registry has undergone quite a decided change recently. "At first our registered nurses protested our taking on practicals, now they are glad to have them helping." "Professional nurses for the most part accept them and realize they fill a real need in our community." "I had to do considerable 'educating' before our graduates would work with practical nurses. I've had no complaints in a long time." "We couldn't get along without them!"

REGISTRY PROCEDURES WITH RELATION TO PRACTICAL NURSES

The procedure outlined here is a summary of those described by the registrars in fourteen professional registries visited by the writer in 1944 and 1945 and the recommendations of the American Nurses' Association (25).

Not more than 200 practical nurses were registered in any one of these registries.*

* In New Jersey in 1937, 800 practical nurses were working in 26 agencies. This obviously was only a portion of those employed in the state.

Enrollment

When the nonprofessional registrant* applies to the professional registry, besides supplying the usual identifying data she must give evidence of preparation and training, history of experience with names and addresses of two recent employers, and two references as to her character and ability (to be secured in writing directly by the registrar). No requirement is stated regarding licensure or graduation from a school of practical nursing or number of years of experience. A registry may, of course, define, raise, or make additions to these standards.

Following is an outline of enrollment procedure.

Personal interview; explanation of rules

Check on credentials through correspondence, including, when available, state license and school graduation

Investigation of work through previous employers, doctors, and hospitals. This may be by telephone or correspondence. Only two or three calls may be made, or five, six, or more

Review of letters from two references given by applicant

General health; not checked by medical examination by doctor of registry's choice (for exception see page 295), but report is usually secured from a doctor

Acceptance of applicant for trial

Check with employer and doctor after nurse leaves case, usually by telephone. This check may be routine for quite a long period of time, only once, or only when there is a complaint. Home visits by registry staff to secure a report of service are now almost nonexistent

Current record of cases nursed, length of service, fee charged, comment if any from doctor or patient, general impression of registrant

Occasional personal conference at registry. Invitation to meetings, lectures, etc.

Fees

Employment agencies are usually licensed under state law and pay $25 or thereabouts a year for license. Commerical registries usually are permitted by law to ask 10 per cent of the first month's salary.

---

* "A non-professional registrant is a worker listed with a nurses' professional registry to give bedside care where skilled nursing is not needed and to assume necessary nonprofessional and household obligations" (26).

Practical nurses have paid as much as $240 a year to a commercial registry for repeated short-term placements (27).

The professional registry fee paid by practical nurses ranges from $5 to $25 a year. Most of the registries make the same charge for the registration of the practical nurse as for the registered nurse because the same machinery is used in placing both.

Charges for Service

The pay for home service for practical nurses placed by the professional registries visited by the writer was $3.50 to $6.00 for eight-hour duty, $5.00 to $7.00 for ten to twelve-hour duty, and $6.00 to $10.00 for twenty-hour duty (28). The highest rates were found in New York and California. At that time professional nurses' charges in these registries were $6.00 to $8.00 for eight-hour duty, $7.00 to $10.00 for twelve-hour duty, and 8.00 to $12.00 for twenty-hour duty. Charges for registered nurses for the care of communicable diseases, mental patients, and more than one patient in a family were slightly higher.*

Obviously, if a patient is sick enough to require three eight-hour shifts of professional nursing service at home, the cost of $168 a week (and one meal for each nurse) is prohibitive for most families. The substitution of a practical nurse during one, then two, shifts would help a little—but very little. In Washington, D.C., for example, on February 8, 1945, if a registered nurse took the 11 P.M. to 7 A.M. shift and two practicals the 7 A.M. to 11 P.M. shifts, the patient would still be paying $18 a day or $126 a week.

Selection of Cases

In 1943, 106 professional registries reported to the American Nurses' Association regarding their placement of practical nurses (called nonprofessional workers in the reports). Thirty-six of them placed this type of nurse, and 30 supplied detailed data (30). It is thought that many more than 36 registries are now listing practical nurses.

These 30 registries received 20,583 calls for nonprofessional nurses, 10 per cent from hospitals and 90 per cent for home service. They filled

---

* It must be remembered that charges change constantly and vary greatly in different sections of the country. Compare these charges with rates found in 1943 (29).

62 per cent of the hospital calls and 56 per cent of those for home service.* About half the calls from homes included both nursing and housekeeping duties.

The percentage distribution of the home calls according to type of case was as follows:

Medical	72 per cent
Obstetrical	15 per cent
Surgical	6 per cent
Well persons	5 per cent
Psychiatric	2 per cent

According to condition of patient it was:

Seriously ill	30 per cent
Convalescent	27 per cent
Mildly ill	19 per cent
Chronic	19 per cent
Well	5 per cent

It is of interest, in view of the field of service of the practical nurse, that 30 per cent of the home calls for her care came from seriously ill patients. Whether the classification of "seriously ill" was based on the report of the doctor, family, or nurse is not known. Nor can we be sure that the situation called for orders and treatments which only a registered nurse should perform. It could well be that the early stages of grippe, influenza, accidents, or other conditions, while alarming to the family and causing the patient great discomfort, might not have presented any problems beyond the skill of a practical nurse. On the other hand, some of the patients called "mildly ill" by the family might in reality have been critically ill and in need of the experienced observation only a professional nurse can give. Furthermore, although the doctor may have accurate knowledge of the patient's condition and immediate environment, he cannot always know the household regime, the family's habits and attitudes toward the sick person—all affecting the ease with which nursing care can be given. Occasionally, with the best intentions the family gives the registrar an optimistic view over the telephone: "The doctor says she just needs to be kept in bed and given good nursing." It may not be until the practical nurse is actually on the case that complications develop and conditions

---

* Many registries reported to the writer that it is easier to fill hospital positions.

change for the worse. The busy doctor may not have been in touch with the registry and had just assumed that a professional nurse would be sent. Quite evidently, the judgment of a registrar, arrived at through telephoned reports, cannot be infallible, and when she can classify the condition of the patient as "seriously" or "mildly" ill she would seem to be little short of clairvoyant. In all cases where the doctor is uncertain as to the type of care he wants or the family's report is vague, a preliminary home visit by a professional nurse would seem to be an essential precaution in giving safe service from a registry.*

EMPLOYMENT PROBLEMS

Employment agencies of all types have their own difficulties in rendering service, especially in wartime. Some of those cited to the writer include the effort of doctors to teach skilled treatments to practical nurses (31), the refusal of both professional and practical nurses to accept cases where care of the household is involved, dislike of long-term "uninteresting" cases, and the fairly constant request of registrants to raise their charges and shorten their hours.

"Registries," said Jean Barthe, president of the Registered Nurses Directory in Oakland, California (32), "have 50 per cent salable products, 50 per cent non-salable, but you have to sell them all." The director of the bureau of Manhattan and the Bronx pointed out the really staggering problem of picking the right nurse for the right patient and the crying need to guide, select, assist, and teach the registrants, adding that their personal qualities are often most important (33). This leads to one of the fundamental needs in the registry field —qualified placement secretaries.

The registered nurse registrar who is assuming the responsibility of placing practical nurses in homes and hospitals needs an unusually wide background of experience. She must understand thoroughly and be up to date on the usual treatments called for by medical and surgical conditions, the degree of skill needed in these and in nursing various types and stages of disease; she must know the local physician's routines, preferences, specialties; the hospital situations; and in so far as possible, the home conditions of the patient. Familiarity with the city

* In this connection, the experience of the Ontario Registered Nurses Association of Canada in promoting practical nursing service through its professional registries is of interest (see page 352).

is essential. She should be a skilled interviewer, a wise and patient counsellor and friend, familiar with the techniques of vocational guidance and placement. She should know the schools from which the practical nurses come, the hospitals to which they go. She should be sensitive to community attitudes, and up to date on professional trends in employment. Hers is no light task.

The conception of a registry as a community nursing bureau, run as a community service under the auspices of a representative board of citizens and members of the medical and nursing professions, including hospital administrators, has been familiar to national and state nurses associations for some twenty years (34), but its realization has been approached in only five or six cities and in none to the complete satisfaction of the promoters. The problems are multiple as they relate to both the professional and the practical nurse. There is, for instance, the wide gap between eight-hour duty and hourly service. The visiting nurse associations try to cover the latter as do some of the registries. Practical nurses, with the exception of those going out from visiting nurse associations, usually serve by the day—and yet, "If the nurse who goes into the home for an hour at a time is more efficient, more adequately paid, and better supervised, and if her patients are better served as a result of organization, one wonders if the same thing might not be true of the nurse who goes in for eight hours, and of her patients" (35). The patient whose needs consume less than eight hours a day of either professional or practical nurse's time would be less wastefully served if nursing time could be purchased by the hour, an end which might be more nearly attained by a pooling of all types of nurses in one bureau.

This idea of a community nursing bureau which would serve primarily the needs of the community and not the profession will not take root quickly, especially as it includes the conception of using a practical nurse instead of a registered nurse whenever a practical nurse may be used safely. In 1936, the director of a large registry stated: "Practical nurses are never sent [from the registry] when a family can afford a professional nurse. . . . The bureau protects its own profession." The writer goes on to say that, of course, if the family cannot pay, then "it is only common humanity to help them get the best of the practical nurses." Yet, in the same article she adds, "There is an increasing demand for the competent nurse who is willing to assume lighter household tasks. . . . It is a problem we are as yet unable to solve (36).

"The remedy," wrote Richards M. Bradley in April, 1938, "does not lie in special legislation or shortening hours, but in organizing all types of nursing service to fit patients' needs and pocketbooks." If an infinitesimal part of the money bestowed on educating nurses were spent on placement, things would be very different, he said. The number of nurses trained in both fields must be related to the demands. In Brattleboro, Vermont, as evidence of what organization can do, the reduction in the cost of private duty nursing offered to families under an insurance plan nearly trebled the demand for such service (37).

The criterion for rendering service on the basis of whether or not the patient can pay is not in accordance with the best traditions of medicine and nursing which grew out of a desire to serve others and to bring needed care to the sick under all conditions. Community nursing bureaus would look beyond the economic status of the patient, beyond the effort to give employment to the registrants, beyond support from the fees of registrants, to a service which exists through community support to bring nursing service to those who need it regardless of their ability to pay. Such has been the aim of the visiting nurses' associations for more than fifty years. The community nursing bureau is simply an enlargement of that conception for the provision of all types of nursing service in any amount needed.

It is evident from the scope of activities of many professional registries that their main concern is restricted to keeping their registrants employed and satisfied with their jobs. Their service to the public is superior to that of commercial registries in that greater pains are taken to investigate registrants, satisfy patients, limit charges, and promote a high quality of service without regard to profit, but so far as attempting to size up and fill the total community need for skilled nursing services of various types or of spreading the service available so far as possible or of supervising the service assigned to private homes, little has been done and that only by a handful of professional registries. "It is noteworthy that the districts which have the strongest registries are those which have encouraged the development of a community and professional program" (38).

Some dozen communities* have attempted to get at this problem of centralizing and distributing all types of nursing service through com-

---

* Alameda County and Los Angeles, Calif.; New Haven, Conn.; Rochester and Rhinebeck, N.Y.; Essex County, N.J.; Philadelphia, Pa.; Saginaw, Battle Creek, Flint, Kalamazoo, and Detroit, Mich.; South Bend, Ind.; and Washington, D.C.

munity nursing councils, health councils, or committees of the Council of Social Agencies (39). The national nursing organizations have studied, surveyed, and made voluminous recommendations on this subject (40) ever since the findings of the Grading Committee in 1926 exposed the shortcomings in overproduction, uneven distribution, and lack of organization among registered nurses (41). The early suggestions for organizing local nursing councils contained no reference to auxiliary workers or practical nurses, to the need of representation from this group on committees to study this type of nursing care in a community, or to an effort to size up their numbers (42). These omissions have been corrected in later outlines, however, and the newest schedules for the survey of community nursing needs have a substantial section on the auxiliary worker (43). In 1940, the American Nurses' Association recommended to state nurses' associations that a study of the practical nursing situation be made in each state and a schedule—now out of date and superseded by the newer one—was provided to states wishing to proceed (44). New Jersey, New York, Pennsylvania, and California were among the states which made such studies between 1937 and 1940.

In 1938, following the study of practical nurses in New Jersey, Ella Hasenjaeger, chairman of the committee, wrote, "It appears that the service of the subsidiary worker [practical nurse] will be utilized increasingly each year, therefore it behooves us to consider action toward the establishment of community nursing bureaus which will control and guide the distribution of nursing service" (45).

A WAY OUT

Viewing the distribution of all types of nursing service as a community enterprise at once suggests the amalgamation of the present professional and hospital registries with the visiting nurse association, or, where there is no professional registry, the development of such a bureau within the visiting nurse association. The names of some of these associations already fit such an expansion: Family Nursing Service, Community Health Association. This idea also is far from new (46).

Under such an arrangement practical and registered nurses who preferred to continue as private duty or free lance workers could do so, but they would probably find it desirable to have the backing of the bureau as Mr. and Mrs. Public came to realize that they were taking chances in engaging nonregistrants. The purpose of the bureau, however, would not be the protection or promotion of the nursing profession, but adequate nursing care of the public—nursing in its broadest sense of health supervision, health education, the prevention of disease and its cure through appropriate and skilled nursing service under medical direction. Visiting nurse associations have already seen considerable reduction in the number of home visits to acutely ill patients (largely due to more complete hospitalization) and an increasing proportion of their calls coming from the chronic and convalescent group. Some curtailment of professional nursing staff has already resulted and the employment of practical nurses begun.* Is not the time ripe for the next great development in the field of their community health service—the acceptance of responsibility for the distribution of all nursing service?

There are cogent reasons why such a step is desirable and would not involve revolutionary changes in the associations:

Many of the desirable features of a well-run placement bureau are already in action in visiting nurse associations, such as machinery for the registration and investigation of applicants; a qualified supervisory staff; in-service training programs; statistical departments for the study of visits, time, and costs; experience in the selection of cases; and a wide knowledge of community resources. "Nurses themselves are the best qualified to determine at what point the need for skilled care may give way to the adequacy of unskilled care" (47).

Representative community boards are responsible for the policies of these agencies and already have support for free and part-pay service through public taxes and private donations.

Consultants in the special phases of nursing are provided when needed and opportunities for self-improvement are offered staff members.

Staffs of competent supervisors are employed in all associations.

A concurrent educational and interpretive publicity program assures growth in the demand for service. This activity is more appropriately carried by a lay group than by the employed professional staff of a registry as at present.

Connection with a community nursing bureau would be greatly to the advantage of practical nurses, affording them professional recogni-

* Boston, New York and Detroit have reported this situation.

tion and backing, more continuous employment, and the assistance of constructive supervision of the kind from which public health nurses have benefited for many years. The orientation programs would assist them in adjusting to this new type of work.

The few community nursing bureaus now functioning make it a special point to see that nursing care is the primary reason for employing practical nurses. It is a fact that families frequently ask the impossible of practical nurses, and they must be protected from such heavy household duties as family washing, general housecleaning, and the entertainment of guests. One bureau found it necessary to explain to the family that the practical nurse could not be expected to milk the cows. Most professional employment agencies have stated rules of service which are fully explained to new registrants and to the families of patients.

The Detroit Community Nursing Bureau (and others of similar type) sends the family the name of their nurse, terms of care, and charges and urges calling the Bureau at any time for advice or help. The family is asked to see that the nurse on full-time duty has a separate bed or cot, rest, and time off duty in the daytime, especially if she is having broken nights. It is stated that light washing (baby clothes), the invalid's bedgowns, and the like may be done by the nurse but not heavy laundry. The nurse in her turn is expected to keep in close touch with the Bureau, respond to a call at once, and notify the Bureau if she herself is sick. A nurse refusing a case agrees to have her name dropped to the end of the list of those on call. She agrees to charge only the fee set by the Bureau—an overcharge may mean dismissal from the roster. Both family and nurse are free to call the supervisor if things are not running smoothly.

A bureau with the backing of "lay" men and women would be in a position to seek contracts for service, not only with industry,* but also in the various group medical care clinics, hospitalization plans, and insurance programs being developed nationally as well as locally. The place of both the registered and the practical nurse in future insurance plans is as yet vague (48), but there is general agreement that nursing must be tied into the provisions for medical and hospital care and not offered by itself (49). The bureau would become the

---

* Compare the contracts for part time nursing service now in force between visiting nurse associations and small industries.

promotional agent for nursing service with all such agencies and plans.

There are naturally in an untried experiment many unanswered questions relating to the place and use of practical nurses and their adjustment to supervision. For example: Should community nursing bureaus insist on a license for all practical nurses in states without legislative control? If the registrant is without a license, what should be accepted as a basis of training or an equivalent? Should there be a minimum of experience required? What responsibility does a bureau assume—ethically and legally—for the placement of unlicensed practical nurses? What type of supervision can be offered and by whom, and how can its expense be met?

One of the most disturbing features in the development of practical nursing service in the last five years has been the ever-rising cost, putting the service beyond the reach of many families who have problems of chronic illness or long-time convalescence. The solution of the problem will probably have to be the same as it was for professional nursing service: the distribution of service through an organization or agency provided with public funds (gifts or taxes) to meet the cost of free or part-pay service to those unable to pay the full fee, or the evolution of health insurance plans, compulsory or otherwise, to take care of the problem on a prepayment basis. The community nursing bureau, the visiting nurse association, or another agency selected to administer the service should be the recipient of such funds and employ the necessary personnel. Many feel that a community nursing bureau developed in conjunction with if not as an integral part of the visiting nurse association should employ practical nurses, instruct, supervise, and assign them for full or part time to families, imbuing this group with the same fine spirit of service associated with visiting nursing and maintaining their high standards of performance. Should such a joint service be developed, the fear that practical nurses will overstep their field, compete for fees with private duty registered nurses, or menace the public's safety would be largely overcome.

It has been suggested that more professional registries be established and that the placement of practical nurses be included in all these new bureaus. Would it not be more effective from the community standpoint to start by uniting the scattered hospital registries already in existence, combining them with a community nursing bureau which would include—or join—the visiting nursing association? A true community nursing bureau of this type, centralizing all nursing resources, would enable an employer to call just one telephone number when he wishes to engage a nurse.

The distributing center for nursing service is a vital point at which the service of practical nurses must be controlled. State legislation is an important preliminary, but making the licensee available to all under safe conditions is equally important and is the responsibility of those who know what safe nursing is and what the community needs. If the profession does not promote community action to set up adequate machinery for furnishing qualified practical nurses to selected cases under professional supervision, who will? The answer is clear—the practical nurses will establish their own employment bureaus or will continue to enrich the coffers of the commercial agencies. Under either plan, the public is exposed to uncontrolled, professionally unsupervised, and potentially dangerous practice (50).

Unfortunately, only a few of the present professional registries are in a position to develop into true community nursing bureaus. Most of them have not welcomed the principles of supervision, of community support for free service, of consumer representation in formulating policies, or of enrolling subsidiary workers. That they have not even been successful as business enterprises the unfilled calls for all types of nurses and their declining income prove. In a community nursing bureau, the business end of the service would be carried by experts in the field of management, while registered nurses would function where they are most necessary and best prepared to serve: in guidance and placement of the nurses, selection of cases, and supervision of service.

One advantage in any pooling of resources and the fullest use of services is usually a reduction in operating costs with better returns to the employee and better service to the consumer. The public would surely gain by being able to find all types of nursing service in one place, with a business office through which to deal instead of an individual.

In addition to all the business advantages of a central bureau, is it not possible that, if she knows the nursing bureau is eager and willing to find a nurse to suit her needs at a price she can pay, the patient will call a nurse earlier in illness, stay in bed until completely recovered, and be relieved of much fatigue during the illness of other members of her family? The bureau would thus serve the interests of public health as well as the needs of the acutely ill.

The art and profession of nursing have far outstripped its organization. We do not have satisfactory means of bringing nurse and patient together. It is not greatly to our discredit, for we are only just emerging as a profession, and our time and thought have rightly been absorbed in creating a body of knowledge worthy of that distinction. But we must not allow the lag to continue and we must recognize that the business setup necessary to the distribution of a product is a specialized undertaking in itself. There are few successful surgeons who are also successful administrators of large hospitals. Business is a mystery to the majority of nurses and with all due respect to dozens of competent nurse registrars, it must be admitted that professional registries have failed to develop their market, increase and improve their services, or fill the crying needs of their communities.

"A considered and courageous plan is needed," wrote Dr. Winslow, "to coordinate all available nursing services and to utilize subsidiary nursing service where such service is desirable under adequate safeguards of supervision and control" (51). "The real difficulties are psychological and inhere in the fears and hesitations, the suspicions and jealousies of the human beings concerned—nurses" (52).

This is a just indictment. It is time we forgot ourselves and planned for the good of the community.

"We are dreaming," wrote Miss Fox in 1929, "of a miracle in social engineering which some of us believe can actually come to pass" (53).

REFERENCES

1 Lists of nurses checked in 1945 in the classified telephone directories of four cities of over 500,000 showed 400 to 900 names. In two of these cities there were listed six nurse registries (commercial), the "official" or professional registry, and the visiting nurse association. In the Rochester, New York, classified telephone directory the RN's were not designated in a list of some 600 "nurses." Most of the visiting nurse associations offer "registered nurses by the hour or on a visit basis." The classified telephone directory in Detroit listed (p. 404), in January 1945, six registries but the Community Nursing Bureau (professional) occupied a 3 by 5 inch space, centered, and stated that it was "the only Detroit Registry officially approved by the Profes-

sional Nursing Organization. A nonprofit making organization. Home Nursing aides (practical nurses) holding certificates from the State Board of Control for Vocational Education—Supervision by graduate registered nurses. Men nurses—registered and practical. Hourly appointment nursing service in cooperation with the Visiting Nurse Association." See also typical list reported in *Study of the subsidiary worker in nursing service in Pennsylvania, 1939–1940,* State Nurses' Association, pp. 21, 39.

2 For up-to-date list, see advertising section, *American Journal of Nursing.* The list appears each month.

3 In 1925–26, 21 per cent of 389 registries said the demand for practical nurses was growing and that was true of small as well as large cities. May Ayres Burgess, *Nurses, patients and pocketbooks;* report of a study of the economics of nursing by the Committee on the Grading of Nursing Schools, New York, the Committee, 1928, p. 30. At that time 121 of these registries were enrolling practical nurses. P. 73.

4 Schools in Cleveland and Boston are examples of this arrangement and schools connected with Y.W.C.A.'s usually use the Y's employment bureau as in New York and Brooklyn.

5 Precedence for this practice can be found in the very early schools of nursing. Isabel M. Stewart, *The education of nurses; historical foundations and modern trends,* New York, Macmillan, 1943, p. 98.

6 Grace L. Reid, "Councils in community nursing; a step toward better community nursing service," *Public Health Nursing* 30:28–30, January 1938.

7 Burgess (note 3), p. 80.

8 "Nurses listed with *professional* registries for placement have had their credentials investigated and their qualifications are recorded in the files. Institutions and doctors who call upon them may be reasonably assured that safeguards have been provided." Editorial, "Some thoughts about registries," *New York State Nurse* 16:50, April 1944. This statement referred to *registered* nurses. See also "Miss Merling explains the registry," *American Journal of Nursing* 40:543–545, May 1940, at p. 545.

9 Florence Dakin and E. M. Thompson, *Simplified nursing,* 4th ed., Philadelphia, Lippincott, 1941, p. xiv.

10 "Community nursing service for all," *Public Health Nursing* 32: 283–284, May 1940.

11 See reports of Nurse Placement Service, Chicago, a nationally approved placement service since 1936.

12 Anna L. Tittman, "Employment in nursing today," *American Journal of Nursing* 39:46–50, January 1939; "Registry relationships classi-

fied by WMC order," *American Journal of Nursing* 44:762, August 1944.

13 There are a few commercial registries which do not follow this practice, however. See Dorothy D. Bromley, "The crisis in nursing," *Harpers Magazine* 161:164, July 1930.

14 It is interesting to note here the comment made by Dr. Sale who remarked that doctors often question whether it is possible for the registrar to select the right nurse for the job. Llewellyn Sale, "Can you send me a nurse?" *American Journal of Nursing* 38:1113–1114, October 1938.

15 Wendell Berge, "Justice and the future of medicine," *Public Health Reports* 60:1–16, January 5, 1945, at p. 10. Mr. Berge is Assistant Attorney General of the United States.

16 Sale (note 14), p. 1114.

17 Josephine Goldmark, *Nursing and nursing education in the United States,* report of the Committee for the Study of Nursing Education, New York, Macmillan, 1923, p. 16.

18 The American Hospital Association recommended "strongly" that "Nurse registries and employment bureaus of all kinds which supply nurse attendants to the public, be licensed and that the matter of local license for all non-graduate nurses be kept in view as a goal to be reached as soon as practicable." *Report of the Committee to Study the Nursing Problem,* Philadelphia, the Association, 1916, p. 20.

19 Consultant service on registry problems and an interpretation of standards, procedures, and organization setup are available from the American Nurses' Association, 1790 Broadway, New York 19, N.Y. A variety of folders and forms for registry use are available to the professional registries approved by state nurses' associations, to chairmen of private-duty sections, and to other representative groups. Requests for material should be sent to the state nurses' associations.

20 See "A.N.A. Board of Directors, Digest of Minutes, June 1944," *American Journal of Nursing* 44:908–914, September 1944, at p. 911.

21 Mary M. Roberts has referred to the fears of nurses "of the inroads of social service on public health nursing, and of the encroachment of the subsidiary worker on the fields of the institutional and private duty groups." And to offset such fears she has urged the flexible distribution of nursing care based on a knowledge of facts and needs. Mary M. Roberts, "Current events and trends in nursing," *American Journal of Nursing* 39:1–8, January 1939, at p. 6.

22 Editorial, *New York State Nurse* (note 8).

23 This is the general description of the function of the professional

registry as it appears in material prepared by the American Nurses' Association for registry use. Subcommittee on Registries, *The minimum standards for nurses' professional registries* (*tentative*), (revised 1943), pp. 3, 5.

24 "A.N.A. Board of Directors" (note 20), p. 911.

25 American Nurses' Association (note 23).

26 "What do practical nurses do?" *American Journal of Nursing* 40: 889, August 1940.

27 Mary C. Jarrett, *A brief study of counseling and placement of practical nurses in New York state,* New York, Committee for Recruitment and Education of Practical Nurses of New York, 1945.

28 See also Dorothy Deming, "Practical nurses—a professional responsibility," *American Journal of Nursing* 44:36–43, January 1944.

29 Deming (note 28), p. 37.

30 "Calls for non-professional workers increase," *American Journal of Nursing* 44:478, May 1944.

31 For actual reports of what doctors tell practical nurses, see Katharine Shepard, "The attendant in the home," *Public Health Nurse* 11:259–260, April 1919. See also Grace E. Allison, "Shall attendants be trained and registered," *American Journal of Nursing* 12:930, August 1912.

32 Quoted by Alice E. Snyder, "The nursing bureau of today," *American Journal of Nursing* 36:568–573, June 1936, at p. 570.

33 Snyder (note 32), p. 568.

34 Daisy Dean Urch, "Reducing nursing costs by means of organized nursing service," *Modern Hospital* 35:152, 154, November 1930, at p. 154. See also "Community funds for professional registries," *American Journal of Nursing* 45:216, March 1945; "Recommendations of the registrars conference," *American Journal of Nursing* 45: 217, March 1945, items 1, 2, and 6.

35 C.-E. A. Winslow, "Nurses show the way," *Survey Graphic* 23:159, April 1934.

36 Snyder (note 32), pp. 572, 573. This conception of a registry is not limited to our country. The secretary of the Royal British Nurses' Club is quoted as saying, "The secret of a good cooperation [the British term for registry] is to accept only the number and kind of nurses you can place." Mary M. Roberts, "Some impressions," *American Journal of Nursing* 31:928, August 1931.

37 Richards M. Bradley, "The attendant and the graduate nurse," *American Journal of Nursing* 38:474–475, April 1938, at p. 475. Speaking of the disadvantages to the registered nurse and the patient

of the "individualistic system" of private duty, Miss Fox wrote in 1929: "Private duty nurses must face the truth—their failure to fill the patients' needs prepares the fertile field for practical nurses." Appropriate cases selected for them calling for their special skill would bring more satisfactory results all around. "Nursing is gravely in need of organization"; Elizabeth G. Fox, "The economics of nursing," *Trained Nurse* 83:337–342, September 1929, and *American Journal of Nursing* 29:1043, September 1929. "Organize," continued Miss Fox, "the provision of nursing care for the sick as a public service coordinated under one central body, such coordination with a salaried staff should be community owned, representative of the general public, the taxpayer, the consumer, the donor to the community chest and professional groups."

38 Editorial, *New York State Nurse* (note 8), p. 50.
39 See also C.-E. A. Winslow, "Organizing for better community service," *American Journal of Nursing* 38:761–767, July 1938; Marion Wetzel and Beatrice Tremper, "Community nursing service; an interesting experiment in northern Dutchess County, New York," *American Journal of Nursing* 40:40–46, January 1940. For a description of the Detroit Council on Community Nursing, a community effort backed by a representative lay and professional group with 38 cooperating agencies, see "Detroit Council on Community Nursing; thirty-eight agencies cooperate to provide nursing service for their community," *American Journal of Nursing* 41:310–313, March 1941.
40 See reports of the Joint Committee on the Distribution of Nursing Service, 1930–1934, which was succeeded in 1935 by the Joint Committee on Community Nursing Service of the American Nurses' Association, 1790 Broadway, New York 19, N.Y. References will be found under the heading "Joint committees" in the annual index of the *American Journal of Nursing*.
41 Burgess (note 3), chapters II, III. See also Dr. Winslow's comment: "Private duty nursing as operated at present [1938] is extraordinarily inefficient because of irregular employment, because of waste in the employment of nurses on full time when hourly service would often be adequate and because of ineffectiveness of home nursing where hospital care is really needed." C.-E. A. Winslow, "Nursing and the community," *Public Health Nursing* 30:230–237, April 1938, at p. 233.
42 See "Suggestions for the organization of local nursing councils (from the Subcommittee on Councils of the Joint Committee on Distribu-

tion of Nursing Service)," *Public Health Nursing* 23:351–353, July 1931. Nor did many of the books dealing with community organization for health and welfare include reference to practical nurse; for example, *Community health organization,* edited by Ira V. Hiscock, 3d ed., New York, Commonwealth Fund, 1939, mentions only visiting housekeepers, p. 252.

43 Reid (note 6). See also *Schedule for a survey of community nursing service* (1945), National Organization for Public Health Nursing, 1790 Broadway, New York 19, N.Y. The cost of the complete schedule with sections on registry service and the community picture is $1.00.

44 Reports of studies are on file in the office of the state nurses associations. For addresses, see the advertising section of the *American Journal of Nursing*.

45 Ella Hasenjaeger, "The subsidiary worker," *American Journal of Nursing* 38:772–776, July 1938, at p. 776.

46 Mrs. John H. Lowman, "The possible amalgamation of visiting, hourly and household nursing," *American Journal of Nursing* 15:975–984, August 1915. Winslow (note 35), p. 159. See also the union in July 1944 of the Visiting Nurse Association of Greater Lansing, Michigan, and the Nurses Official Registry.

47 American Hospital Association and National League of Nursing Education, *Manual of the essentials of good hospital nursing service,* Chicago and New York, the Associations, 1942, p. 64.

48 Margaret C. Klem, "Is prepaid nursing care possible?" *American Journal of Nursing* 44:1154–1160, December 1944, at p. 1155.

49 Winslow (note 39), p. 764. See also Marion G. Randall, "Nursing in health service plans," *Public Health Nursing* 36:311–317, July 1944; Helen H. Avnet, *Voluntary medical insurance in the United States,* New York, Medical Administration Service, 1944, p. 92.

50 England's experience in finding unregistered and untrained "nurses" working for "cooperatives" (registries) and commercial interests serves as a warning to us that health insurance plans, group cooperatives, and industrial medical services can and do employ unlicensed practical nurses. "This state of affairs is obviously contrary to the public interest." Editorial, "Nursing problems; report by British Medical Association on questions raised by the College of Nursing," *British Medical Journal,* supplement, June 26, 1937, pp. 410–413.

51 Winslow (note 41), p. 235.

52 Winslow (note 39), p. 766.

53 Fox (note 37), p. 1044.

CHAPTER EIGHTEEN

Next Steps

SINCE THE day when Florence Nightingale proclaimed nursing as "the finest of the fine arts" and pointed out that a body of knowledge and professional skill was necessary to its practice, nursing has gone forward into more and more difficult and specialized fields (1). It stands alone now, a profession in its own right, no longer any more dependent upon the medical profession than the medical profession is upon nursing, but joined to it in an equal partnership of mutual respect and confidence, working for a common goal.

There is every reason to expect that there will be a scaling up of the demands made on professional nurses as the years go by. "I can see no escape from the proposition that increasingly the nurse will take over the physician's routine work," wrote Alden B. Mills in 1934 (2), and within the last ten years directors of nurses in hospitals everywhere have seen, to an amazing degree, the transference of physicians' treatments to professional nurses—accelerated by the wartime shortage of doctors. As there is no reason to think that these duties will be withdrawn in the years after the war, a wider and wider gap will appear between professional and elementary nursing, a gap into which the trained practical nurse should step. The need for such service will be more evident as the enrollment of professional student nurses drops back to a peacetime level.

There would be an even greater demand for the service of practical nurses if hospital patients were distributed according to their nursing needs. If those in convalescence were separated from the acutely ill, if those needing merely custodial and protective care were removed from the convalescents, not only would the patients benefit but the cost of care would be proportionate to the skill of the worker, and nurses and doctors alike would find their work much easier. This would be a safe way to stretch the public's dollar.

The suggestion has even been made to public health nurses that an advanced type of education be required of selected groups of public health nurses who would serve as medical "assistants" to relieve the doctor of many of his routine jobs (3). Replacement of these workers might well start at the bottom of the scale by the addition of licensed practical nurses to relieve the "assistants to the doctor" of routine bedside care.

The filling of these "gaps" in service, the caring for an increasing number of patients needing simple nursing care, and the full acceptance of a "second level" worker in homes and hospitals by the majority of professional nurses do not, even taken together, justify, the writer believes, an indiscriminate rush to prepare practical nurses in great numbers for postwar positions. There are very good reasons for this conclusion. They are:

For the first five years after the war there should be enough nurses of all types to fill immediate needs—the largest number of registered nurses and nurses' aides in the country's history.

The existing approved schools of practical nursing can treble their present class enrollment and still have room for expansion, therefore new schools need not be precipitated upon unprepared communities but can be placed according to need and their practice fields can be developed and staffed with qualified instructors.

We have no studies or evidence to tell us how many practical nurses are actually needed in all the fields open to them.

We have some evidence that practical nurses will not find postwar conditions quite as favorable as conditions of the war years or as those of us who believe in the service would wish. Hospitals, visiting nurse associations, and professional nurses who welcomed these workers during the war now may indeed "reconvert" in the wrong direction. "The vast unselfishness of wartime gives way, and gives way abruptly, to something very different indeed when peace is declared" (4), especially if bread and butter are at stake. We would be doing practical nurses the worst possible favor if we created machinery, established schools, and encouraged wide enrollment of students only to have them find competition for jobs so keen and professional nurses so numerous that they could not make a living.

For nearly a hundred years we have been well aware of this enigma of the untrained nurse. In all that time we have not established real control of those who nurse for hire, except in New York state where pending mandatory legislation has yet to become effective. The few states now controlling title only should be introducing mandatory legislation and the states without laws to license practical nurses should initiate preliminary legislation. To turn out unlimited numbers of practical nurses without some form of legal control of their practice is like allowing flood waters to pour down the rivers without flood gates, levees, or storage lakes. The water may be useful and needed, but it is destructive and harmful when allowed to rush freely anywhere. Logically, provisions for state licensure should precede any intensive, nationwide campaign to produce large numbers of practical nurses. We have survived many years of struggle with this problem. Ten more years devoted to legislative and investigative efforts will not be a fatal delay and should result in a far better control of the supply, more uniform distribution of service, and safer care of patients.

From those who have trained and supervised some thousands of practical nurses and have been in close touch with hundreds of others comes a warning not to travel ahead of the public's understanding of this new phase in the development of practical nursing care. When a practical nurse tells her patient she is as good as a registered nurse (and charges a registered nurse's fee), she is as far "off the beam" as the registered nurse who presumes to diagnose a patient's disease—but the family may not know it. A well publicized campaign for licensing the trained practical nurse and vigorous efforts to make clear the difference between the two types of nurses should precede the production of thousands more nonprofessional nurses. At present, it is not quantity so much as controlled quality that we need in the field of practical nursing.

Let us also remember that the lower cost of service from practical nurses does not alone justify their training—low cost professional home nursing service is already available to many from visiting nurse associations and may be provided everywhere on a widespread scale in the future through some form of insurance plan. The justification for increasing the supply is the existence of an entirely distinct and separate service need. That this service is not so costly as professional nursing is one of its great assets. It should not be allowed to become costly, but it should not be less safe or less available in order to remain cheap.

The establishment of the practical nurse as a trained and licensed worker in the field of sickness and health will require more than just passive acceptance of the idea and the passage of laws. Actually, the education of the public in the recognition and use of the practical nurse only starts with the legislative campaign. It must be carried on through every known source of publicity, and every opportunity must be developed to interpret her function as distinguished from that of the registered professional nurse. It will not be enough for a few schools, state boards of nurse examiners, and practical nurses' associations to back such a campaign. The effort should be initiated by the two nursing groups, professional and practical, through their representative national and local bodies, assisted vigorously and intelligently by the medical profession and organized men's and women's groups throughout the country. As state after state falls into line with appropriate legislation, a program of public education and interpretation should be planned and financed to accompany every step on the way from the first draft of the bill, through its enactment into law, and on through the years until the groups concerned are satisfied that the place and practice of the practical nurse are understood by the public and that her services are being wisely and widely used and are as thoroughly accepted as are the services of the professional nurse today. The responsibility for the earliest publicity and organization of efforts will probably rest with the legislative committee sponsoring the bill. Thereafter, money to promote understanding, raise standards, approve schools, and increase the number of prepared and licensed practical nurses in proportion to their need should be provided not only under the law to enable the state board of nurse examiners to do an effective job, but also by the professional and practical nursing associations, local, state, and national. So long as the public can hire cheap "nursing" and do not know there are better trained and licensed practical nurses, so long as they do not recognize the difference between the skills of those whom they hire, the job of interpretation must be constantly pressed. The public has learned to call for a "trained," registered, "graduate" professional nurse. It ought not to be very difficult to teach people the lesson: if you hire a practical nurse, be sure she is licensed.

A program of public education, then, is one of the vital accompaniments to legislation and to sound growth and continuing use of this service.

Surveys, studies, appraisals, or evaluations, whatever one calls the process of finding out about a field of service, are desperately needed in practical nursing. National postwar plans include such studies. Among the state postwar plans, Pennsylvania's is of interest (5); the State Nurses' Association plans to study the subprofessional nursing groups (definition, clarification of needed preparation, working relationships), and the immediate plans are:

To review the reports from Red Cross Chapters in Pennsylvania as to the
number of volunteer nurse aides who are active; the possible activity of this group in the postwar period; the possible percentage
that might remain in this field of work on a paid basis

To ascertain the number of paid auxiliary workers that might be absorbed in state and private hospitals including institutions for
chronic illness, mental hospitals, general hospitals without schools
of nursing, and general hospitals with schools of nursing, assuming that graduate nurses would be employed on the same
basis as before the war

To review reports from public health agencies to determine the degree to
which these workers could be employed

To assist in revision of classification of auxiliary workers to include new
groups

To assist in the differentiation of functions of professional and auxiliary
nursing groups

To draft a nurse practice bill to meet the need for auxiliary nursing groups
in Pennsylvania, covering definition and preparation

The program for the subprofessional worker provides:

That the curriculum as set up for attendants be changed to meet modern
trends

That the name be changed from "licensed attendant" to one suitable for
the subprofessional worker

That steps be taken for the organization and registration of subprofessional workers (5)

To these steps might be added studies on costs of service, education,
and placement, and an appraisal of the place of the practical nurse in
health insurance plans.

A thoroughgoing analysis of the postwar outlook for the employment of women as practical nurses or attendants in homes, hospitals,
and institutions has been prepared by the Women's Bureau of the
United States Department of Labor (6). In general, its conclusions
anticipate an increasing demand for the services of this group. The report cites in support of this forecast:

The firmly established habit of people to want and use a practical nurse

The growing load of chronic illness in an aging population

The replacement of volunteer nurses' aides in our hospitals by licensed
practical nurses

The assistance needed by parents in the care of their babies and little children

The employment of practical nurses in visiting nurse associations

The demand for home care by those dismissed from hospitals early in convalescence

The need of veterans for long-time care

The increasing census in mental institutions

The interest of professional registries in placing practical nurses

Recognition of the value of the practical nurse in the care of subacute illness by a variety of institutions, doctors, and lay people

To these hopeful signs the writer would add:

There is more professional interest in this group than at any other previous period in our nursing history

There is organized activity among the practical nurses themselves

Official recognition and leadership are being offered from national and federal bodies*

Actual testimony from many hospitals and agencies favors a permanent place for practical nurses as nurses' assistants and the expectation of retaining such service in the future

There is growing opportunity for more effective distribution of practical nursing service through community nursing bureaus

A wider postwar selection of candidates applying to the schools should result in a better selection of a more highly qualified student who in turn will command more skills and have greater chances of employment and advancement

The great problem of the future is two-fold: how fast will the opportunities develop to enable practical nurses to make a decent living, and in what numbers should practical nurses be trained? If vocational schools spring up with a vigorous, attractive, and far-reaching recruiting program offering free training, women from industries and the armed forces may sign up in great numbers (7). Will the profession be ready to train and work with the graduates? Will the public be able to absorb as many as are prepared? Studies of need should precede the establishment of new schools.

Possible limitations to job opportunities within the next five years would seem to the writer to counsel making speed very slowly. Noth-

---

* To those already mentioned in this chapter should be added the National Nursing Council for War Service and the General Federation of Women's Clubs.

ing would be more fatal to the acceptance of the practical nurse by the medical and nursing professions than to find a surplus of this type of worker clamoring for employment and competing for professional positions. Possible adverse developments affecting the rate of their postwar employment might be:

A surplus of registered nurses, many with veterans' preference, which must be absorbed before practical nurses will be really sought after by the hospitals (8)

The limitation to veterans of attendant positions in federal, state, and municipal institutions under Civil Service

A residue of reluctance on the part of registered nurses to accept practical nurses because of the past record, a record of poor training, competition for jobs, exorbitant charges, and desire to be thought of as registered nurses. Hospital administrators offered a choice between registered and practical nurses may prefer the former

Most of the positions for practical nurses and attendants in the new governmental hospitals will be suitable for men rather than for women

The competition of WAC and WAVES corpsmen from the medical departments of the Army and Navy, with veterans' preference, may be strong for positions in private institutions, especially in states without legislative control of all who nurse for hire

It will be seen from this summary that the possibilities of finding satisfying employment for the increased number of licensed practical nurses outweigh, in number at least, the factors against it. One may also deduce from these statements that it will be important in the future to train more men as practical nurses, certainly many more than are available at present.

Predictions are uncertain and unwise in a field as uncontrolled and disorganized as that of practical nursing. The march of world events and our national economic status in the postwar years as much as any one thing may influence doctors and nurses in deciding whether or not to give whole-hearted support to measures which will protect the public and at the same time develop a type of nurse prepared to share in improving the care of sick people.

Looking into the future to the time when normal demands express themselves and the disrupted labor market is a thing of the past, it will be essential to determine the number of registered nurses needed, to adjust production accordingly, and to decide where practical nurses may serve safely and how many are needed. These estimates are parts of one study.* So long as practical nurses are considered necessary only when registered nurses are not available, just so long will we withhold a place for them in the care of the sick and fail in our obligation to bring to the public skilled and safe nursing care for those who are not seriously ill.

The unsolved problems and the needed studies in this field are reminiscent of the early days of professional nursing. For example, we very much need experiments in developing a series of training centers around a central school. Which will be the first college to sponsor facilities for the preparation of directors and teachers for schools of practical nursing? Where will we find the first county health department installing a staff of qualified practical nurses to assist in clinics and visit bedside care cases under the supervision of the public health nursing staff? Who will study the opportunities in industry? Which registry and visiting nurse association will combine to provide all types of nursing service in homes in a community? Where will practical nurses take their place beside professionals in national insurance plans (9)? In group medical care units?

Immediate and constructive steps to be taken for the future healthy growth of this new form of an old service would appear to the writer to be:

1. Mandatory legislation in every state of the Union to license all those who nurse for hire, preferably incorporated in one nurse practice act

2. Development of modern testing methods for selecting candidates for the schools of practical nursing, requiring completion of eighth grade schooling as a minimum but playing down graduation from high school as a desideratum

3. Preparation and promotion by the National League of Nursing Education, National Association for Practical Nurse Education, and U. S. Office of Education of a curriculum adapted to the country as a whole and recommended to the state boards of nurse examiners as standard in schools from which graduates are to be accepted for state licensure

4. Determination of desirable standards for schools relating to size, place,

---

* Ideally, such a study should precede postwar recruitment of students for either the professional or the practical field.

qualifications of faculty, equipment, length of course, and practice fields. In the study of the latter, such problems as size of hospital, type, supervision, and integration with theory are important. New schools should be established only after a survey of needs and resources in the areas

5. Studies in representative communities—urban, rural, east, west, north, south—of the need for practical nurses, attempting to adjust supply to demand as soon as feasible and to discriminate between the two levels of service as offered in institutions, hospitals, and homes

6. Establishment of community nursing bureaus as a central source of qualified nurses under professional supervision. As the supply of service is a community problem, it falls logically under the program of the National Organization for Public Health Nursing

7. Investigation of the place of practical nurses in the prepaid insurance and health service plans

8. Development in connection with steps 1, 2, 6, and 7 of appropriate publicity and public interpretation programs, aimed especially at the medical profession and organized women's groups as well as the general public

9. When steps 1, 3, 4, 5, and 6 are well under way, accreditation of schools for practical nursing by the National League of Nursing Education, taking over the activities now handled by the National Association of Practical Nurse Education

10. When steps 1 to 9 are well under way, the organization of state and local organizations and in due time a national organization of licensed practical nurses

Many of these activities will be completely joint ventures of professional and practical nurses, working through their membership bodies; a few will profit by federal cooperation; a few will necessitate outside support from foundations or fund raising agencies, such as community chests. Representatives of the medical profession, hospital administrators, and lay people should be invited to participate as consultants, board and committee members, and interpreters of the service. Practical nursing is a *community* problem. It has outgrown its childhood in the home.

These steps will take the better part of the next ten years. That should not deter us from starting at once to straighten out the existing chaos. The National Nursing Planning Committee of the National Nursing Council for War Service adopted in September 1944 as one of its ten objectives a purpose really inclusive of all the other health goals to "promote, develop and establish standards to guard the public and the nurse" (10).

These can remain vague, comfortable-sounding words so far as practical nursing is concerned, or they can be made to include the pursuit of all the ten steps just cited—and many others—in behalf of improved nursing care of patients. The issue is squarely up to the profession of nursing.

REFERENCES

1 Isabel M. Stewart, *The education of nurses; historical foundations and modern trends,* New York, Macmillan, 1943, p. 365.

2 Alden B. Mills, "Need for subsidiary workers in nursing services," *40th Annual Report of the National League of Nursing Education,* New York, 1934, p. 159.

3 Hugh Cabot, "Future of nursing education," *Modern Hospital* 60: 47–48, February 1943; Hugh Cabot, "The place of nursing in health service," *Public Health Nursing* 35:181–184, April 1943.

4 Alan Gregg, "Adaptation for survival; reflections on our postwar problems," *American Journal of Nursing* 44:923–927, October 1944.

5 Program of the Pennsylvania State Nurses Association, accepted by House of Delegates, October 24–25, 1944, pp. 7, 10–11.

6 United States Women's Bureau, *The outlook for women in occupations in the medical services; practical nurses and hospital attendants,* Washington, Government Printing Office, 1945 (Bulletin 203, No. 5), pp. 12–13.

7 Joseph W. Mountin, "Suggestions to nurses on postwar adjustments," *American Journal of Nursing* 44:321–325, April 1944.

8 Dorothy Deming, "War and postwar needs for nurses," *Medical Care* 4:103–114, May 1944.

9 If, for example, insurance plans decide to include professional nursing service at $5 a day at home or in the hospital over a given period, why could not an alternative in suitable cases—or an additional period of service—be made available for practical nurses at $4? For professional considerations, see Marian G. Randall, "Nursing in health service plans," *Public Health Nursing* 36:311–317, July 1944.

10 "Planning committee defines objectives," *Public Health Nursing* 36: 497, October 1944. See also "A comprehensive program for nationwide action," *American Journal of Nursing* 45:707–713, September 1945.

APPENDIX

Annotated List of Textbooks and Instruction Outlines

This list of textbooks and material describing duties and techniques in the field of practical nursing does not include the dozens of books prepared for courses in physiology, anatomy, personal hygiene, community health, and sanitation given in high schools and colleges. Some of these books are used in schools of practical nursing, but few of them contain elementary nursing procedures. A good example of this type of textbook is *Health for you*, by Katharine B. Crisp (Philadelphia, Lippincott, 1944). The main headings are "Your health and personal appearance," "Your health and well being," "Your health and personality," "Your health and safety."

Aikens, Charlotte A., *Home nurse's handbook of practical nursing*, Philadelphia, Saunders, 1913; 4th ed., 1927. Out of date, but interesting historically.

American National Red Cross, *First aid text-book*, rev. ed., Philadelphia, Blakiston, 1945.

American National Red Cross, *Textbook on Red Cross home nursing*, Philadelphia, Blakiston, 1942. For use in teaching home nursing to high school girls and older women.

American Nurses' Association, Joint Committee with the National League of Nursing Education and the National Organization for Public Health Nursing, *Subsidiary workers in the care of the sick*, New York, 1940; revised June 1941. A list of duties and some accepted policies. In need of revision in the light of wartime experiences.

Brownell, Kathryn O., *Textbook of practical nursing*, 2d ed. rev., Philadelphia, Saunders, 1944. One of the currently used textbooks, written especially for practical nursing.

Dakin, Florence, and E. M. Thompson, *Simplified nursing*, 4th ed., Philadelphia, Lippincott, 1941. Also a basic textbook planned for practical nurses.

Douglas, George Margaretta, *Health and home nursing*, New York, Putnam, 1936. Written for the home; nursing in the absence of a professional or trained practical nurse.

Fitzsimmons, Laura W., *Manual for training attendants in mental hospitals*, New York, American Psychiatric Association, 1945. Procedures and instructions as well as general approach to training problems.

Gilbert, Norma S., *Home care of the sick*, Philadelphia, Saunders, 1929. Out of date.

"The household nurse," a series of articles in *The New York Sunday American*, December 1911. Said to be by Esther Robertson, of Bellevue Hospital. Of historical interest only.

Lippett, Louisa C., *Hygiene and home nursing*, Yonkers-on-Hudson, World Book Co., 1940. Not a textbook but a series of articles; incomplete from this reviewer's standpoint.

Lowry, E. B., *The home nurse*, Chicago, Forbes & Co., 1919. Interesting only historically.

Mohs, Emma L., *Principles of home nursing; a text-book for college students*, 3d ed. rev., Philadelphia, Saunders, 1931. Formerly used as a textbook. Needs revision.

Norlin, Elinor E., and B. M. Donaldson, *Everyday nursing for the everyday home*, New York, Macmillan, 1942. Well expressed. Assumes subacute illness cared for by the family. Not intended for practical nurses only but to teach high school age group simple nursing and health rules.

Olson, Lyla Mae, *Improvised equipment in the home care of the sick*, 3d ed., Philadelphia, Saunders, 1939. Not a textbook, but used in many schools as illustrative of adaptations used in home care of the sick.

Orbison, Katherine Barnard, *A handbook for nurse's aides*, New York, Devin-Adair, 1943. Helpful suggestions for nonprofessional nursing in hospitals.

Read, Charles F., *Manual for hospital attendants*, revised, Elgin, Illinois, State Department of Public Welfare, 1939. Handbook for attendants in mental hospitals.

Shepard, Katharine, and C. H. Lawrence, *Textbook of attendant nursing*, New York, Macmillan, 1935. Widely used textbook designed for practical nurses, based on the twenty-five years' experience of the staff of the Household Nursing Association of Boston.

Stern, Edith M., *The attendant's guide*, New York, Commonwealth Fund, 1945. Brief, direct, and readable description of attendants' responsibilities in mental hospitals. No techniques. An important contribution to the field.

Stewart, Isabel M., *Lessons in home nursing*, Teacher's College Bulletin, Ninth series, No. 2, Education Bulletins, No. 32, September

1917. Simple, very brief, fundamentally sound list of procedures for the home nurse in wartime emergencies, as of World War I.

Swartout, H. O., and B. Harter, *Home nursing made easy,* Mountain View, California, Pacific Press Publishing Association, 1942. Articles. Not useful as text material, more for the general public.

U. S. Public Health Service, "Home care of the sick," *Public Health Reports* 55:1865–1868, October 11, 1940. Very brief outline of a few essential steps in home care.

U. S. Veterans Administration, *Instructions for hospital attendants in Veterans Administration facilities,* revised, October 1941.

Wagner, Betty Quinn, *Art of home nursing;* simple technics and practical procedures, Philadelphia, Davis, 1945. For the untrained home "nurse." Does not contain much more than the Red Cross home nursing textbook and is confusing in its presentation of subject matter.

Wheeler, Mary Wright, *Practical instruction for the home nurse,* Home Institute, Inc., 1939. Incomplete from the point of view of practical nursing.

The Approved Schools of Practical Nursing

Each of the following 46 schools for training practical nurses or licensed attendants had been approved as of July 1945 by the state board of nurse examiners or other legally appointed authority in the state in which it is located.

CALIFORNIA

Berkeley General Hospital, Berkeley
Fairmont Hospital, San Leandro
Japanese Relocation Center in Manzanar
Riverside County Hospital and Sherman Institute, Arlington
St. John Hospital, San Francisco
Seaside Memorial Hospital, Long Beach

CONNECTICUT

Home Memorial Hospital, New London
Manchester Memorial Hospital, Manchester
State Trade School, New Britain

MARYLAND

Baltimore City Hospitals, Baltimore
Crownsville State Hospital, Crownsville
Eudowood Sanatorium, Towson
Hebrew Home for the Aged, Baltimore
Home for Incurables, Baltimore
Jenkins Memorial Hospital, Baltimore
Maryland Tuberculosis Sanatorium, Frederick
Spring Grove State Hospital, Catonsville
Springfield State Hospital, Sykesville

MASSACHUSETTS

Beverly Hospital Course for Attendant Nurses, Beverly (course not functioning)
Community School for Nursing Attendants, Springfield
Evangeline Booth Hospital, Boston
Harley Hospital Training School for Attendant Nurses, Dorchester
Holden District Hospital School of Attendant Nursing, Holden
Holy Ghost Hospital, Cambridge
Household Nursing Association School of Attendant Nursing, Boston

Robert B. Brigham Hospital Training School for Attendant Nurses, Boston

Tewksbury State Hospital and Infirmary School for Nursing Attendants, Tewksbury

Winthrop Community Hospital, Winthrop

NEW YORK

Albany Training School for Practical Nurses, Albany
Ballard School (Y.W.C.A. Central Branch), New York
Brooklyn Y.W.C.A., Central Branch, School of Practical Nurses, Brooklyn
Caledonian Hospital School for Practical Nurses, Brooklyn
Child's Hospital School for Practical Nurses, Albany
Department of Hospitals, New York
Harlem Y.W.C.A. School for Practical Nurses (for colored women), New York
Montefiore Hospital, Bronx, New York
N. Y. State Technical Institute, Delhi
N. Y. State Technical Institute, Morrisville
Rochester School of Practical Nursing, Rochester
William Booth Memorial Hospital, New York

PENNSYLVANIA

D. T. Watson Home for Crippled Children, Leetsdale
Harrisburg State Hospital, Harrisburg
Stetson Hospital, Philadelphia State Hospital (course discontinued)

VIRGINIA

Raiford Hospital, Franklin
Sheltering Arms General Hospital, Richmond
Westbrook Sanatorium, Richmond

Not all of these schools were admitting classes in 1945.

The following 6 schools have been approved by the National Association for Practical Nurse Education. All were functioning in 1945.

OHIO

Family Health Association, Course for Home Nursing Attendants, Cleveland

MICHIGAN

Detroit Council on Community Nursing, Detroit

MINNESOTA
Vocational Hospital, South, Minneapolis

NEW JERSEY
Essex County Vocational High School, Newark

VERMONT
Thompson School for Training Attendants, Brattleboro

WASHINGTON
Edison Vocational School, Practical Nursing Training, Seattle

Practical Nurses in Visiting Nurse Associations

The writer made the following list in March 1945. Approximately 45 practical nurses were employed in all these agencies. The list does not pretend to be complete as all the agencies in the United States were not circularized. It differs from that of the National Organization for Public Health Nursing as it does not include agencies responsible for practical nurses in institutions.

Hamden, Connecticut, Public Health and Visiting Nurse Association

Watertown, Connecticut, Public Health Nursing Association

Des Moines, Iowa, Public Health Nursing Association

Boston, Massachusetts, Visiting Nurse Association

Detroit, Michigan, Visiting Nurse Association

Hennepin County, Minnesota, working under the Minneapolis Community Health Service

Minneapolis, Minnesota, Visiting Nurse Association

St. Paul, Minnesota, Family Nursing Service

Collingwood, New Jersey, Community Nursing Service

Brooklyn, New York, Visiting Nurse Association

Millbrook, New York, Visiting Nurse Committee

New Rochelle, New York, Visiting Nurse Association

New York, New York, Visiting Nurse Service

Ossining, New York, District Nursing Association

Ardmore, Pennsylvania, Community Health and Civic Association

Practical Nursing Service through Professional Registries in Ontario, Canada

The Ontario Registered Nurses Association of Canada, besides being much interested in sponsoring courses for practical nurses (see page 247), has developed unusually forward-looking registries in some 20 cities which approach the ideal of a centralized service in a community nursing bureau—the name, for example, of the London registry is London Community Nursing Registry. The Ontario Association maintains a full time consultant service for registries in the Province, with an adviser who visits each registry from time to time and assists in initiating the organization of new community nursing registries. These registries enroll qualified practical nurses.

During the month of December 1944 the registry at London (population 75,000) had a list of 30 practical nurses and 185 registered nurses. Twelve calls for practical nurses were filled, twelve were unfilled. Fifteen of the 30 practical nurses were on cases in December and were not called by the registry. It will be noted that this is a far better percentage of calls filled than in the States (see page 46).

The cases taken by the practical nurses were arthritis 4, paralysis 3, cardiac condition 3, cancer 2, neurosis 1, and senility 2. All these patients were at home and needed the nurse for one to four weeks or longer.

The types of cases which were not filled were obstetrical, arthritic, paralytic, cardiac, and a child convalescing from burns.

As to length of service asked of practical nurses, the London Registry reports that 11 nurses were on cases less than one month; 7 were on cases one month to three months; 7 were on cases three months to eight months; and 3 were on cases eight months or more. Two nurses were ill at the time of this review.

This would seem to be a typical picture of the demand for longterm services, quite unsuited to the level of preparation of registered nurses.

Types of calls filled through the professional registries visited by the writer in the States consisted in postmaternity cases, chronic cases such as cancer, paralysis, fractures, cardiac conditions, and all stages of convalescence from acute illness. Maternity cases were not as a rule cared for until after the third day, but there were many exceptions to this.

The boards of the professional registries in Ontario have representation from laymen, doctors, professional and practical nurses. Committees deal with such subjects as the needs of the community, publicity for the registry service, education and welfare of registrants, and financing (pages 6–7, Article 7, Standing Committees of Constitution and By-laws, 1942).

In November 1944 charges were as follows:

Practical nurses	8 hour day, $18 per week
	12 hour day, $21 per week
	20 hour day, $24.50 per week
Professional nurses	8–12 hour day, $6–$8 a day
	20 hour day, $42 a week

It will be seen from this that the cost of practical nursing service has been kept decidedly below that of professional care in Canada.

The information given here was obtained through personal observation during visits in Ontario arranged through the courtesy of members of the Ontario Registered Nurses Association. Special thanks are due Madalene Baker, Registry Adviser, who supplied data and answers to many questions. See also Isabel M. MacIntosh, "A review of the present status of the nursing profession in Ontario," *Hospital Progress* 16:429, December 1935.

Past Opinions Regarding State Licensure
of Practical Nurses

For their historical interest, a few expressions of opinion regarding state legal control of practical nurses through licensure are quoted here.

In a discussion of the place of the attendant nurse at a meeting of the Nurses Association Alumnae of the United States in 1906, a representative from Indiana reported the need of legal recognition of this group: "A drayman must have a license before he can carry your trunk from one depot to another. . . . We have grades of teachers." Remarks by Mrs. Fournier, following address by Sister Ignatius Feeney, "How may a nurse charge below her price without lowering her standard?" *American Journal of Nursing* 6:771, July 1906. See also Ida Washburn, "Are nurses being overtrained," *ibid.*, pp. 799–805.

"I want," wrote Annie W. Goodrich in 1912, "to make an earnest plea for compulsory legislation, not who may practice as a registered nurse, or who shall practice as a graduate, trained or registered, but who shall practice as a *nurse*. . . . I make a plea for such registration; not for the protection of the nurse, but of the community." *The social and ethical significance of nursing; a series of addresses,* New York, Macmillan, 1932, p. 166. See also Grace E. Allison (taking the affirmative), "Shall attendants be trained and registered?" *American Journal of Nursing* 12:928–931, August 1912.

In 1912 one writer made the naive suggestion that, rather than license practical nurses, professional nurses should offer a sliding scale of charges—more for an acute case, less for a chronic—to prevent the encroachment of the practical nurses. The central registry was to determine the charges. Editorial Comment: "The small hospital, the attendant question and the sliding scale," *American Journal of Nursing* 12:280–281, January 1912.

Retta Johnson feared more than one standard of nursing care. She thought legal recognition would be the entering wedge to undermine "the foundations of our professional life. . . . Second class physicians are not called on cases for a smaller fee, why two standards of nurses?" Report of the Fifteenth Annual Convention of the American Nurses' Association, June 1912, *American Journal of Nursing* 12:933–934, August 1912.

In 1916 the American Hospital Association felt that state registration of practical nurses might be "a hindrance" to their use. Improvement in the service will come *"by close personal supervision over workers in this field* and adaptation to local needs" (the italics are the Committee's). Both the best and the worst of doctors have been known to monopolize the services of a few good practical nurses, teaching them as many skilled nursing procedures as their cases call for, until some of these doctors vociferously proclaim, "Practical nurses are as good as registered nurses, so why bother with a nurse practice act?" *Report of the Committee to Study the Nursing Problem,* Philadelphia, American Hospital Association, 1916, p. 20. See also the comments made by physicians in 1925–1926 when they were circularized by the Committee on the Grading of Nursing Schools; May Ayres Burgess, *Nurses, patients and pocketbooks,* New York, the Committee, 1928, pp. 153–181.

"Our efforts at present should be confined to keeping the attendant out of legislation for nurses. . . . We must establish some recognized standards first." Edith M. Ambrose, "How and where should attendants be trained?" *American Journal of Nursing* 17:993–1002, October 1917, at p. 997. This is a very complete discussion, giving contemporary points of view.

In 1918, in discussing a paper presented at the American Nurses' Association convention in Cleveland, Miss Goodrich is quoted as saying there was "need for two classes of women to care for the sick and the simple and clear thing would be to license one class as nurses and the other class as attendants." "Position of attendants," *American Journal of Nursing* 18:1008, October 1918.

In 1929, Elizabeth G. Fox felt that organization should come before legislation. "The economics of nursing," *American Journal of Nursing* 29:1043, September 1929.

A few registered nurses have been deeply disturbed by the problem of a name for the practical nurse. They ask: Does not licensing a second group of workers whose title includes the word "nurse" or "nursing" confuse the public? Should not the law protect the title "nurse" and restrict it to the professional registered nurse? In answer to them Effie J. Taylor wrote that the control of the word "nurse" has not been successfully accomplished in any state, and added that it has been used too long in the household and by nonprofessional people to hope that it can ever be protected by law. Public opinion would not support its restriction. "The auxiliary worker in the care of the sick," *I.C.N. International Nursing Review* 13:314–321, December 1939, at pp. 317–319. See also editorial, "Is a nursing craft needed?" *American Journal of Nursing* 43:521–522, June 1943.

Registered nurses in at least one state, when the practical nurses asked the state nurses' association to help them secure legislation, voted against such a move; "Washington nurses consider legislation," *American Journal of Nursing* 39:212–213, February 1939. See also Eleanor McGarvah, "Our changing attitudes toward legislation for nurse registration," *Trained Nurse and Hospital Review* 100:397–403, April 1938.

Index

Accreditation of schools of practical nursing, 232, 264, 293, 341

Age of practical nurses
entering schools of practical nursing, 19–20, 21, 197, 218
in camp nursing, 208
in cancer hospitals, 134
in Civil Service, 188
in public health, 166, 173
in tuberculosis hospitals, 188

Aged, care of. *See* Chronically ill and aged, care of

American College of Surgeons, 225

American Hospital Association, 44, 225, 255, 268

American Journal of Nursing, ix, 30, 43, 65, 82, 164, 272, 298, 299

American Medical Association, 29, 62, 88, 225

American Nurses' Association, 44, 284, 292, 317
approval of registries, 313–314
attitude toward correspondence schools, 230
attitude toward licensure of practical nurses, 6, 297–298, 302
attitude toward practical nursing schools in same institution as professional nursing schools, 6
duties of subsidiary workers defined, 66
practical nurses as advisers to professional registries recommended, 315
registry procedures suggested, 315–319
regrading of professional nurses advocated, 191
study of auxiliary workers, 30, 33, 89–90, 101
study of practical nurses recommended, 322

American Psychiatric Association, 93, 95, 97

American Public Health Association, 148–149

American Red Cross, 44, 145, 156
volunteers. *See* Red Cross Volunteer Nurses' Aides

American Trudeau Society, 102, 104

Appointment service, 3, 50

Approval of practical nurses. *See* Attitude toward practical nurses

Approved schools of practical nursing, list, 348–350

Assistant nurse, 15

Associations of practical nurses, 6–7, 341

Attendant nurse
as title for practical nurse, 15
licensure, 285

Attendants, 15, 29, 88
in government services, 186, 189
in industry, 149–151
in mental hospitals, 88–96
in visiting nurse associations, 164–165
salaries in tuberculosis hospitals, 111

Attitude of practical nurses
in general hospitals, 80–81
in public health work, 174
toward homemaking, 256
toward legislation, 287
toward supervision, 55

Attitude toward legislation, 6, 297–300, 302, 336, 354–356

Attitude toward practical nurses, 4–7
in industry, 158–160
of general hospitals, 23, 61–62, 63, 72, 77
of medical profession, 4, 11–12, 54, 61, 62, 76, 111, 174
of patients, 131
of professional nurses. *See under* Professional nurses
of registries, 314–315
of tuberculosis hospitals, 111–112
of visiting nurse associations, 174, 181

Auxiliary workers
confusion in duties, 77–78, 154

Titles in This Series

14   Annette Fiske. *First Fifty Years of the Waltham Training School for Nurses.* New York, 1984. BOUND WITH Alfred Worcester. "The Shortage of Nurses—Reminiscences of Alfred Worcester '83." *Harvard Medical Alumni Bulletin 23*, 1949.

15   Virginia Henderson et al. *Nursing Studies Index, 1900–1959.* Philadelphia, 1963, 1966, 1970, 1972.

16   Darlene Clark Hine, editor. *Black Women in Nursing: An Anthology of Historical Sources.*

17   Ellen N. LaMotte. *The Tuberculosis Nurse.* New York, 1915.

18   Barbara Melosh, editor. *American Nurses in Fiction: An Anthology of Short Stories.*

19   Mary Adelaide Nutting. *A Sound Economic Basis for Schools of Nursing.* New York, 1926.

20   Sara E. Parsons. *Nursing Problems and Obligations.* Boston, 1916.

21   Juanita Redmond. *I Served on Bataan.* Philadelphia, 1943.

22   Susan Reverby, editor. *The East Harlem Health Center Demonstration: An Anthology of Pamphlets.*

23   Isabel Hampton Robb. *Educational Standards for Nurses.* Cleveland, 1907.

24   Sister M. Theophane Shoemaker. *History of Nurse-Midwifery in the United States.* Washington, D.C., 1947.

25   Isabel M. Stewart. *Education of Nurses.* New York, 1943.

26   Virginia S. Thatcher. *History of Anesthesia with Emphasis on the Nurse Specialist.* Philadelphia, 1953.

27   Adah H. Thoms. *Pathfinders—A History of the Progress of Colored Graduate Nurses.* New York, 1929.

28   Clara S. Weeks-Shaw. *A Text-Book of Nursing for the Use of Training Schools, Families, and Private Students.* New York, 1885.

29   Writers Program of the WPA in Kansas, compilers. *Lamps on the Prairie: A History of Nursing in Kansas.* Topeka, 1942.